Trauma and Dissociation in a Cross-Cultural Perspective: Not Just a North American Phenomenon

Trauma and Dissociation in a Cross-Cultural Perspective: Not Just a North American Phenomenon has been co-published simultaneously as *Journal of Trauma Practice,* Volume 4, Numbers 1/2 and 3/4 2005.

Monographic Separates from the *Journal of Trauma Practice*™

For additional information on these and other Haworth Press titles, including descriptions, tables of contents, reviews, and prices, use the QuickSearch catalog at http://www.HaworthPress.com.

Trauma and Dissociation in a Cross-Cultural Perspective: Not Just a North American Phenomenon, edited by George F. Rhoades, Jr., PhD, and Vedat Sar, MD (Vol. 4, No. 1/2 and 3/4, 2005). *Examines the psychological, sociological, political, and cultural aspects of trauma and its consequences on people around the world.*

Prostitution, Trafficking, and Traumatic Stress, edited by Melissa Farley, PhD (Vol. 2, No. 3/4 2003). Prostitution, Trafficking, and Traumatic Stress *documents the violence that runs like a constant thread throughout all types of prostitution, including escort, brothel, trafficking, strip club, and street prostitution. The book presents clinical examples, analysis, and original research, counteracting common myths about the harmlessness of prostitution. It explores the connections between prostitution, incest, sexual harassment, rape, and battering; looks at peer support programs for women escaping prostitution; examines clinical symptoms common among prostitutes; and much more.*

Trauma Practice in the Wake of September 11, 2001, edited by Steven N. Gold, PhD, and Jan Faust, PhD (Vol. 1, No. 3/4, 2002). *"Extraordinarily timely and important. . . . It is now a different world that confronts mental health professionals. This book presents both broad theoretical perspectives and the personal accounts of some who have required care and those who provide it. It begins to help us understand the changes of the post 9/11 era–how domestic terrorism has affected the national psyche as well as individuals, inflicting new wounds and awakening old hurts." (James A. Chu, MD, Director, Trauma and Dissociative Disorders Program, McLean Hospital, Belmont, Massachusetts; Editor,* Journal of Trauma & Dissociation*)*

Trauma and Dissociation in a Cross-Cultural Perspective: Not Just a North American Phenomenon

George F. Rhoades, Jr., PhD
Vedat Sar, MD
Editors

Trauma and Dissociation in a Cross-Cultural Perspective: Not Just a North American Phenomenon has been co-published simultaneously as *Journal of Trauma Practice,* Volume 4, Numbers 1/2 and 3/4 2005.

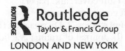
Routledge
Taylor & Francis Group

LONDON AND NEW YORK

Published by
The Haworth Maltreatment & Trauma Press, 10 Alice Street, Binghamton, NY 13904-1580
USA.
The Haworth Maltreatment & Trauma Press is an imprint of The Haworth Press, Inc., 10 Alice
Street, Binghamton, NY 13904-1580 USA.

Trauma and Dissociation in a Cross-Cultural Perspective: Not Just a North American Phenomenon has been co-published simultaneously as *Journal of Trauma Practice,* Volume 4, Numbers 1/2 and 3/4 2005.

The development, preparation, and publication of this work has been undertaken with great care. However, the publisher, employees, editors, and agents of The Haworth Press and all imprints of The
Haworth Press, Inc., including The Haworth Medical Press® and The Pharmaceutical Products Press®,
are not responsible for any errors contained herein or for consequences that may ensue from use of ma-
terials or information contained in this work. With regard to case studies, identities and circumstances
of individuals discussed herein have been changed to protect confidentiality. Any resemblance to actual
persons, living or dead, is entirely coincidental.

The Haworth Press is committed to the dissemination of ideas and information according to the highest
standards of intellectual freedom and the free exchange of ideas. Statements made and opinions expressed in this publication do not necessarily reflect the views of the Publisher, Directors, management,
or staff of The Haworth Press, Inc., or an endorsement by them.

Cover design by Karen Lowe.

Library of Congress Cataloging-in-Publication Data

Trauma and dissociation in a cross-cultural perspective: not just a North American phenomenon /
George F. Rhoades, Jr., Vedat Sar, editors
     p. cm.
    "Co-published simultaneously as Journal of trauma practice, volume 4, numbers 1/2/3/4 2005."
    Includes bibliographical references and index.
    ISBN-13: 978-0-7890-3407-6 (alk. paper)
    ISBN-10: 0-7890-3407-7 (alk. paper)
    ISBN-13: 978-0-7890-3408-3 (soft cover: alk. paper)
    ISBN-10: 0-7890-3408-5 (soft cover: alk. paper)
    1. Psychic trauma–Cross-cultural studies. 2. Dissociation (Psychology)–Cross-cultural studies.
I. Rhoades, George F. II. Sar, Vedat. III. Journal of trauma practice.
RC552.T7R46 2006
362.196'8521–dc22

            2006014297

Indexing, Abstracting & Website/Internet Coverage

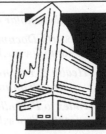

This section provides you with a list of major indexing & abstracting services and other tools for bibliographic access. That is to say, each service began covering this periodical during the year noted in the right column. Most Websites which are listed below have indicated that they will either post, disseminate, compile, archive, cite or alert their own Website users with research-based content from this work. (This list is as current as the copyright date of this publication.)

Abstracting, Website/Indexing Coverage . . . . Year When Coverage Began
- *(IBR) International Bibliography of Book Reviews on the Humanities and Social Sciences (Thomson) <http://www.saur.de>* 2006
- *(IBZ) International Bibliography of Periodical Literature on the Humanities and Social Science (Thomson) <http://www.saur.de>* . . . 2006
- *Biological Sciences Database (Cambridge Scientific Abstracts) <http://www.csa.com>* 2006
- *Cambridge Scientific Abstracts (A leading publisher of scientific information in print journals, online databases, CD-ROM and via the Internet) <http://www.csa.com>* 2002
- *CINAHL (Cumulative Index to Nursing & Allied Health Literature), (EBSCO) <http://www.cinahl.com>* 2003
- *Contemporary Women's Issues* 2002
- *Criminal Justice Abstracts (Sage)* 2002
- *Drug Policy Information Clearinghouse* 2002
- *EBSCOhost Electronic Journals Service (EJS) <http://ejournals.ebsco.com>* 2002
- *Elsevier Eflow-I* 2006
- *Elsevier Scopus <http://www.info.scopus.com>* 2005
- *Environmental Sciences and Pollution Management (Cambridge Scientific Abstracts International Database Service) <http://www.csa.com>* 2006
- *Family & Society Studies Worldwide (NISC) <http://www.nisc.com>* . . 2001
- *Family Index Database <http://www.familyscholar.com>* 2004
- *Family Violence & Sexual Assault Bulletin* 2002
- *Google <http://www.google.com>* 2004

(continued)

*Special Bibliographic Notes related to special journal issues
(separates) and indexing/abstracting:*

- indexing/abstracting services in this list will also cover material in any "separate" that is co-published simultaneously with Haworth's special thematic journal issue or DocuSerial. Indexing/abstracting usually covers material at the article/chapter level.
- monographic co-editions are intended for either non-subscribers or libraries which intend to purchase a second copy for their circulating collections.
- monographic co-editions are reported to all jobbers/wholesalers/approval plans. The source journal is listed as the "series" to assist the prevention of duplicate purchasing in the same manner utilized for books-in-series.
- to facilitate user/access services all indexing/abstracting services are encouraged to utilize the co-indexing entry note indicated at the bottom of the first page of each article/chapter/contribution.
- this is intended to assist a library user of any reference tool (whether print, electronic, online, or CD-ROM) to locate the monographic version if the library has purchased this version but not a subscription to the source journal.
- individual articles/chapters in any Haworth publication are also available through the Haworth Document Delivery Service (HDDS).

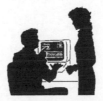

ABOUT THE EDITORS

George F. Rhoades, Jr., PhD, practices and lives in Hawaii as a clinical psychologist. Hawaii is known as the "melting pot" of the Pacific wherein the application of cross-cultural principles of psychotherapy is both practical and necessary. Dr. Rhoades is both the Founder and Director of Ola Hou Clinic, Aiea, Hawaii and Adjunct Psychology Faculty at Wayland Baptist University. He was Chairman of the Psychology/Counseling Department at the International College and Graduate School from 1989 to 1997. He is an international author and speaker conducting workshops/trainings in Hawaii, USA, Canada, Europe, Asia, and the Middle East on anger management, trauma, dissociation, and Satanic Ritual Abuse. Dr. Rhoades worked in trauma counseling/workshops in Sri Lanka, Russia, Northern Ireland, and Iran. He was Consulting Editor for Corsini Dictionary of Psychology, radio host for four radio stations in Honolulu, Fellow with the International Society for Study of Dissociation (ISSD), Chair of ISSD World listserv, and Co-Chair of ISSD International Conference in Los Angeles.

Vedat Sar, MD, is a psychiatrist and Clinical Professor in Istanbul University Istanbul Medical School. He is founder and director of the Clinical Psychotherapy Section and Dissociative Disorders Program in the Department of Psychiatry at the Istanbul University Medical Faculty Hospital. A fellow member and former International Director of the International Society for the Study of Dissociation (ISSD), Dr. Sar has served as Co-Chair of the DSM-V Research Planning Conference sponsored by the ISSD. He is a fellow member of the International Society for the Study of Dissociation (ISSD) and has been honored by the ISSD with the David Caul Memorial Award in 1995 and 1999, the Morton Prince Scientific Achievement Award in 2001, and the Cornelia Wilbur Award in 2004. Dr. Sar has published more than 100 papers in peer-reveiewed journals, book chapters, and special journal issues in Turkish and English. He sits on the editorial board of the *Journal of Trauma & Dissociation.*

Trauma and Dissociation in a Cross-Cultural Perspective: Not Just a North American Phenomenon

CONTENTS

Foreword:
Is Affect Dysregulation a Factor
That Corresponds Across Cultures
with the Presence
of Dissociative Processes?

How does a mind work? What genetic and environmental factors contribute to the "happening" of a thought or feeling? How does a mind deal with adversity or stress that's so great that it alters how that mind functions for a moment or for as long as a person lives? What are the modes of experience that spice the particular cultural broth in which a mind grows and then influence the flavor of human relatedness? What does culture have to do with how a mind hides from itself? How are dissociative processes related to these kinds of conscious and unconscious experiences?

I am far from being convinced that we will answer these questions completely in my lifetime. Nevertheless, I am reassured that we are in an age where these questions are being addressed relentlessly and with a sense of urgency that takes offense at the outrage of attributing the "nervous" conditions of the survivors of domestic, military, and natural disasters/violence to inadequacies in the people who have been wounded by life (as our German colleagues point out in their essay in this book).

Address correspondence to: Richard A. Chefetz, MD, 4612 49th Street N.W., Washington, DC 20016 (E-mail: r.a.chefetz@psychsense.net).

[Haworth co-indexing entry note]: "Foreword: Is Affect Dysregulation a Factor That Corresponds Across Cultures with the Presence of Dissociative Processes?." Chefetz, Richard A. Co-published simultaneously in *Journal of Trauma Practice* (The Haworth Maltreatment & Trauma Press, an imprint of The Haworth Press, Inc.) Vol. 4, No. 1/2, 2005, pp. xix-xxvi; and: *Trauma and Dissociation in a Cross-Cultural Perspective: Not Just a North American Phenomenon* (ed: George F. Rhoades, Jr., and Vedat Sar) The Haworth Maltreatment & Trauma Press, an imprint of The Haworth Press, Inc., 2005, pp. xv-xxii. Single or multiple copies of this article are available for a fee from The Haworth Document Delivery Service [1-800-HAWORTH, 9:00 a.m. - 5:00 p.m. (EST). E-mail address: docdelivery@haworthpress.com].

Available online at http://jtp.haworthpress.com

In this age of automated violence, there are few questions more pressing than how to help a person heal from traumatic experience. There is no person reading this who cannot be impressed by the wide diversity of both natural and un-natural disasters that afflict the people of this world. What better work is there than to attempt to heal the wounded, and by doing so, interrupt the intergenerational cycles of violence that threaten us all?

In this collection of articles by a guest list of serious clinicians who have managed to pursue their interests in human traumatic experience and the dissociative disorders I have a sense of being a witness to these authors having all had an experience of standing in the middle of a crowded society and shouting out to the people gathered around them: "Hey, don't you get it?! They've been hurt, wounded! It's not some weakness of their minds. They're hurt! We can help them. Just pay attention to the wound, please. Can't you see it? It's there, right there. What's wrong? Why can't you see it? Look. Look where I'm pointing!" Why are these clinicians pointing and shouting? What are they looking at that others find so hard to see or even acknowledge might be there?

As you read these words, are you not familiar with a longing to not read more about violence, tragedy, and suffering? Have you not ever dreaded a return to your work after a good enough vacation? Remember, we clinicians are the ones with our eyes already open! What of those who learned to close their eyes as children? How eager would they be as adults to understand or even notice the wounds in the people who surround them?

Seeking an understanding of cross-cultural similarities and differences in the human response to severe adverse experience is a fine tool to use in the service of discovering basic human responses to emotional and physical trauma. It can remove the cultural packaging of individual and group behaviors and teach us all about the basics of being human. Basic assumptions of a given culture hide the rationales for cultural events that seem to elude a culture's members. Of course, there is a tax to be levied on any person who persists in opening their eyes: you get to see the world as it is: wonderful and terrible. Both conditions, wonderful and terrible, exist, simultaneously, sequentially, and inescapably. It is a sad reality. Yes, it has more or less always been this way for us humans. We are adaptable. BUT, the breadth and depth of the violent outcomes for human life that are arrayed before us in the beginning of the 21st Century are truly breathtaking. Let's consider a short list:

1. Global warming that will make the oceans rise, at some point and cover land occupied at this moment by 100 million people
2. Climatic changes from global warming that threaten everyone with more violent weather patterns even while temperatures rise minimally, on the average
3. Terrorist threats that randomly destroy human lives in both highly civilized and less civilized nations
4. Nuclear holocaust potentials
5. AIDS/HIV and the threat of the loss of whole populations of young and middle aged adults in some nations.
6. Predictions of an Avian flu pandemic
7. Pollution of the sky, water, and land to the extent that heavy metal and toxic chemical accumulations will gradually poison sources of human food and make them unfit for consumption without the risk of illness

If I am going to maintain my sense of well-being I have to find ways to escape consciousness for these world-wide disasters in progress (not in the making). Are you uncomfortable yet? I am. And I'm hoping you are too because then maybe you, like me, will try to figure out how to deal with some of these problems and apply yourself toward some solutions. And in this little list of some of the world's problems I have not addressed any of the interpersonal issues that have a well documented cumulative negative effect on psychological and physical health (Felitti, 1998). We must find ways of better understanding how to grow healthy minds, and how to help heal and repair those minds

The seventeen articles in this book provide you with two kinds of information that are not available elsewhere. First, in some of these articles, you will hear about the particular shape of psychological syndromes that have some of the hallmarks of dissociative processes such as dissociative amnesia, disremembered behaviors, possession beliefs, and spontaneous trance, amongst others. Second, you will learn about the state of the art in dissociative disorders studies and the struggles that exist in different societies as consciousness for the dissociative disorders tries to make its way into the thinking of mental health professionals throughout the world. There is no other comprehensive source for this information. It is a remarkable collection of efforts by many individuals and organizations. Equally important is that only fifteen years ago, just a handful of these authors were nearing professional recognition as experts in their field. Dissociative Disorders Studies are maturing and spreading throughout the world. This collection of papers is well worth your time in taking the pulse and learning the rhythms of views of dissociative processes across many cultures.

WHAT ARE SOME UNDERLYING COMMON THEMES ASSOCIATED WITH DISSOCIATIVE PROCESSES ACROSS CULTURES?

As a psychoanalytically attuned psychiatrist, who is also trained in techniques such as hypnosis, eye movement densensitization reprocessing, and short-term dynamic psychotherapy, I have found it useful to try and identify common thematic elements of all these treatments. I suppose this is an aftereffect of my ten years of practicing medicine in a rural Virginia community, a town of two hundred people, in a county of ten-thousand, nestled against the east side of the Blue Ridge Mountains. I say this because I was born and raised in New York City, went to medical school in Richmond, Virginia, and did a residency in family practice in rural Blackstone, Virginia. It's been necessary, for this clinician, to look beyond the cultural differences between a cosmopolitan New York upbringing, the "southern charm" of Richmond, Virginia, the capital city of the Confederate States of America, and the provincialism of a rural, Baptist, Blue Ridge, farming community. In all these communities I met and befriended a number of wonderful people. In order to provide good medical care, I had to be aware of the individual beliefs that ran in families, as well as the local practices of different religious groups. For example, the risk of venereal disease was a part of the accepted risk taking behaviors of young adults in the era preceding AIDS/HIV in Richmond. However, the same infection was more often a major crisis in the life of a young adult in rural Virginia. Likewise, a diagnosis of cancer was very often felt to be a personal failing and a sign of un-cleanliness in the person who fell ill. Illness was thus associated with tremendous shame, despair, and secondary depression. The presence of a psychiatric disorder and a visit to a psychiatrist was much better tolerated in a large city than in a small town in rural Virginia. Thus, the function of a family physician was often similar to that of the head of a local place of worship; doctors and ministers were counselors as much as anything else they did. The shame of mental illness was too often viewed as a weakness of the soul, or culturally disowned as the work of "the devil." In other words, the feelings that people had about being ill more often than not determined the extent to which they could engage in their treatment, and succeed in proper management or cure of their illness. This is doubly true about psychiatric problems.

What then can a clinician discern about psychiatric illness through the lens of dissociation as we scan across many cultures? I believe that what shows up inevitably is the role of affect, and affect dysregulation at the root of disturbances for all the individual cases described. Is affect dysregulation a factor which is present as a problem across cultures when mental illness is present, and especially when there is dissociative process? The authors in this book don't go out of their way to make this point, but if we look between the lines, and not even all that hard, I think this becomes obvious.

Let's look at a few examples. One of the more consistent cultural themes is the notion of demon possession, or simply possession by an outside entity. What are the properties and characteristics of these possession states? Thoughts, feelings, and motivations of the demons are anathema to the culture involved. Violent feelings and wishes to perpetrate violence, sexual feelings and wishes to engage sexually are part of what is routinely disowned in many cultures. [While the emphasis in this text is intentionally from outside North America, possession beliefs have included people living in the United States, as indicated in the infamous Salem Witch Trials of 1692 (http://www.salemweb.com/guide/witches.shtml].) Aggressive feelings are part of the demons who possess persons, in these reports. These are "Not-Me" experiences (Chefetz, 2004). Shame feelings are also very much at the core of intense emotional pain that is visible in many cultures where there is possession (see the papers from Iranian, Pacific Rim, and Hispanic cultures). The emphasis in the cure of possession experience is on the exorcism of these thoughts and feelings as embodied in the demon spirit. In a psychoanalytic therapy, the emphasis is on acceptance of these feelings representing a human response to living in adversity and reacting to the world around us. Feelings are distinguished from actions. However, for example, Catholicism has made a point of telling people that to have a thought or feeling that might be called criminal is equivalent to committing the crime. These kinds of beliefs make having discordant thoughts and feeling not just inimical to one's stability or acceptability in a social group, but run the risk of shunning or excommunication from a life giving social setting. It is this kind of threat that "stray" affects, wishes, motives, and thoughts presents to the one who beholds these experiences.

The work of Alan Schore, Mary Main, Karlen Lyons-Ruth, and many others (Schore, 2003) (Main, 1996) (Lyons-Ruth, 2003) (Beebe, 1997) makes clear that it is in the interaction between infant and parent that the growing child develops their capacity to emote and to manage affective experience. Knowing feelings is a relationally based experience, a skill that is taught by interactive and unconscious implicit processes from the early moments of life onward. Listen to the histories of people with the illness described as "amok." The unmanageable rage is visible. This is also the case in some other culture bound syndromes with violent and amnestic episodes. This is the case in "latah," where there is a hypersensitivity to fright. "Ataque" seems to be related to symptoms of panic. In my experience, panic is related to fear of intense affects such as anger and shame. The affects cannot be consciously tolerated, and instead there is a dissociation of the manifest physiology of the affect from the knowledge of the named emotion that would result if the feeling was able to be felt. Somatization, as described in the work of Henry Krystal, is the somatic manifestation of an affect state that lacks translation from the affective physiological roots of emotional response to the felt and lived experience of a feeling (Krystal, 1988) (in this discussion an affect is the not-conscious psychophysiologic tension out of which lived, conscious feelings emerge to which we assign the name of an emotion). Somatization is a frequent corresponding symptom in people with culture-bound dissociative processes.

Support for the contention that we could track the affect regulatory styles between cultures as a way to understand culture bound psychiatric syndromes comes from cross-cultural attachment studies. In a chapter on the individual differences that occur in personality between persons, the authors describe the results of some attachment research (Oatley, 2006). They cite data in comparison to norms in English speaking countries where they state that 65% of infants are secure, 20% avoidant, and 15% ambivalent (this obviously leaves out data on what was formerly known as the "unresolved" or disorganized/disoriented classification that a vast majority of children show when their parent is frightened, frightening, or unresponsive (Schuengel, 1999)). Israeli Strange Situation studies showed a higher proportion of children who were ambivalent (Sagi, 1985), German studies showed that nearly 50% were avoidant (Grossman, 1985), and in Japan there were no avoidant children (Miyake, 1985). As Oatley and colleagues speculate "children . . . are likely to vary in how frequently they experience separation . . . [how parents] value independence . . . [how parents encourage] expression of fear and sadness . . . [and, how often parents] encourage bodily contact" (p. 297). How parents manage and communicate affect has a profound influence on the growth and development of a child, and reflects culturally sanctioned and enforced modes of affective communication and behavior. Dissociative process, in this view, is fundamentally a result of the relational aspects of familial styles of affect regulation. Family styles of affect regulation are guided by cultural sanctions.

CONCLUSION

Whether you agree or not about the role that affect regulation, or the lack of it, plays in the genesis of culture bound syndromes related to dissociation, or to dissociation itself, my challenge to you is to track *something* of interest to you as you read through these pages and develop your own hypotheses that can lead to your own formulation of some meta-theory, some organizing principles, that allow you to translate what you read into what you can take with you to talk about with your patients. There is little that is as important as educating ourselves in the service of increasing our understanding of what it is to be human. The study of dissociative processes, their manifestations in different cultures, and the particulars of "the shapes, colors, and sizes" of these manifestations have a lot to teach us about each of our own cultures and the minds that are grown within. As you read through the pages that follow, I hope you will take the time to speculate about your own observations and the observations of others who study dissociative processes. If you do, then at least some of the wishes of the dedicated clinicians who have written about their observations will come true, and make a difference in this wonderful and terrible world in which we all try to live.

Some weeks ago, as I made preliminary plans to write this foreword, I came across these words, the source for which I've lost. I believe this is a fitting way to close my contribution to his book:

> In a small, ancient cemetery in Celigny, Switzerland, there is a gravestone
>
> with this message from the deceased occupant of the plot:
>
> "Listen my friends: There is still time for you to help change the world".

Richard A. Chefetz

REFERENCES

Beebe, B. (1997). *Developmental factors of hatred: Co-constructing mother-infant distress.* Hatred and Its Rewards, Bethesda, Maryland.

Chefetz, R. A., & Bromberg, P.M. (2004). "Talking with "me" and not-me." *Contemporary Psychoanalysis, 40*(3): 409-464.

Felitti, V. J., Anda, R.F., Nordenberg, D., Williamson, D.F., Spitz, A.M., Edwards, V., Koss, M.P., Marks, J.S. (1998). "Relationship of childhood abuse and household dysfunction to many of the leading causes of death in adults. The Adverse Childhood Experiences (ACE) Study." *American Journal of Preventive Medicine, 14*(4): 245-258.

Grossman, K. E., Grossman, K. et al. (1985). "Maternal sensitivity and newborn orientation responses as related to quality of attachment in northern Germany." *Monographs of the Society for Research in Child Development, 50*(1-2, Serial #209): 233-256.

Krystal, H. (1988). *Integration and Self Healing: Affect, Alexithymia, and Trauma.* Hillsdale, N.J., Analytic Press.

Lyons-Ruth, K. (2003). "Dissociation and the parent-infant dialogue: A longitudinal perspective from attachment research." *Journal of the American Psychoanalytic Association 51*(3): 883-911.

Main, M., & Morgan, Hillary (1996). Disorganization and disorientation in infant strange situation behavior: Phenotypic resemblance to dissociative states. *Handbook of Dissociation: Theoretical, Empirical, and Clinical Perspectives.* L. K. Michelson, and Ray, William J. New York, Plenum Press: 107-138.

Miyake, K., Chen, S.-J., & Campos, J.J. (1985). "Infant temperament, mother's mode of interaction, and attachment in Japan: An interim report." In I. Bretherton & E. Waters (Eds.) Growing points of attachment theory and research. *Monographs of the Society for Research in Child Development, 50*(1-2, Serial #209): 276-297.

Oatley, K., Keltner, D., & Jenkins, J.M. (2006). *Understanding Emotions.* Malden, Massachusetts, Blackwell.

Sagi, A. et al. (1985). "Security of infant-mother, -father, metaplet attachments amongst kibbutz-reared Israeli children." *Monographs of the Society for Research in Child Development, 50*(1-2 Serial #209): 257-276.

Schore, A. N. (2003). *Affect Regulation and Repair of the Self.* New York, W.W. Norton & Co.

Schuengel, C., Bakermans-Kranenberg, Marian J., van IJzendoorn, Marinus H., & Blom, Marjolijn (1999). Unresolved loss and infant disorganization: Links to frightening maternal behavior. *Attachment Disorganization.* J. Solomon, George, Carol. New York, Guilford: 71-94.

PART I

Introduction

George F. Rhoades, Jr.
Vedat Sar

It was 9:00 a.m. on the eastern shores/beaches of Sri Lanka, December 26, 2004. Without warning, the first tsunami wave hit, only to be followed by two even more devastating waves. People called the next town to warn them and as they were still on the phone, the wave came into sight of the new victims. It only took minutes, but 800,000 persons lost their homes and over 38,000 lost their lives. The tsunami was no respecter of persons; both locals and tourists, rich and poor were equally devastated.

The first author personally visited Sri Lanka approximately a month-and-a-half after the event and was astonished by the contrasts in the wake of this so-called natural disaster. One site visited was the empty passenger train that had come from Colombo (the capital city) on that fateful day. The train had over 1,000 people on board, but swelled to almost 2,000 as people climbed aboard to seek shelter from the killer waves; they all drowned. Four family members clung to a coconut tree and were able to survive. A father told of holding two children in his arms to only have one ripped from him and then the other child as well. The author met a fisherman in the southern city of Galle who lost all 11 members of his family in minutes: his wife, children, and grandchildren. He wondered why he was left behind. A camp leader (refugee camp) told of his 13-year-old daughter who was swept away by the fast mov-

[Haworth co-indexing entry note]: "Introduction." Rhoades, George F., Jr., and Vedat Sar. Co-published simultaneously in *Journal of Trauma Practice* (The Haworth Maltreatment & Trauma Press, an imprint of The Haworth Press, Inc.) Vol. 4, No. 1/2, 2005, pp. 3-5; and: *Trauma and Dissociation in a Cross-Cultural Perspective: Not Just a North American Phenomenon* (ed: George F. Rhoades, Jr., and Vedat Sar) The Haworth Maltreatment & Trauma Press, an imprint of The Haworth Press, Inc., 2005, pp. 3-5. Single or multiple copies of this article are available for a fee from The Haworth Document Delivery Service [1-800-HAWORTH, 9:00 a.m. - 5:00 p.m. (EST). E-mail address: docdelivery@haworthpress.com].

ing waters. He later found her dead in the mud; he cleaned her up and then carried her on a board, on his back to the hospital. The hospital refused to return the body for a burial.

Some people reportedly became greedy and started cutting off ear lobes and fingers to steal the jewelry and even tried to sell the bodies to the families. Due to these reasons and the need to maintain community health standards, the government decided to intervene and did mass burials, continuing the trauma for the families. They now lost their loved ones twice, once in death and then in not being able to say goodbye in a memorial service.

In a period of a month-and-a-half, the number of homeless has been reduced to around 400,000, with multiple refugee camps around the country. The camps are housed in Buddhist monasteries, Catholic schools/grounds and government-sponsored areas. Many of the camps are guarded by the Sri Lankan military, to provide order within and without the camp. The overcrowding, lack of water/resources in some camps and the overwhelming grief of the refugees extend the trauma of the tsunami and create daily dissociation. The refugees desire to have memorials for their loved ones, permanent homes, and to return to work.

In contrast, the inland of Sri Lanka has continued in many ways as it was before the tsunami. The streets of the cities/towns are very busy with a menagerie of vehicles and animals. Driving up the left side of a street in central Sri Lanka (traveling to Kandy) the author was passed by an elephant on the right side, along with buses, cars, trucks, "three-wheelers," "free" cows, goats, and dogs. Roadside vendors are smiling and ready to sell seasonal fruits and delicious locally-grown cashews. People work hard, parents are seen walking their children to school each morning and have celebrations such as weddings.

The people of Sri Lanka had never experienced a trauma as universal and devastating as the tsunami. They have responded to the trauma in a way unique to Sri Lanka, but also in common with other nations and peoples of the world. They have sought understanding of the trauma according to their religious beliefs (Buddhist, Hindu, Muslim, and Christian) and have tried to recover according to their cultural practices. They have also experienced intense grief, survivor's guilt, and the dissociation that is seen among trauma survivors around the world. The commonly seen anger in such situations is beginning to surface as the Sri Lankan survivors move out of the emotional numbness/dissociation into a more full realization of their losses. The dissociation of the rest of the country is similar to other countries dealing with tremendous losses and even individuals that want to dissociate from pain and trauma to live their lives.

The people of Sri Lanka are a strong, proud people that will come through this crisis with the help of their families, their religious faith, fellow citizens, the government, and millions of concerned individuals and organizations throughout the world. We are truly an international community in times of crises. It is also increasingly apparent that we are also an international community in the experiencing of trauma and the resulting effects of that trauma.

This international mosaic of pieces has been formed through selection of the individual content by the authors themselves. The editors did not perceive any necessity to guide the authors in order to prevent repetitions as the chapters had a complementary nature already. It is noteworthy that so many contributors have perceived trauma and dissociation as a socio-psychological phenomenon and referred to sociological and even political aspects of long-lasting traumatization in various countries. In fact, besides man-made traumas such as childhood abuse and neglect, terror, and war, even the prevention of devastating effects of natural disasters has economic and political dimensions. An example would be the impact of the Marmara area earthquake in Northwestern Turkey in 1999, which led to twenty thousand casualties. The devastation could have been limited by more rational urbanization policies and human-centered economic investment.

This volume will look at international trauma around the world, including the uniqueness and the similarities of that trauma, both to the particular nation presented and the world at large. We will examine trauma and dissociation in the United Kingdom, Northern Ireland, France, Germany, Turkey, Iran, Israel, Africa, China, Japan, Philippines, Australia, New Zealand, Hawaii, Puerto Rico, Columbia, and Argentina. The book has purposely not included North America to show that trauma and dissociation is not just a "North American phenomenon."

What Is Trauma and Dissociation?

Vedat Sar

Erdinc Ozturk

SUMMARY. Although the official term of posttraumatic stress disorder implies the opposite, trauma is not identical with the noxious event itself. An adequate definition of trauma would require the inclusion of both the objective and subjective components of a traumatic experience. Moreover, trauma is not limited solely to the traumatic situation, but is better defined as a socio-psychological process which can be completed in the course of time, if at all. The superposition of multiple trauma processes throughout a person's life span can make this task even more complex. We propose that what turns an experience to be traumatic is not only the interruption of information processing, but the activation of a maladaptive process, i.e., trauma is a threatening experience which turns an adaptive process to a maladaptive one. The six concepts of traumatic double-bind, traumatic turning point, completion expectancy, traumatic time perception, traumatic obsessions, and traumatic whirlpool are presented to better clarify this maladaptive process. Traumatic experiences and the consequently altered self-perceptions contribute to the impairment of the mutuality between internal world and external reality of the affected person. This is accompanied by a renewed percep-

Vedat Sar, MD, and Erdinc Ozturk, PhD, are affiliated with Istanbul University, Istanbul, Turkey.

Address correspondence to: Prof. Dr. Vedat Sar, Istanbul Tip Fakultesi Psikiyatri Klinigi 34390, Capa Istanbul, Turkey (E-mail: vsar@istanbul.edu.tr).

[Haworth co-indexing entry note]: "What Is Trauma and Dissociation?" Sar, Vedat, and Erdinc Ozturk. Co-published simultaneously in *Journal of Trauma Practice* (The Haworth Maltreatment & Trauma Press, an imprint of The Haworth Press, Inc.) Vol. 4, No. 1/2, 2005, pp. 7-20; and: *Trauma and Dissociation in a Cross-Cultural Perspective: Not Just a North American Phenomenon* (ed: George F. Rhoades, Jr., and Vedat Sar) The Haworth Maltreatment & Trauma Press, an imprint of The Haworth Press, Inc., 2005, pp. 7-20. Single or multiple copies of this article are available for a fee from The Haworth Document Delivery Service [1-800-HAWORTH, 9:00 a.m. - 5:00 p.m. (EST). E-mail address: docdelivery@haworthpress.com].

Available online at http://jtp.haworthpress.com
doi:10.1300/J189v04n01_02

tion of the self in context of a different reality accompanied by an alteration in vigilance, awareness, control, and sense of concentration. Depersonalization is the core clinical element of this resulting condition which is called dissociation. *[Article copies available for a fee from The Haworth Document Delivery Service: 1-800-HAWORTH. E-mail address: <docdelivery@haworthpress.com> Website: <http://www.HaworthPress.com> © 2005 by The Haworth Press, Inc. All rights reserved.]*

KEYWORDS. Trauma, dissociation, cognition, time dimension, society

Trauma is not limited to or identical with a noxious event. Thus, the term posttraumatic stress disorder is a misleading one. Trauma is, in fact, an experience which is related to both the subjective and objective components of a situation. Accordingly, Fischer and Riedesser (1999) have defined trauma as the experience of vital discrepancy between threatening factors in a situation and individual coping abilities. Moreover, trauma is not merely a situational phenomenon, but a longitudinal socio-psychological process which develops in time and follows a course.

The resolution of traumatic experience is comprised of multiple components. The hallmark of trauma resolution is the ability and opportunity of the subject to respond to traumatic experience adequately. The available responses in a traumatic situation, however, may be rather limited. First, a person may escape from the traumatic situation. Second, the subject may process the situation until it is resolved. A third possibility is to deny some aspects of the experience. The latter results in the inadequate processing of the traumatic experience. Fischer and Riedesser (1999) even assert that, by definition, a traumatic situation is a condition where an adequate response is not possible despite existential threat. This inherent paradox, however, drives the trauma process.

Without immediate resolution of the traumatic experience, the subject will devote extensive energy for processing of the trauma after an interval following traumatic experience. Past trauma is then repeatedly handled in the context of present time in the person's active memory (Horowitz, 1986). This repetition is inevitable and different psychological realities emerge following each repetition. The new psychological realities contain cognitions which are designed to provide solutions for the perceived traumatic impasse. However, these cognitions usually have a self-destructive character, i.e., they do not lead to resolution of the impasse. In contrast to that, the subject who is able to process the traumatic experience immediately has no need to produce further versions of realities or to distort realities in order to find solutions.

These repetitions only cease when the contents held in present, active memory have been terminated by the completion of the cognitive processing of the trauma. The word 'ukde' of everyday language in Turkey, which means 'knot' etymologically, refers to the inner experience about an unforgotten upsetting past event that the subject was not able to respond adequately and timely. The word 'ukde,' with both its meanings, accurately describes the situation of a traumatized person.

INNER WORLD AND EXTERNAL REALITY

The goal of the trauma process is the continuity of the traumatic experience with other life memories, and the reintegration of personal goals. However, a traumatic life event is, by definition, one that is not fully in accord with a person's usual inner working models (Horowitz, 1986). Thus, the continual revision of relatively enduring structures of meaning is necessary to bring these inner models into accord with current reality. They can then guide decisions toward the next most effective possible actions.

The harmony or synthesis of an organism and environment may be illustrated by internal regulation systems called schemas (Piaget, 1947). Schemas have the two functions of assimilation and accommodation. When there is no problem, the schema is active. It assimilates the constellation of the external world into a personalized environment. In this case, the environment does not resist the reproduction of the schema. If there is a problem, the schema needs to be transformed until the problem is solved through effective action. The accommodation process then involves an active modification of the person's schemas to allow the incorporation of the new experience or information. When the process of accommodation is successful, the environmental situation can then be assimilated (Fischer & Riedesser, 1999).

Relationship schemas contain cognitions, emotions, affects, wishes, and moods. General schemas which coordinate other schemas are called scripts. Persons in a healthy mental state maintain a variety of inner working models or 'cognitive maps' of basic factors in their lives. These factors include their body image, various other self-concepts, role relationship models, scripts and agendas, spatial layouts of their repeated environmental circumstances, and other schemata that help them organize their perceptions and plan their future actions (Horowitz, 1986). Traumatic experiences which can not be integrated to the whole system of schemas remain as dissociated schemas, contradicting coordination rules, and scripts. There may be trauma-compensation schemas as well (Fischer & Riedesser, 1999).

INTERRUPTED PROCESS AND COMPLETION TENDENCY

The need to match new information with inner models based on older information, and the revision of both until they agree, can be called a completion tendency (Horowitz, 1986). The completion principle summarizes the human mind's intrinsic ability to continue to process new information in order to bring up to date the inner schemata of the self and the world.

Lewin (1935) stated that any intention to reach a goal produces a tension system that is preserved until a goal is reached. It was this theory that led to the prediction of the Zeigarnik effect, i.e., a tendency for interrupted, uncompleted tasks (not performed under stressful situations) to be better remembered than completed tasks. Mandler (1964) suggested that in addition to the completion tendency of initiated plans, interruption may lead to a state of increased arousal that is distressing and is maintained until the plans have been completed. The organism thus favors completion in order to end this distress.

Completion requires the resolution of differences between new information and enduring mental models. Every repetition may be a confrontation with a major difference between what is and what was gratifying and may invoke various responsive emotional states such as fear, anxiety, rage, panic, or guilt. If these emotional responses are likely to increase beyond the limits of toleration, the result may be overwhelmed states of mind. To avoid entry into such states of mind, therefore, control mechanisms are activated that will modify the cognitive processes (Horowitz, 1979).

WHAT IS TRAUMATIC?

According to the DSM-III's definition (criterion A) of Post-Traumatic Stress Disorder, a traumatic event creates significant stress symptoms and is outside of usual human experience (American Psychiatric Association, APA, 1980). The assumption was that the severity and unusualness of the event would lead to similar symptoms for an average person with similar sociocultural values and under similar conditions. However, this requires a decision by clinician as to what would be outside of the usual human experience and the the subjective experience of the person affected was not taken into account. In DSM-IV, for an event to be traumatic, "unusualness" was no more required and subjective experience was taken into account (APA, 1994). The criterion A was separated into two parts: (1) The person experienced, witnessed, or was confronted with an event or events that involved actual or theatened death or serious injury, or a threat to the physical integrity of self or others, and (2) the person's response involved intense fear, helplessness, or horror. Although this revision led to a more balanced view, as a phenomenological definition, it does not refer to the main psychopathological point what makes an event traumatic for a certain person.

Traumatic Obsessions and Completion Expectancy

The subject who has not resolved a traumatic process needs to work on the unmetabolized traumatic experience repeatedly. These repetitions may eventually take the form of 'traumatic obsessions.' From a psychopathological point of view, the traumatic impact of a noxious event depends on the activation of a maladaptive process. The starting point of this maladaptive process is the conversion of traumatic obsessions into a "traumatic whirlpool" The intensive urge to maintain the development of the life goals established before the traumatic experience is called 'completion expectancy.'

One of the most important aspects of processing trauma is not the issue of whether an adequate response was possible or not, but the degree of the preoccupation about developing an adequate response. The subject liberates all his or her devoted energy for this preoccupation and maintains an expectancy for the complete metabolization/resolution of the trauma. This expectancy of an exhaustive metabolization leads, in fact, to resistance against processing trauma in psychotherapy as well. Herman (1992) wrote that the "resolution of the trauma is never final and recovery is never complete." Nevertheless, the expectancy of completion of trauma process remains.

The completion expectancy is different than the completion tendency. The completion tendency is seen as the drive to complete an interrupted process. The completion expectancy consists of positive predictions, that one can or will be able to complete the goals/process of one's life. This is interrupted by traumatic experience suddenly and definitely. This intensive and involuntary urge (i.e., the completion expectancy) and the repetition tendency of the information (which is interrupted by traumatic obsessions) end up in a traumatic whirlpool. It is crucial to stop the obsessions and to take the person from this maladaptive process to an adaptive one.

Unpredicted Possibility and Being an Object

The traumatic event would have been seen as an 'unpredicted possibility' (Öztürk, 2004a). The development of the fear response and its maintenance among human and animals are related to the unpredicted and/or uncontrollable nature of the stressor (Basoglu & Mineka, 1992). People tend to inquire into the causes of and attempt to understand stressful events in order to better predict and control them (Harvey & Weary, 1985; Weiner, 1986). The traumatic experience interferes with the ability to attribute meaning, diminishes associative capacities and leads to the temporary loss of control.

Trauma is often characterized by loss of control which may be experienced by the subject as helplessness (Fischer & Riedesser, 1999). As such, the person may be seen as merely an object of the unpredicted traumatic situation rather than being a subject, because the person can not save himself/herself. The person can not possess mastery about the experience. This may be seen as the main reason that a situation becomes traumatic. The traumatized individual often experiences anger. The person is at the center of this feeling at the beginning. The anger generalizes afterwords to involve the people in their life and can reach the level of rage. This generalized anger may be seen as the main motive of repeated suicide attempts and self-destructive behavior (Öztürk, 2004b).

These circumstances prevent the traumatic experience from being processed. The unprocessed traumatic experience leads to a dysregulation in the responsiveness of the individual. The person's behavorial reactions tend to polarize on a spectrum from unresponsiveness to excessive reactivity (Öztürk, 2004b). The person is seen as more fragile after the traumatic experience, i.e., more unprotected against external influences. The subject then tends to lose the leading capacity in their circle of life. Thus, the incomplete trauma process has the three clinical consequence of loss of temperance, loss of sense of control, and a sense of increased or diminished interpersonal distance in their life circle.

TRAUMATIC EXPERIENCE AND PERCEPTION OF TIME

Time is one component of the background which influences all perception (Beere, 1995). All experience, all perception occurs in and over time: the present moment comes from a past which leads to a future (Merleau-Ponty, 1962, as cited in Beere 1995; Levine, 1997; Stern, 2004). A traumatic situation does not end in the objective time, or not per se when the traumatic event ends (Fischer & Riedesser, 1999). On the other hand, the experience is not intially conceived as trauma when the noxious event is still happening. It becomes psychologically traumatic when the event becomes past. Each moment that the trauma is processed becomes the present whereas the traumatic experience remains in the past. Normal time perception is replaced by "traumatic time perception" during the trauma process.

Traumatic Obsessions and Time Perception

In the processing of the traumatic experience, the subject's concentration on the past traumatic experience is done in the present. The main difference between past trauma experience and its version(s) in the present time are related to both time and context. The traumatic experience which remains in the past tends to create new and distorted perceptions of reality. The existence of multiple versions of perceived reality make the processing of the originial trauma difficult. The current versions of the trauma may differ after each repetition and may detach from its original form gradually. The most recent version remains as the final form for a certain period of time. New versions of reality and new cognitions form according to the moment when the processing of the trauma is interrupted and according to the phase of the process in which the subject is stuck. These cognitions typically suggest that a solution is not possible or they do not provide one. Consequently, the subject is unable to complete the trauma process.

These traumatic obsessions dualize the perception of present time. Each traumatic obsession is an infiltration of the past into present. Although the traumatic experience belongs to the past, the subject experiences the present time as infiltated by the past due to these intrusions without being aware (Van der Kolk & Van der Hart, 1991). This phenomenon interferes with the integration capacity and leads to a loss of ability.

The traumatic experience is then characterized by a vast proliferation (inflation) of operational options in the subject's mind. They are based on representations of inadequate operations in other past problematical experiences of the subject. One of these options takes the priority to deal with the trauma experience. This option, however, does not usually lead to a solution. The repetition of the representations of these operations in the active memory is an attempt to solve the trauma. All other operations which are excluded (from the perspective of time dimension that remain in the past) are transferred to inactive memory during these repetitions, either partially or totally.

The excluded operations may then lay the foundation for the immediate or future development of alter personalities seen among dissociative subjects. The various solution methods for recurrent traumatic experiences and repeated cognitions detach from each other. They become autonomous and reveal separate domains. They are transformed to alter personalities. Excluded operations, when formed alter personalities, are then tried to be utilized as solution methods in further domains of life problems.

Traumatic Turning Point and the Most Upsetting Traumatic Experience

Traumatic experiences interrupt the linear process of the complete psychological development throughout a person's life . These interruptions interfere with several capacities of the individual, e.g., social adjustment, defense mechanisms, problem solving and coping skills. At the same time, these interuptions can cause inadequacies in the person's intellectual and affective personality dimensions (Öztürk, 2003).

Traumatic experiences, that occur in childhood in particular, are unpredicted and unexpected. Thus, early traumatic experiences cause more intense interruptions in the aimed psychological integration more intensively. The traumatized individual has two life periods around the traumatic turning point: one life period before the traumatic experience and one after. The traumatic turning point does not refer to the first trauma which the subject has experienced, remembers, or realizes in time, but rather the most upsetting experience which happened most likely in childhood. The traumatic turning point refers to the most upsetting traumatic experience which takes a major role in the development of trauma schemata (Öztürk, 2004a).

The traumatic turning point may be perceived as a double-bind that interferes with the completion expectancy of a person's life. The traumatic event divides life in two parts. The expectancy and aim of a complete and whole life mostly consists of positive predictions. A person's positive predictions of the future helps provide assistance in overcoming current frustrations. The expectancy of a complete life and positive predictions are correlated with the psychological structure of the person; they are fundamental elements and/or locomotives. The rise of psychopathology after a traumatic turning point leads the person who continues to be exposed to acute or chronic trauma to a more intensive and exhausting struggle for saving his or her former more positive psychological structure.

The person is no more himself/herself. This turning point may lead to a psychological dividedness which may markedly interfere with the person's integrative and associative capacities. After the turning point, the person will detach and estrange from himself/herself, which he/she wants to save and own (Öztürk, 2004b). The most upsetting traumatic experience at the turning point is the most difficult, if possible, traumatic experience(s) to metabolize. When a traumatic experience is not metabolized, the person's self-perception begins to change. The different versions of external reality in the internal world which were developed through distortion of internal and external realities after trauma change the self-perception (Öztürk, 2004b). The changes in self-perception then continue to destroy the mutuality of internal world and external reality.

Dualization of Time and the Traumatic Whirlpool

Time perception turns into a dual one after traumatic experience and is known as traumatic time perception. The traumatized person perceives him/herself being controlled by their weaknesses, leading to helplessness, fearfulness, and loss of control of themselves and their environment. The traumatic obsessions may then turn into a traumatic whirlpool. The person's associative capacities, awareness and attribution of meaning are wounded. The inability to use previous coping ways after the traumatic experience may lead to further maladaptive thoughts, emotions and behavior.

The trauma-related aspect of the self lags behind the present time, i.e., it is related to past. It has a sense of present time which is shaded by the past. This present time is affixed to traumatic experience and it differs from real present time. Thus, time is divided by traumatic experience: time determined by traumatic experience and the real time. Trauma-related cognitions are distorted due to the effect of time as well. Throughout this process, the subject reveals different cognitions in the time dimension infiltrated by the traumatic experience and in the real time.

In its most extreme form, the traumatized subject can not experience past, presence and future; the time perception is distorted. In fact, the person's sense of time is lost (timelessness, loss of time feeling). The subject who detaches from the present moment is alienated to time; this is detemporalization (Beere, 1995). This means, nevertheless, that he or she is alienated to everything. Detemporalization is the hallmark of all alienation. Alienation to time facilitates the development of alter personalities among dissociative subjects.

When a traumatic experience is reevaluated by the subject in the present time, reality distortions may also interfere with the individual's consciousness, i.e., consciousness, control, vigilance, and awareness may alter. The subject may even alienate against his or her own traumatic experience. Psychotherapeutic interventions can not work in these conditions. The processing of trauma and elimination of the pathological formations require an adequate level of consciousness. In the psychotherapy of stress response syndromes, the process of using conscious awareness of change is of central importance (Horowitz, 1986).

TRAUMA AND DISSOCIATION

Basseches (1980, as cited by Fischer and Riedesser, 1999) defined an additional cognitive developmental stage subsequent to Piaget's (1947) formal operations phase, i.e., the stage of dialectical operations. This is an integrative style of thought which analyzes cognitive contradictions and resolves them through forming concepts of higher rank. This is the force behind the development of a coherent self-system. The subject can develop meta-schemas which coordinate schemata specific to situation in order to establish a continuity of action in the personal life story. Trauma distrupts these integrating schemas.

Trauma and Double-Bind

Double-bind is a message containing two contradictory instructions. It is a concept developed originally to describe a dysfunctional communication style which was believed to be common among families of schizophrenic patients (Bateson, Jackson, Haley, & Weakland, 1956; Cattell, & Schmahl-Cattell, 1974). We propose that all traumatic events (interpersonal or impersonal) have the inherent character of a double-bind (Sar & Ozturk, in press).

Double-bind creates multiple perceptions of reality, i.e., various versions of reality are created in the internal world (Sar & Ozturk). The traumatized subject perceives himself/herself from the perspective of these multiple versions of reality (Bromberg,1998) and developes isolated subjectivities (Chefetz & Bromberg, 2004). Although these perceptions may create opportunities for progression in a few matters, they lead to impasses and negative cognitions in many areas. To cope with this, the traumatic fact (person, idea, situation, etc.) is kept at a distance, or, alternatively, the subject remains in an oscillating relationship with it. Clinical studies have demonstrated that at least a subgroup of patients remain in an ambivalent attitude about their traumatic childhood (Sar, Akyuz, Kundakci, Kiziltan, & Dogan, 2004; Sar, Akyuz, & Ozturk, 2004), i.e., they tend to minimize them.

If the subject can enter a dialectical process in the face of trauma, he/she may have the power of turning the situation to his/her favor in a limited extent. Otherwise, this incomplete process may lead to the generalization of the previously experienced double-bind to his or her entire life (Sar, 2004). The multiple simultaneous perceptions of reality destroy personalization, i.e., one's experience that all psychological faculties (perception, body perception, memory retrieval, imagination, thought, feeling, etc.) belong to oneself (Jaspers,1913). Depersonalization is the core element of clinical categories which are considered to be trauma-related conditions, e.g., dissociative disorders, Borderline Personality Disorder, or Conversion Disorder (Sar et al., 2004; Sar, Akyuz, & Ozturk, 2004).

Trauma and Dissociation: A Sociopsychological Response

Trauma makes both the subject's conceptualizations of the self and the world questionable (Fischer & Riedesser, 1999). The trauma process is not only an individual but a social endeavor as well. Thus, the problem brought up by the traumatic event can not be solved by the individual solely, because the traumatized individual does not stand alone. Recovery can take place only within the context of relationships; it cannot occur in isolation (Herman,1992). It is important how the community responds to the misery of the individual (Fischer & Riedesser, 1999).

Trauma process is a socio-psychological response. We believe that the completion tendency (Horowitz, 1986) has a further meaning for relationship traumas in particular: the subject has the need to express his or her opinions and emotions related to the past trauma experience. The incomplete processing of trauma disturbs the subject's responsiveness to the world. This damaged responsiveness may manifest as not being able to respond adequately to the situation or a choice to not respond at all. This manifestation may infiltrate all areas of the person's life. It is thus an important function of psychotherapy to help a person develop responsiveness to individuals and to society.

The ability to distinguish between destructive and helpful environmental stimuli becomes difficult after a traumatic experience. The therapist has to support the ability of the subject to differentiate destructive from helpful environmental stimuli (Fischer & Riedesser, 1999). Every subject maintains interpersonal distances in concentric trajectories in everyday life. Dissociation turns this life circle to a "pool system," i.e., concentric trajectories of interpersonal distances disappear. The subject is then relatively unprotected against destructive attacks. This can end up in a closed system characterized by self-help and social withdrawal, i.e., relationships with the external world are diminished (Blizard, 2003; Howell, 2003). Thus, the dissociative disorders may be seen as a noninteractive solution (Crandell, Morrison, & Willis, 2002; Sar, Ozturk, & Kundakci, 2002).

In our view, trauma should be defined as a threatening experience which turns an adaptive process to a maladaptive one. This is the condition when upsetting and unpredicted situational and/or continuous factors interrupt the psychosociological experiencing suddenly and significantly, and interfere with the coping capacity of the person for a moment or a period of time. The impact of this interference depends on the severity of these factors and the quality of the person's previous experiences. A definition of dissociation based on our elaborations should be as follows: traumatic experiences and consequently altered self-perceptions contribute to the impairment of the mutuality between internal world and external reality. This is accompanied by a renewed perception of the self in the context of a different reality accompanied by altered vigilance, awareness, control, and sense of concentration. Depersonalization is the core clinical element of this condition.

REFERENCES

American Psychiatric Association. (1980). *Diagnostic and Statistical Manual of Mental Disorders: DSM-III* (3rd ed.). Washington DC: Author.
American Psychiatric Association. (1994). *Diagnostic and Statistical Manual of Mental Disorders: DSM-IV* (4th ed.). Washington DC: Author.

Basoglu, M., & Mineka, S. (1992). The role of uncontrollable and unpredictable stress in post-traumatic stress responses in torture survivors. In M. Basoglu (Ed.) *Torture and its consequences: Current treatment approaches*. Cambridge: Cambridge University Press.

Basseches, M. (1980, cited in G. Fischer and P. Riedesser, 1999). Dialectical schemata: A framework for the empirical study of the development of dialectical thinking. *Human Development*, *23*, 400-421.

Bateson, G., Jackson, D.D., Haley, J., & Weakland, J.H. (1956). Toward a theory of schizophrenia. *Behavioral Science*, *1*, 251-264.

Beere, D. (1995). Loss of 'background': A perceptual theory of dissociation. *Dissociation*, *8*, 165-174.

Blizard, R.A. (2003). Disorganized attachment, development of dissociative self-states, and a relational approach to treatment. *Journal of Trauma and Dissociation*, *4(3)*, 27-50.

Bromberg, P.M. (1998). *Standing in the spaces. Essays on clinical process trauma & dissociation*. Hilsdale, NJ: The Analytic Press.

Cattell, J.P., & Schmahl-Cattell, J. (1974). Depersonalization: Psychological and social perspectives. In S. Arieti (Ed.) *American handbook of psychiatry*, Vol. 3, (pp. 766-799). New York: Basic Books.

Chefetz, A.R., & Bromberg, P.M. (2004). Talking with 'me' and 'not-me.' A dialogue. *Comtemporary Psychoanalysis, 40*, 409-464.

Crandell, J., Morrison. R., & Willis, K. (2002). Using psychomotor to treat Dissociative Identity Disorder. *Dissociation, 3*, 57-80.

Fischer, G., & Riedesser P (1999). *Lehrbuch der Psychotraumatologie* (Textbook of psychotraumathology). München: Ernst Reinhardt Verlag.

Harvey, J.H., & Weary, G. (1985). *Attribution: Basic issues and application*. Orlando: Academic Press.

Herman, J.L. (1992). *Trauma and recovery*. New York: Basic Books.

Horowitz, M.J. (1986). *Stress response syndromes* (2nd ed.). Northwale NJ: Jason Aronson Inc.

Horowitz, M.J. (1979). *States of mind*. New York: Plenum.

Howell, E.F. (2003). Narcissism, a relational aspect of dissociation. *Journal of Trauma and Dissociation*, *4*, 51-71.

Jaspers, K. (1913). *Allgemeine Psychopathologie* (General psychopathology), Berlin: Springer Verlag.

Levine, P.A. (1997). *Waking the tiger. Healing trauma*. Berkeley, CA: North Atlantic Books.

Lewin, K. (1935, cited in M.J. Horowitz, 1976/1986). The conflict between Aristotelian and Galilean modes of though in contemporary psychology. In *A dynamic theory of personality* (pp. 1-43). New York: McGraw Hill.

Mandler, G. (1964, cited in M.J. Horowitz, 1976/1986).). The interruption of behavior. *Nebraska symposium on motivation. 12* (pp. 163-220). Lincoln: University of Nebraska Press.

Merleau-Ponty, M. (1962, cited in D. Beere, 1995). *Phenomenology of perception*. New York: The Humanities Press, Routledge & Kegan Paul.

Öztürk, E. (2003). Travma kökenli dissosiyatif bozukluk vakalarinin aile bireylerindeki çocukluk çagi travmalari (Childhood traumata in the first degree relatives of traumatized dissociative patients). *Doctoral Dissertation*, Istanbul: Istanbul University Institute of Forensic Medicine, Department of Social Sciences.

Öztürk, E. (2004a). Ruhsal bölünme: Dissosiyasyon ve dissosiyatif bozukluklar, (Psychological dividedness: Dissociation and dissociative disorders). *Paper presented at the XIII. Annual Conference of the Turkish Psychological Association*, Istanbul.

Öztürk, E. (2004b). Psikoterapide travmatik kendilik ve kendilesme (Traumatic self and getting himself/herself in psychotherapy). *Presentation at the Symposium: Self, Traumatic Reality, and Psychotherapy (Chair: V. Sar) in the VIII. Annual Spring Conference of the Psychiatric Association of Turkey*, Antalya.

Piaget, J. (1947). *Psychologie der Intelligenz* (Psychology of intelligence). Zürich: Rascher.

Sar, V. (2004). Travmatik gerçeklik karsisinda kendilik. (Self exposed to traumatic reality). *Presentation at the symposium 'Self, traumatic reality, and psychotherapy' (Chair: V. Sar) in the VIII Annual Spring Conference of the Psychiatric Association of Turkey*, Antalya.

Sar, V., Akyuz, G., Kundakci, T., Kiziltan, E, & Dogan, O. (2004). Childhood trauma, dissociation, and psychiatric comorbidity in patients with conversion disorder. *American Journal of Psychiatry, 161(12)*, 2271-2276.

Sar, V., Akyuz, G., & Öztürk, E. (2004). Axis-I dissociative disorder comorbidity of borderline personality disorder and its impact on reports of childhood trauma. *Paper presented at the 21th Annual Conference of the International Society for the Study of Dissociation*, New Orleans.

Sar, V., Öztürk, E., & Kundakci, T. (2002). Psychotherapy of an adolesent with Dissociative Identity Disorder: Changes in Rorschach patterns. *Journal of Trauma and Dissociation, 3*, 81-95.

Sar, V. & Öztürk, E. (in press). Psychotic presentations of Dissociative Identity Disorder. In P. Dell & J. O'Neill (eds): *Dissociation and the dissociative disorders: DSM-V and beyond.*

Stern, D.N. (2004). *The present moment in psychotherapy and everyday life.* New York: Norton Company.

Van der Kolk, B.A., & Van der Hart, O. (1991). The intrusive past: The flexibility of memory and the engraving of trauma. *American Imago, 48 (4)*, 425-252.

Weiner, B. (1986). *An attributional theory of motivation and emotion.* New York: Springer Verlag.

Cross-Cultural Aspects
of Trauma and Dissociation

George F. Rhoades, Jr.

SUMMARY. The importance of culture and the cross-cultural manifestations of trauma and dissociation was presented. A discussion of culture and psychopathology was shown, noting that although psychiatric disorders appear in all cultures, their form and expression may vary often in a way that is linked to cultural belief systems. The Culture-Bound Syndromes of *amok, ataque de Nervios, falling out or blacking out, latah, nervios, pibloktoq, qi-gong psychotic reaction, shin-byung, spell, susto,* and *zar,* seen as having dissociative symptoms, were then presented with relevant research. The Possession Trance Disorder was also presented as a cultural disorder. Finally, therapeutic considerations to better facilitate cultural sensitivity were noted. *[Article copies available for a fee from The Haworth Document Delivery Service: 1-800-HAWORTH. E-mail address: <docdelivery@haworthpress.com> Website: <http://www.HaworthPress.com> © 2005 by The Haworth Press, Inc. All rights reserved.]*

KEYWORDS. Cross-Cultural Therapy, trauma, dissociation, Culture-Bound Syndromes, amok, ataque de Nervios, falling out or blacking out,

George F. Rhoades, Jr., PhD, is Director, Ola Hou Clinic, 98-1247 Kaahumanu Street, Suite 223, Aiea, HI 96701 (Email: rhoades@pdchawaii.com)

[Haworth co-indexing entry note]: "Cross-Cultural Aspects of Trauma and Dissociation." Rhoades, George F., Jr. Co-published simultaneously in *Journal of Trauma Practice* (The Haworth Maltreatment & Trauma Press, an imprint of The Haworth Press, Inc.) Vol. 4, No. 1/2, 2005, pp. 21-33; and: *Trauma and Dissociation in a Cross-Cultural Perspective: Not Just a North American Phenomenon* (ed: George F. Rhoades, Jr., and Vedat Sar) The Haworth Maltreatment & Trauma Press, an imprint of The Haworth Press, Inc., 2005, pp. 21-33. Single or multiple copies of this article are available for a fee from The Haworth Document Delivery Service [1-800-HAWORTH, 9:00 a.m. - 5:00 p.m. (EST). E-mail address: docdelivery@haworthpress. com].

doi:10.1300/J189v04n01_03

latah, nervios, pibloktoq, qi-gong psychotic reaction, shin-byung, spell, Susto, Zar, Possession Trance Disorder

The recent tsunami of December 26, 2004 in South East Asia was devastating in the loss of life, property and the traumatizing effect on millions of persons. The world felt the trauma through electronic and written media and responded in kind with financial and other needed support. An important lesson from the tsunami was that we are an international community and the trauma experienced there has and will affect the entire world. Another critical lesson is that the reaction to trauma will be both unique according to a person's culture and similar in aspects to the experiences of others around the world.

Traumatic events may be defined as "very stressful, often emotionally arousing situations that an individual directly experiences and that have immediate consequences for the individual's unfolding life" (Brown, Scheflin, & Hammond, 1998, p. 154). A response to trauma is often dissociation.

To "associate" is to connect or to bring into a relationship. Dissociation is thus the breaking or splitting off of that connection. In mental health, we often look at dissociation as the splitting off of certain mental (physical, emotional) processes from the main body of consciousness. Dissociation can thus cause a lack of association with one's inner world or even outer world. Dissociation can be a normal coping skill to an abnormal situation/stressor, such as trauma. The dissociation may then become dysfunctional for the person in their personal and interpersonal lives.

This chapter will look at trauma and dissociation in the context of culture and how they may be manifested in culture bound syndromes and possession trance disorder. The author will also focus on therapeutic principles/considerations to provide counseling for persons of a different culture.

CULTURE AND PSYCHOPATHOLOGY

It is important to note that what is considered healthy in one society may be viewed unhealthy in another. Although psychiatric disorders appear in all cultures, their form and expression may vary often in a way that is linked to cultural belief systems (Ritts, 1999). Castro (1998) noted that "the subjective experience of traditional illness is shaped both by the cultural background of individuals, and by the sociological features of the setting where these individuals live" (p. 203).

CULTURE-BOUND SYNDROMES

The American Psychiatric Association (2000), in the *Diagnostic and Statistical Manual of Mental Disorders-Fourth Edition-Text Revision (DSM-IV-TR), has defined Culture-Bound Syndromes (CBS) as, recurrent, locality-specific patterns of aberrant behavior and troubling experience that may or may not be linked to a particular DSM-IV diagnostic category. Many of these patterns are indigenously considered to be "illnesses," or at least afflictions, and most have local names (p. 898).*

Rhoades (2003a, b) noted that at least 11 of the 25 CBS listed in the DSM-IV-TR (2000) may be seen as possibly involving dissociative symptoms. These syndromes and the typical country/culture where they are manifested included amok (Malaysia), ataque de nervios (Caribbean), falling out or blacking out (Southern United States and Caribbean), latah (Malaysia or Indonesia), nervios (Latin America), pibloktoq (Arctic and subarctic Eskimos), qi-gong psychotic reaction (China), shin-byung (Korea), spell (Southern United States), susto (Latin America), and Zar (North African and Middle Eastern Societies).

The CBS of amok has been known for many centuries in the Malaysian culture (Knecht, 1999). The syndrome has been defined as an episode of dissociation (Suryani & Jensen, 1993) and is often characterized by "a sudden rampage, usually including homicide, ending in exhaustion and amnesia" (Hatta, 1996). Typically seen as a Malaysian CBS, amok has been further documented in India, New Guinea, North America, and Britain (Kon, 1994).

The legal defense of amok was utilized for a Filipino-American that had killed five people and injured three others in Hawaii. Orlando Ganal, Sr. (HonoluluAdvertiser.com, 1999) was enraged by his wife's reported relationship with another man, shot and killed his wife's parents and wounded his own wife and son. Ganal continued to firebomb the home of the other man's brother, Michael Touchette, killing Michael, Michael's two children and badly burning his wife, Wendy Touchette. Ganal was seen as a mild mannered man, until the stress grew and he finally "ran amok."

Ataque de Nervios is a CBS that may or may not involve amnesia has been found by Latinos from the Caribbean, Latin America, and Latin Mediterranean groups.

Commonly reported symptoms include uncontrollable shouting, attacks of crying, trembling, heat in the chest rising to the head, and verbal or physical aggression. Dissociative experiences, seizure-like or fainting episodes, and suicidal gestures are prominent in some attacks but absent in others. A general feature of an ataque de nervios is being out of control. Ataque de nervios frequently occur as a result of a stressful event relating to the family. (DSM-IV-TR, 2000, p. 899)

In contrast to another CBS–*Hwa-byung* (Korean) which is seen as a syndrome of repressed anger, *ataque de nervios* is an episode of expressed anger that has built up over time.

Schechter et al. (2000) studied 70 treatment-seeking Hispanics and concluded that "in some Hispanic individuals, ataque represents a culturally sanctioned expression of extreme affect dysregulation associated with childhood trauma." Schechter et al. (2000) conducted a mother-infant case study of ataque de nervios and concluded that the syndrome was associated with childhood trauma and dissociation. Steinberg (1990) recommended the consideration of the diagnosis of Multiple Personality Disorder (now called Dissociative Identity Disorder) with Ataque de Nervios patients.

In a study of 29 Puerto Rican Psychiatric outpatients that had experienced ataque de nervios, Lewis-Fernandez et al. (2002) found that dissociative symptoms (as measured by the Dissociative Experiences Scale) increased as the frequency of ataque de nervios increased.

The syndrome has been described as "a culturally condoned expression of distress that is most frequently seen in Hispanic women" (Oquendo, 1995), up to 80% (Liebowitz et al., 1994).

The ataque de nervios may be seen as the expression of three core themes (Guarnaccia, DeLaCancela & Carrillo, 1989):

1. emotions of anger/rage, grief, and fear of being alone;
2. problems in key family relationships between spouses and between parents and children; and
3. the social experiences of [the] death of a loved one, intergenerational conflict, and abuse by a close family member. (p. 47)

Guarnaccia (1993) called the syndrome that "popular illness," rather than a "culture-bound syndrome" (p. 157). In addition, in a study of 145 survivors of a 1985 flood disaster in Puerto Rico, Guarnaccia, Canino,

Rubio-Stipec, and Bravo (1993) found the survivors to be more likely "female, older, less educated, and formerly married" (p. 157).

Falling Out or Blacking Out primarily occurs in the Southern United States and the Caribbean, and is described as,

> a sudden collapse, which sometimes occurs without warning, but sometimes preceded by feelings of dizziness or "swimming" in the head. The individual's eyes are usually open, but the person claims an inability to see. The person usually hears and understands what is occurring around him or her, but feels powerless to move. This may correspond to a diagnosis of Conversion Disorder or a Dissociative Disorder. (DSM-IV-TR, 2000, p. 900)

The CBS of Latah is a Malaysian or Indonesian term (DSM-IV-TR, 2000), but the condition has been found in other parts of the world under different names, i.e., Siberia (Amurakh, Irkunii, Ikota, Olan, Myriachit, and Menkeiti); Thailand (Bah-tschi, Bah-tsi, and Baah-ji); Japan (Imu); and Philippines (Mali-mali and Silok). Latah is described as a,

> Hypersensitivity to sudden fright, often with echopraxia, echolalia, command obedience, and dissociative or trancelike behavior. The term *latah* is of Malaysian or Indonesian origin, but the syndrome has been found in many parts of the world. In Malaysia it is more frequent in middle-aged. (DSM-IV-TR, 2000, p. 901)

Bartholomew (1994) reviewed 37 cases of Latah and surmised that Latah could be seen as an infrequent, culturally conditioned habit or even malingering and fraud. Should we only look at these cultural illnesses through Western eyes and/or accept them as realities within their cultures? Our concept of a cultural illness will thus affect our treatment of same.

Nervios, similar to nevra (Greece), is a common CBS found among Latinos in the United States and Latin America. This CBS is seen as,

> both a general state of vulnerability to stressful life experiences and to a syndrome brought on by difficult life circumstances. The term nervios includes a wide range of symptoms of emotional distress, somatic disturbance, and inability to function. Common symptoms include headaches and "brain aches," irritability, stomach disturbances, sleep difficulties, nervousness, easy tearfulness, inability to concentrate, trembling, tingling sensations, and mareos

(dizziness with occasional vertigo-like exacerbations). Nervios tends to be an ongoing problem, although variable in the degree of disability manifested. (DSM-IV-TR, 2000, p. 901)

Jenkins (1988) found that Mexican-Americans could view Schizophrenia as a manifestation of nervios. This view would thus allow a reduction of the stigma of the schizophrenic diagnosis, a strengthening of family bonds and the tolerant inclusion of the mentally ill family member. The author saw this use of a "folk label" as helping to mediate the course and outcome of the Schizophrenic disorder.

Ecuadorian Andes children experience this disorder with varied symptoms such as melancholy and anger. This disorder is often said to strike when the children are separated from their parents, especially their fathers (Pribilsky, 2001). Mexican rural communities showed a prevalence of 15.5% in the general population for the diagnosis of nervios. Women had a prevalence of 20.8% to that of 9.5% for men.

Pibloktoq has been found primarily in the Arctic and sub-Arctic Eskimo communities (DSM-IV-TR). This syndrome has been described as,

> An abrupt dissociative episode accompanied by extreme excitement of up to 30 minutes' duration and frequently followed by convulsive seizures and coma lasting up to 12 hours. This is observed primarily in arctic and subarctic Eskimo communities, although regional variations in name exist. The individual may be withdrawn or mildly irritable for a period of hours or days before the attack and will typically report complete amnesia for the attack. During the attack, the individual may tear off his or her clothing, break furniture, shout obscenities, eat feces, flee from protective shelters, or perform other irrational or dangerous acts. (DSM-IV-TR, 2000, p. 901)

A Qi-Gong Psychotic Reaction may occur when a person participates in the Chinese folk health-enhancing practice of Qi-Gong. A person is seen as more vulnerable when they are "overly involved" in the practice which is seen as an "exercise of vital energy" (DSM-IV-TR, 2000, p. 902). This psychotic reaction is seen as "an acute, time-limited episode characterized by dissociative, paranoid, or other psychotic or nonpsychotic symptoms" (p. 902).

Qi-Gong is a Chinese folk health-enhancing practice which consists of controlled breathing and body movements (Lim & Lin, 1996). Qi-Gong may be seen as a form of hypnosis, an offshoot of martial arts. The operator projects an invisible force (chi) from his body to that of the subject to restore that person's balance of the two opposing elements of chi (Mackett, 1989). Qi-Gong has been accepted as one of the many common psycho-physiological gymnastic exercises in China for 2000 years (Shan, 2000). Shan noted that Chinese Qi-Gong is "an important cultural heritage of China and a part of traditional Chinese medicine" (2000, p. 12). He cautioned, however, that the practice could "lead to abnormal phenomena or even mental disorders, especially if practiced inappropriately" (p. 12).

Shin-Byung is "a Korean label for a syndrome in which initial phases are characterized by anxiety and somatic complaints" (DSM-IV-TR, 2000, p. 902). The somatic complaints consist of general weakness, dizziness, fear, anorexia, insomnia, and gastrointestinal problems. The patient subsequently manifests with "dissociation and possession by ancestral spirits" (p. 902).

Shin-Byung is known as "god illness" or "divine illness." Yi (2000) described a Western and Korean treatment of the syndrome involving the following elements: (1)Visiting a Shaman in Korea, (2) Completed eight months of psychotherapy in United States, (3) Became immersed in shamanic rituals, and (4) 100-day prayer ritual. Yi reported that subsequent to above treatments, psychotherapy was sporadic and there was significant symptom improvement.

A trance state that is more typically seen among African Americans and European Americans in the southern United States is called a spell. In the trance state, the individual tends to have brief periods of personality change and is reportedly able to communicate with deceased relatives or with spirits. This culturally specific syndrome would not typically receive a medical/psychiatric diagnosis, "but may be misconstrued clinically as a psychotic episode" (DSM-IV-TR, 2000, p. 903).

Another cultural bound syndrome that is commonly seen among Latinos in America and people in Mexico, Central and South America is called Susto.

> Susto is also referred to as *espanto, pasmo, tripa ida, perdida del alma*, or *chibih. Susto* is an illness attributed to a frightening event that causes the soul to leave the body, and results in unhappiness and sickness. Individuals with susto also experience significant strains in key social roles. Symptoms may appear any time from days to years after the fright is experienced. It is believed that in

extreme cases, susto may result in death. Typical symptoms include appetite disturbances, inadequate or excessive sleep, troubled sleep or dreams, feeling of sadness, lack of motivation to do anything, and feelings of low self-worth, or dirtiness. Somatic symptoms accompanying susto include muscle aches and pains, headache, stomachache, and diarrhea. Ritual healings are focused on calling the soul back to the body and cleansing the person to restore bodily and spiritual balance. (DSM-IV-TR, 2000, p. 903)

A case study of susto involved a Chilean political refugee living in Tasmania, who became disabled after an industrial accident. Holloway (1994) noted that immigrant clients tended to exacerbate their situations by overconforming to traditional medical practices. Treatment then involved "removing victims from the medical system and desocializing them from their roles as victims" (Holloway, 1994, p. 989). Baer and Penzell (1993) investigated 30 farm workers in Florida who were exposed to pesticide poisoning. The patients who identified their illness as susto complained of more residual symptoms. Logan (1993) has presented a case for susto as a "widelyspread ethnomedical belief diverse in its manifestation. It crosscuts age, gender, ethnic, and class lines, and is patterned in its occurrence" (p. 189).

The last CBS to be presented is that of Zar, a syndrome that is found in Ethiopia, Somalia, Sudan, Egypt, Iran, and other North American and Middle Eastern societies. The person experiencing Zar is,

possessed by a spirit [and] may experience dissociative episodes that may include shouting, laughing, hitting the head against a wall, singing, or weeping. Individuals may show apathy and withdrawal, refusing to eat or carry out daily tasks, or may develop a long-term relationship with the possessing spirit. Such behavior is not necessarily considered pathological locally. (DSM-IV-TR, 2000, p. 903)

A 45-year-old woman who had emigrated from Ethiopia to Israel and was referred to an emergency room for internal pain, due to a reported punishment from the Zar. The patient was diagnosed with Obsessive Compulsive Disorder and given medication, but the patient did not improve. The "patient's situation improved once her cultural context and background were considered" (Grisaru, Budowski & Witztum, 1997).

POSSESSION TRANCE DISORDER

The Possession Trance Disorder (DSM-IV-TR, 2000) is a single or episodic replacement of a person's personal identity with a new identity. This new identity is attributed to the influence of a spirit, deity, power or another person. This influence is indicated by either culturally determined or stereotyped behaviors, or a sense that the person is controlled by the possessing agent. The person also has full or partial amnesia for the event. The possession trance disorder causes significant distress in important areas of functioning such as social and occupational and is not seen as a normal part of the collective culture or religious practice.

Examples of possession trance disorder have been noted in Judaism (Somer, 2004), South Asia (Suryani & Jensen, 1993; Castillo, 1994a, 1994b), and in Northern Sudan (Boddy, 1988). The possession trance disorder was regarded as one of criteria sets and axes included in DSM-IV-TR (2000) for further study.

CULTURE AND THERAPY

To have effective counseling/therapy with persons of different cultures, the therapist must be aware of culture-bound syndromes, possession trance disorder and be culturally sensitive. Zayas, Torres, Malcolm, and DesRosiers (1996) surveyed 150 nonminority psychologists and social workers and found the following four overlapping dimensions in becoming culturally sensitive:

1. Being aware of the existence of differences.
2. Having knowledge of the client's culture.
3. Distinguishing between culture and pathology in assessment.
4. Taking culture into account in therapy. (p. 78)

It is also important to learn how to raise the issue of race and ethnicity in the process of therapy. Cardemil and Battle (2003) noted six important areas. First, that it was important to suspend preconceptions about clients' race/ethnicity and that of their family members. Second, recognize that clients may be quite different from other members of their racial/ethnic group. Third, consider how racial/ethnic differences between therapist and client might affect psychotherapy. Fourth, acknowledge that power, privilege, and racism might affect interactions with clients. Fifth, when in doubt about the importance of race and ethnicity in treatment, be willing to discuss the issues and to take risks in the area of culture with clients. The sixth area was to keep learning. It is better to acknowledge that you may not know your client's culture and to be willing to learn from the client about that culture.

In my clinical work in Hawaii, it is common to have clients of many different races and cultures. It is important to first determine what "generation" the person is, i.e., a first generation Japanese was born in Japan and immigrated to Hawaii. The assumption is that first generation clients are more traditional in their cultural practice. The second question is how traditional is the person in the practice of their culture. It is possible for a first generation client to want to become more like people in his new country, almost to the point of denouncing his or her past homeland culture. In contrast, it is possible for a fourth generation client (three generations born in the new land/country) to have a desire to be traditional and to exhibit many characteristics of their ancestral heritage.

It is also important to note that there are several layers or levels of cross-cultural work in any society. The first level is that of the indigenous peoples of the land. A second group of people would be persons born in the country, but that are not of indigenous heritage. The third group is the individuals that have immigrated with the intention to permanently live in the new land. A fourth group are speciality groups of persons, i.e., the military or temporary hires, that live and work in the new land, but who typically move back to their homes after a pre-determined period of time. Each of these groups may have special needs and concerns when in treatment for trauma and dissociation.

Therapists that are involved in cross cultural counseling should also be aware of the five therapeutic "Cultural Traps" delineated by Schein (2003),

> Trap 1: You assume that good intervention should be based on good diagnosis, and that good diagnosis must be scientifically valid. You therefore choose diagnostic tools that are validated, that are reliable, that are standardized, that have academic credibility. But in making the choice on those criteria, you overlook their impact on the client (p. 76),

> Trap 2: You assume that the client is an individual rather than a set of interconnected individuals and groups who make up a cultural unit (p. 79),

Trap 3: You assume that your client knows what culture is and does, and, worse, you assume that you know what culture is and does (p. 79),

Trap 4: You assume that individual assessment provides valid data for group phenomena (p. 80), and

Trap 5: You assume that you have and should use a standard method of working based on sound theory and past history of success (p. 81).

The process of cross-cultural counseling involves working with an individual who is unique in him/herself, but also part of the culture that he/she was born into and has chosen to live in. It is reasonable that sound clinical assessment and treatment practices developed within one culture may or may not work with the patient of a different culture. Patients who have experienced trauma and dissociation, leading to significant distress in areas of their lives will display that distress within and through their culture. It is thus important for therapists to be aware of the client's culture, culture-bound syndromes, possession trance disorder and to be culturally sensitive in providing treatment.

REFERENCES

American Psychiatric Association (2000). *Diagnostic and statistical manual of mental disorders-text revision (4th ed.)*. Washington, DC: Author.

Baer, R. D. & Penzell, D. (1993). Research report: Susto and pesticide poisoning among Florida farmworkers. *Culture, Medicine & Psychiatry, 17,* 321-327.

Bartholomew, R. E. (1994). Disease, disorder, or deception? Latah as habit in a Malay extended family. *Journal of Nervous and Mental Disease, 182,* 331-338.

Boddy, J. (1988). Spirits and selves in Northern Sudan: The cultural therapeutics of possession and trance. *Transcultural Psychiatric Research Review, 25,* 5-46.

Brown, D., Scheflin, A. W., & Hammond, D. C. (1998). *Memory, trauma treatment, and the law*. New York: W. W. Norton & Company.

Cardemil, E. V. & Battle, C. L. (2003). Guess who's coming to therapy? Getting comfortable with conversations about race and ethnicity in psychotherapy. *Professional Psychology, Research and Practice, 34,* 278-286.

Castillo, R. J. (1994a). Spirit possession in South Asia, dissociation or hysteria? II. Case histories. *Culture, Medicine & Psychiatry, 18,* 141-162.

Castillo, R. J. (1994b). Spirit possession in South Asia, dissociation or hysteria? II. Theoretical background. *Culture, Medicine & Psychiatry, 18,* 1-21.

Grisaru, N., Budowski, D., & Witztum, E. (1997). Possession by the "Zar" among Ethiopian immigrants to Israel: Psychopathology or culture-bound syndrome? *Psychopathology, 30*, 223-233.

Guarnaccia, P. J. (1993). Ataques de nervios in Puerto Rico: Culture-bound syndrome or popular illness? *Medical Anthropology, 15*, 157-170.

Guarnaccia, P. J., Canino, G., Rubio-Stipec, M., & Bravo, M. (1993). The prevalence of Ataques de Nervios in the Puerto Rico Disaster Study: The role of culture in psychiatric epidemiology. *Journal of Nervous & Mental Disease, 181*, 157-165.

Guarnaccia, P. J., DeLaCancela, V., & Carrillo, E. (1989). The multiple meanings of Ataques de Nervios in the Latino community. *Medical Anthropology, 11*, 47-62.

Hatta, S. (1996). A Malay crosscultural worldview and forensic review of Amok. *Australian & New Zealand Journal of Psychiatry, 30*, 505-510.

Holloway, G., (1994). Susto and the career path of the victim of an industrial accident: A sociological case study. *Social Science and Medicine, 38*, 989-997.

HonoluluAdvertiser.com (1999). *Hawaii Multiple Slayings*. Posted on: Wednesday, November 3, 1999. Honolulu: Honolulu Advertiser.

Jenkins, J. H. (1988). Ethnopsychiatric interpretations of schizophrenic illness: The problem of nervios within Mexican-American families. *Culture, Medicine & Psychiatry, 12*, 301-329.

Knecht, T. (1999). *Schweizer Archiv fur Neurologie und Psychiatrie, 150*, 142-148.

Kon, Y. (1994). Amok. *British Journal of Psychiatry, 165*, 685-689.

Lewis-Fernandez, R., Garrido-Castillo, P., Bennasar, M. C., Parrilla, E. M., Laria, A. J., Ma, G., & Petkova, E. (2002). Dissociation, childhood trauma, and Ataque de Nervios among Puerto Rican psychiatric outpatients. *American Journal of Psychiatry, 159*, 1603-1605.

Liebowitz, M. R., Salman, E., Jusino, C. M., Garfinkel, R., Street, L., Cardenas, D. L. et al. (1994). Ataque de Nervios and panic disorder. *American Journal of Psychiatry, 151*, 871-875.

Lim, R. F. & Lin, K.-M. (1996). Cultural formulation of psychiatric diagnosis: Case No. 03: Psychosis following Qi-Gong in a Chinese immigrant. *Culture, Medicine & Psychiatry, 20*, 369-378.

Logan, M. H. (1993). New lines of inquiry on the illness of susto. *Medical Anthropology, 15*, 189-200.

Mackett, J. (1989). Chinese hypnosis. *British Journal of Experimental & Clinical Hypnosis, 6*, 129-130.

Oquendo, M. A. (1995). Differential diagnosis of ataque de nervios. *American Journal of Orthopsychiatry, 65*, 60-65.

Pribilsky, J. (2001). Nervios and 'modern childhood': Migration and shifting contexts of child life in the Ecuadorian Andes. *Childhood: A Global Journal of Child Research, 8*, 251-273.

Rhoades, G. F. Jr. (2003a, May/June). Culture-Bound Syndromes. *The International Society for the Study of Dissociation NEWS*, 21, 3.

Rhoades, G. F. Jr. (2003b, November). Culture-Bound Syndromes and dissociation. Workshop presented at the annual meeting of The International Society for the Study of Dissociation (ISSD), Chicago, Illinois.

Ritts, V. (1999). *Infusing culture into psychopathology: A supplement for psychology instructors*, Retrieved November 1, 2003, from http://www.stlcc.cc.mo.us/mc/users/vritts/psypath.htm

Schechter, D. S., Marshall, R., Salman, E., Goetz, D., Davies, S., & Liebowitz, M. R. (2000). Ataque de Nervois and history of childhood trauma. *Journal of Traumatic Stress, 13*, 529-534.

Schein, E. H. (2003). Five traps for consulting psychologists: Or, how I learned to take culture seriously. *Consulting Psychology Journal: Practice and Research, 55*, 75-83.

Shan, H. H. (2000). Culture-bound psychiatric disorders associated with Qi-Gong practice in China. *Hong Kong Journal of Psychiatry, 10*, 12-14.

Somer, E. (2004). Trance Possession Disorder in Judaism: Sixteenth-Century Dybbuks in the Near East. *Journal of Trauma & Dissociation, 5*, 2004, 131-146.

Steinberg, M. (1990). Transcultural issues in psychiatry: The Ataque and Multiple Personality Disorder. *Dissociation: Progress in the Dissociative Disorders, 3*, 31-33.

Suryani, L. & Jensen, S. (1993). *Trance and possession in Bali: A window on western multiple personality, possession disorder, and suicide.* New York: Oxford University Press.

Yi, K. Y. (2000). Shin-byung (divine illness) in a Korean woman. *Culture, Medicine & Psychiatry, 24*, 471-486.

Zayas, L. H., Torres, J. M., & DesRosiers, F. (1996). *Professional Psychology: Research and Practice, 27*, 78-82.

Coping with Childhood Trauma and Dissociation in Argentina

Sandra Baita

SUMMARY. This piece will review two categories of childhood trauma in Argentina. First, the tragedy of the children kidnapped and missing during the last military government in Argentina (1976-1983). Second, the current occurrence of child sexual abuse and its treatment in this country. The author will show the societal response to these two categories of childhood trauma in the context of the particular cultural background, and discuss the potential damaging impact on the victims. The clinical vignettes will help the reader to better understand to which extent dissociation is present in these societal responses. Issues related to the mental health and legal systems in Argentina are also discussed. *[Article copies available for a fee from The Haworth Document Delivery Service: 1-800-HAWORTH. E-mail address: <docdelivery@haworthpress.com> Website: <http://www.HaworthPress.com> © 2005 by The Haworth Press, Inc. All rights reserved.]*

Sandra Baita, MA, is affiliated with the Department on Women Affairs of the Government of the City of Buenos Aires, Argentina.

Address correspondence to: Sandra Baita, Amenábar 3672 20th Floor Apt. "B," (1429) Ciudad de Buenos Aires, República Argentina (Email: sbcc@ciudad.com.ar).

The author wishes to thank Patricia Visir, MA, for her ideas, her revision of the draft of this paper, and her help with the English version of this piece; the International Society for the Study of Dissociation for the support given to the non-North American members; and Dr. George Rhoades for his trust.

[Haworth co-indexing entry note]: "Coping with Childhood Trauma and Dissociation in Argentina." Baita, Sandra. Co-published simultaneously in *Journal of Trauma Practice* (The Haworth Maltreatment & Trauma Press, an imprint of The Haworth Press, Inc.) Vol. 4, No. 1/2, 2005, pp. 35-53; and: *Trauma and Dissociation in a Cross-Cultural Perspective: Not Just a North American Phenomenon* (ed: George F. Rhoades, Jr., and Vedat Sar) The Haworth Maltreatment & Trauma Press, an imprint of The Haworth Press, Inc., 2005, pp. 35-53. Single or multiple copies of this article are available for a fee from The Haworth Document Delivery Service [1-800-HAWORTH, 9:00 a.m. - 5:00 p.m. (EST). E-mail address: docdelivery@haworthpress.com].

KEYWORDS. Childhood trauma, dissociation, desaparecidos, Argentina

The modern study of psychological trauma in children and the consequences for their future adulthood has primarily focused on the abuse of women in their homes. This research has called attention to the fact that many children were also abused in multiple ways by their caregivers (Cazabat, 2002; Figley, 2002; Herman, 1992; Walker, 2002).

The story of this victimization and traumatization of children, both inside and outside of their families, is as old as humanity (Grosman & Mesterman, 1998; Kempe & Kempe, 1979; Lascaratos & Poulakou-Rebelakou, 2000; Makari, 1998). As stated by deMause (1994), the "history of childhood is a nightmare from which we have just started to awake" (p. 15). Sadly, childhood psychic trauma has historically tended to be minimized, misdiagnosed or even denied in both psychology and psychiatry (Terr, 1990).

The difficulty in understanding the pain and suffering of children is typically related to their ongoing development, and lack of cognitive and verbal skills. Another contributing factor to this difficulty is the tendency for adults to see, understand and explain children's behaviors and emotions from the adult viewpoint (Baita, 2002).

From a sociological point of view, a child matures inside a family constructed with implicit and explicit conceptions, shared by their particular society, and by any sub-cultures supporting that society (Grosman & Mesterman, 1998). The way in which a society views and conceptualizes childhood is especially related both to the ideologies and to the policies that the society supports in the protection and promotion of child welfare (Baratta, 1995). The success of these child protection policies would be determined by the society's interaction with other social constructs (such as the idea of family, marriage, private versus public affairs, etc.). Childhood trauma and the future consequences for the child, would thus be conceptualized–and accepted–within this particular context.

This means that even if there is universal agreement that an event is traumatic, the response to this event would depend on how trauma and childhood are regarded in the society in which the event occurred. As stated by Cazabat (2002) "It's impossible to address a serious study of the consequences of psychological trauma without any social and political support" (p. 38).

The link between childhood trauma and later psychopathology has been well documented (Cook, Blaustein, Spinazzola, & van der Kolk,

2003; Felitti et al., 1998; Terr, 1990), as well as the link between child-hood trauma and dissociative disorders (Barach, 1991; International Society for the Study of Dissociation, ISSD, 2003; Kluft, 1985; Putnam, 1997). The correct recognition of psychic trauma in childhood and the improvement of diagnostic tools and therapeutic approaches should be a priority in every political agenda, in order to decrease the number of potentially disabled adults, diminish the transgenerational transmission of trauma and enhance the quality of life of every human being.

This paper will review two different situations of childhood trauma during the last thirty years in Argentina, and the societal response to them. The conceptualization, understanding and treatment of trauma and dissociation within these two situations, will also be discussed.

A LASTING WOUND:
THE DISAPPEARANCE OF CHILDREN
DURING THE LAST MILITARY GOVERNMENT

"Where are my parents?"(from a little girl to the couple who illegally appropriated her, after she knew the truth of her birth in captivity)

"Allí en el piso nació una hermosa beba a la que se llevaron unas horas después" (from the testimony of a witness of a missing child's birth in a concentration camp)[1]

The Story of the Disappearance of Children

One of the most tragic wounds in the modern history of Argentina was the one left by the last dictatorial military government (1976-1983). Historically, Argentina has had many military governments due to a very unstable political scenario and successive weak democracies. These military types of government were always imposed by force, breaking the existenting democratic regime. At the time period of the last dictatorial military government noted, most of the Latin American countries were also governed by a military regime.

The last military government in Argentina was later known world-wide due to that government's continuous violation of human rights. Extremely violent actions against the population, especially directed against the opponents of the political left, were executed by the military forces. Some of these actions included the disappearance of people–both known or suspected to be political activists–from their homes, their job places, or even the street. The disappearances gave birth to the word *desaparecidos*,[2] a word that internationally acknowledged the country's special political situation. Many years later, the kidnapping and the changing of a child's identity was listed as a new category of child abuse (Bringiotti, 1999; Finkelhor & Korbin, 1988).

The military forces, especially during the dictatorship's first years of power, devoted intense effort in the disappearence and murder of many political opponents,. The National Commission on the Disappearance of Persons (Comisión Nacional por la Desaparición de Personas, CONADEP) was created at the end of the military government to investigate the torture, kidnapping, disappearance and murder of persons during the military government, due to political reasons. The CONADEP (1984) reported 8,960 cases of missing persons that disappeared during this period, with the conclusion that this number was probably underreporting the accurate number of "*desaparecidos*."

Today, almost thirty years after the start of the military government, human rights organizations are still submitting claims for any information about the final destination of their loved ones. This information is needed for the survivors to move on in their grief and to have more closure. Currently most Argentines are resigned to the fact that the persons who disappeared during the military government were murdered.

There is, however, another tragic story inside the tragedy itself. The most innocent victims of this drama were the offspring of the *desaparecidos*. Some of the children were caught and murdered with their parents, while some others were abandoned after the capture of their parents. The abandoned children were fortunately returned by neighbors to their relatives, i.e., grandparents, uncles. A number of these children, however, were definitively separated from their biological families, subsequent to their capture, with the political and ideological purpose to cut off the continuity of the political ideas of their parents. Some of these children were born in captivity–as their mothers had been caught while they were still pregnant–or kidnapped after their parents were illegally captured. While some of them were adopted *bona fide* by families who were totally uncertain about the newborn origins, many of these children were illegally adopted by families who were close to or had some kind of relationship with members of the military forces. In some cases, the "new" father was a person directly involved in the capture or even in the torture or murder of the biological parents, who decided to keep the newborn or the child for himself.

The National Commission for the Right to Identity (Comisión Nacional por el Derecho a la Identidad, CONADI) has reported that 18 children disappeared with their parents, almost 136 were born in captivity, and only 55 have been found and returned to their biological families (Tables 1 and 2). Recently two former missing children were found, while this piece was in process, almost twenty-seven years after their disappearance. The destiny of the children who were born in captivity and the ones who were kidnapped with their parents and haven't yet been found, remain still unknown.

The Delayed Effects of Trauma: Society and the Mental Health System

The identities or names of the children were changed and their biological history was erased to further cover up the disappearances and to further vanquish the parent's political ideas.

Some of these children were later found by a socio-political organization called *Abuelas de Plaza de Mayo*,[3] and were given back their real names. The children then started to live their lives in contact with or inside their biological families. Some of the abandoned children, who were later given to their relatives, had lived hidden lives, due to their families' fear of retaliation from the military forces.

Some of the former vanished children, almost young adults at the time of their discovery, decided that they didn't want to change their histories. These children apparently did not blame their adoptive parents for the way in which they were adopted, and refused every kind of contact with their biological families. One of the most pathetic cases was a set of twins who were kidnapped and adopted by a member of the military forces. The twins were age 11 when the case came to the light and the couple was convicted for crimes against humanity. The twins remained closely allied with their "adoptive" parents (even when they were in jail) and for several years the twins rejected any kind of contact with their biological family.

The CONADEP Report (1984) documented different sequelae in children in the aftermath of trauma. One of the most dramatic cases reported a 12-year-old boy who had witnessed the kidnapping of his parents. The boy was found dead a year later, lying on his grandmother's bed, still waiting for the return of his parents. A girl, almost six years old, had been captured with her mother and sister and was forced to see her father tortured. The child was released to live with her grandparents, but found her pain was so devastating that she committed suicide

TABLE 1. Children who had disappeared during the last military government in Argentina, and were later found (National Commission for the Right to Identity, CONADI, 2004).

AGE AT THE TIME OF KIDNAPPING		AGE AT THE TIME OF LOCATION
Born in captivity =	14	7 found between 5 & 12 y.o. 7 found between 18 & 27 y.o.
Less than 12 months old =	19	1 found within the same month of disappearance 13 found between 5 & 13 y.o. 5 found between 19 & 27 y.o.
From 1 to 5 y.o. =	21	12 found between 4 & 10 y.o. 3 found between 11 & 14 y.o. 6 found between 18 & 26 y.o.
From 6 to 9 y.o. =	3	3 found between 17 & 19 y.o.
TOTAL =	57	57

TABLE 2. People in charge of these children before their location (source: National Commission for the Right to Identity, CONADI, 2004).

MILITARY/POLICE STAFF	19
RELATIVES	15
ADOPTED	14
OTHER PEOPLE	3
NO DATA AVAILABLE	6
TOTAL	**57**

by shooting herself with her grandfather's gun. A third child was born in captivity and was finally freed, along with his mother. The boy was subsequently diagnosed with bilateral deafness. A condition, according to the doctors, caused by the physical tortures his mother had suffered while she was still pregnant and captive.

The psychological aftereffects found in children and adolescents who were forced to see their parents tortured, who were tortured themselves, or even used as a decoy to capture someone else (sometimes a relative, a neighbor, or a friend), have not been described, nor widely documented. In addition, no research about the prevalence of posttraumatic disorders in this population has been conducted.

Many of the human rights organizations at great risk, started their work of healing and restoration with the victims of terror even during the military government. The vanished persons who would later reappear, the families that had someone missing, persons who were desperately looking for the truth and the body of their loved ones, all of them now had someone to talk to. Mental health professionals were devoted to work closely with the missing children who had been found and whom after knowing the truth about their origins, were returned to their biological families.

The predominant theoretical framework for the mental health community in Argentina was psychoanalysis and was the framework wherein the trauma was mainly conceptualized. In the cases of restitution where the children who had been missing and illegally appropriated or adopted, the later brutal confrontation with the truth of their kidnapping and illegal appropriation revealed other traumatic effects. Some of these effects included screaming, crying, temper tantrums, and rejection of the real family. Their denial of the truth that they were forced to see, and the attachment they had to their parents-captors was terribly overwhelming, even for the professionals.

The proceedings in these cases led to the confrontation of two opposite positions in the mental health field on how to communicate the truth to the children. A small group stated that the procedure of communicating the truth to the child at the same moment the judge had ordered the separation from the illegal family and immediate placement with the biological, unknown family, had the same traumatic impact of the child's original kidnapping and illegal appropriation. They suggested a progressive work, trying to create instead of imposing a bond between the child and the biological, legal family. A second, larger group rejected this position and explained the effects of facing the truth in such way as a "rectifying trauma," which was supposed to lead the psychic apparatus to a recomposition (Abuelas de Plaza de Mayo, 1997).

The concept of dissociation as an adaptive response to trauma, or as a defense mechanism used to separate two unconceivable realities, was absent in both mental health positions. Some of the children's stories that came to light, however, show how dissociation, even if unexplained, acted in the children minds. One case involved a little girl who, after returning to her biological family, went for a walk in a park with her grandmother and grandmother's friend. The child began talking like a baby when she entered the park. Her therapist later had found the link between this regressive behavior and the fact that she was kidnapped in this park, with her mother when she was a baby (Lo Giudice, 1997).

Another dramatic picture of the effects of trauma and the dissociation of truth (both in children and in the professionals who worked with their best intention for the children rights) is depicted in this vignette: a little girl was brought to the court by her "adoptive" parents, who were responsible for her illegal appropriation after the birth, to have a first meeting with her biological grandparents. She was still unaware of the truth of her origins as of the existence of a biological, real, legal family. While the judge was still conducting hearings with the different persons involved in the situation (the illegal parents, expert professionals, and the biological relatives), the girl was waiting in another room. She was quite and calm, and spontaneously started playing a game in which she was representing the story of two houses and two girls, with two different names. After this symbolic, simple play, the judge announced to her that from this moment she would no longer live with the persons she called her "parents." She left the court with her biological grandparents, whom she had never seen before (Conte, 1997).

During the military government, terror was so dominant in the lives of people that a great part of the society separated themselves from the situation. Silence, lack of involvement, bias against the *desaparecidos* (i.e., they must have done something bad, so they were responsible for their disappearance), and denial were the main societal responses to the situation. This "cultural dissociation" (Olafson, Corwin, & Summit, 1993, p. 8) reflected a self-protective societal behavior, which increased the power of terror, and left the victims even more isolated from discovery or help.

Some of the places that were later recognized as concentration camps, were located in urban areas, close to highways or big avenues, where ordinary people used to walk and drive. The entire society became accustomed to live with terror as a part of their daily life. Dissociation could be seen as an appropriate explanation for this behavior. Some years later, many people would tell that they were totally unaware of what was going on, even if they had suspected there was something serious enough to justify their silence.

As stated by Herman (1992), "the ordinary response to atrocities is to banish them from consciousness (. . .) atrocities, however, refuse to be buried" (p. 1). The fact that two of these disappeared children have been discovered twenty-seven years later is the evidence of this refusal. Herman noted that "remembering and telling the truth about terrible events are prerequisites both for the restoration of the social order and for the healing of individual victims" (p. 1).

The children who had disappeared during the last military government in Argentina are the evidence of a trauma that is still bleeding across the generations. The little baby born on the floor deserves her real name. Perhaps she's still waiting for it.

THE ONGOING WOUND:
COPING WITH CHILD SEXUAL ABUSE IN ARGENTINA

*"I want to see my father once again just to tell him
that I want a good dad"* S. - 9 y.o.

The Dissociative Denial of Child Sexual Abuse

The historical minimization and denial of child sexual abuse, both as a fact and as a traumatic event, is widely documented (Bringiotti, 1999; deMause, 1994; Herman, 1992; Olafson et al., 1993; Summit, 1988).

Olafson et al. (1993) have described cycles of discovery and suppression in the modern history of child sexual abuse awareness. These cycles represent a process called "cultural dissociation"(p. 8) that parallels society's behavior and the victims' need to protect themselves from pain and terror by the use of denial and dissociation. This cyclical process still exists despite the contemporary research and increasing knowledge about childhood sexual trauma. This societal attitude towards child sexual abuse has also been referred to as a "shared negative" hallucination (Goodwin, 1985, p. 14) or a "societal blind spot" (Summit,1988, p. 51). Whatever the name chosen for the explanation of societal avoidance and denial, it is clear that this attitude lies at the base of the "backlash" movement.

"Backlash" has been defined as a counter reaction against professionals and child protective service workers in the field of child sexual abuse (Conte, 1994). Conte asserts that the backlash is manifested by statements such as *"young children are inaccurate in their report of the abuse experienced,"* or *"adult memories of child sexual abuse can be easily manipulated and implanted by unethical or incompetent therapists"* (p. 228).

Despite the apparent widespread need to deny child sexual trauma, it is important to consider the possible societal differences that might exist due to that society's culture and present situation. The arise of the "false memory syndrome" (fms) as a manifestation of this modern counter-reaction against child sexual abuse, is clearly linked to the possibility of legal proceedings against the alleged perpetrator many years, and even decades, after the abuse had occurred. The current position of the Argentine legal system is also that young children are poor reporters of their own traumatic experiences. False memories, however, are not at the forefront of the legal discussion. Since the statute of limitations is only twelve years after a crime has been committed, most adult survivors of childhood sexual abuse cannot seek prosecution against their abusers. Without the foundation of possible prosecution, the question remains as to why there is a backlash in Argentina.

Child Sexual Abuse, Dissociation, and Backlash in Argentina

Argentina has a population of over 39 million people with the main religion being Catholicism. The Catholic Church has historically had a strong participation in the process of decision making, both on a social and a political level. It is due to this power that married couples were not allowed to legally divorce until 1987, and abortion is illegal except for a few medical reasons that have to be well documented and justified by the intervening doctor. Education about sexuality, except for human reproduction, is still a very controversial matter at schools.

Historically considered a very rich country in Latin America, 44.3% of the population living in urban areas were below the poverty line, as measured during the first semester of 2004 (Instituto Nacional de Estadísticas y Censos, INDEC, 2004). The increasing number of people under the line of poverty is related to several financial crises that have occurred in the last decades.

The local backlash seems to primarily rely on a very strong policy of family preservation (Ganduglia, 2002). The idea that family must be protected at any cost had replaced the concept of child protection in many situations (Malacrea, 1998). This type of thinking has led to two different kinds of action in the child sexual abuse arena, depending on the socioeconomic status of the population to be treated.

In the case of low income groups, the failure of the government to meet the needs of people living under the poverty line was justified with a self-indulgence action of no intervention in family matters, especially any intervention by the legal system. This has led to the mistaken link between poverty and violent behavior as a cause and effect relationship. Within this context neglect is understood as a consequence of the lack of financial resources, physical abuse as an effect of the overwhelming stress derived from indigent life conditions, and sexual abuse as a consequence of many people living in a small room. The lack of personal space was assumed to cause either the lack of or elimination of physical and relational boundaries. This basic assumption supports the idea that the protection of children is possible only when the intervention of government is addressed to solve their basic and real needs (food, education, home, health).

While there is still an academic recognition that child maltreatment is not necessarily related to poverty, real actions are based on the implicit assumption that disadvantaged life conditions from a socioeconomic point of view could be the real causes of maltreatment against children. There is no empirical data that supports this Argentine position.

In these cases the sexual abuse was simply translated into a issue of poverty as a result of the societal context, rather than the family dysfunction or the perpetrators' psychopathology. If the problem is a societal one, the solution must then come from the improvement of the social environment. Thus, even if "misbehavior" is recognized, the problem is no longer defined as child sexual abuse. The denial of risk factors inside the family is the main consequence for this type of response to child sexual abuse. This denial facilitates the transformation of the reality of child sexual abuse for the society to that of a problem with poverty. This minimization of sexual abuse doesn't, however, have the power to vanish the problem itself. On the contrary, it keeps risk factors intact, exposing children to chronic suffering. The pathological condition of child sexual abuse is only socially recognized when cases involving priests (a few) or teachers (more) come to the light with the help of the media.

For the more advantaged social and financial groups of the population, the family preservation ideology shows its real face. Many therapists and even Family Court judges had supported statements such as "*the child needs a father,*" "*we must forgive,*" "*it doesn't matter what he did, he IS the father,*" and addressed reunification processes, even in cases in which a criminal prosecution against the alleged sexual perpetrator was still in process (Baita & Visir, 2004).

In my opinion, the response required by the child in these type of cases is essentially dissociative. The legal system is asking a child to behave in two different ways, to adapt to two different kinds of communication: the Family Court communication, which presents the need for parental reunification no matter what had happened between this father and the child, and the Criminal Court communication, which asks the child to testify against the same father with whom she must relate again, as if the sexual abuse had never happened. In addition, during the reunification process the child is not allowed to talk about the accusation, because the alleged offender has the right to not declare himself guilty. This statement supports the family preservation idea, which then becomes a social need. In many of these controversial cases the lack of contact between a parent and a child has been stated as a risk factor for the psychosocial development of the child (Viar & Lamberti, 2003).

Nevertheless, the discussion about the pathological bond between the parent and the child which led to the sexual abuse was absent.

In these cases the policies of intervention are even more neglectful for the child's best interests, than the policies for the abused child living below the poverty line. The advocates of this premise for those of the financial upper class don't even consider the existence of the sexual abuse, leading to an effect of more severe dissociation, by convincing society that the abusive event never happened.

Dissociation was originally born as a way to cope with the *interpersonal* trauma. When the community is willing to dismiss the abuse altogether, the need of the child to further dissociate from and/or pretend that no abuse occured in order to survive, will be paramount.

Despite the different positions stated above, it remains clear that both positions reinforce the power of the abuser in two ways: first, by confirming his communication to the child of "no one will trust you" and second, by reinforcing the distorted perceptions about the sexual misbehavior found in many abused children, "what is happening is normal, every father does this kind of gestures to his daughter, etc." It is reasonable to assume that an increasing use of dissociative defenses are a potential consequence of the reunification processes that is enacted in spite of a child being sexually abused (Baita & Visir, 2004). The following three clinical vignettes will give some support to this position.

During 2004, I've been directly involved in three cases of child sexual abuse, with an ongoing criminal prosecution, in which the Civil Court had decided to reunificate the child with the alleged perpetrator (the father). In one of these cases, after three years of legal procedures, a formerly Court-ordered reunification process was suspended after the little victim stated to the professional involved in the process that she loved her father but she no longer wanted to go to his house *"because of his bad touching."* The case files were full of these kind of statements from the little victim since she was four years old (now she was almost seven) and many mental health professionals had supported through their reports findings of significant psychological distress *and the presence of dissociative features*. Nevertheless, none of these signs were considered as a reason to suspend the reunification process. The most bizarre feature in this case was that it was the father who asked the suspension of the reunification process, as a legal strategy designed with his counselors, which was agreed to by the judge.

The second case involved a little 5-year-old girl, suspected to have been sexually abused by her father. The Family Court ordered a suspension of any kind of contact between the father and the daughter while the criminal prosecution was ongoing. In the mean time, the mother decided to bring her little girl to a psychotherapist, due to the daughter behaving in a very sexualized and aggressive manner, and having many other symptoms. When the father became aware of this decision, he submitted a motion at the court to suspend the therapy, stating that as his daughter had been treated by a sexual abuse expert therapist, the professional might certainly have "implanted" and "reinforced" a false allegation of a sexual abuse that never happened.

The family court judge decided to accept the father's motion and compelled the mother to suspend any kind of therapeutic treatment, unless she was able to agree with the father to contact a "new" therapist. In the meantime, the father surprisingly appeared near the girl's school, when she was coming home back with her baby sitter, almost a year after the restraint order was in place. He held her in his arms, asked her a few things, whispered something on her ear, asked her not to talk about that meeting with her mom, and after saying "bye" disappeared as surprisingly as he came, into the darkness. No legal action was taken against this father due to the breaking of the restraint order.

The psychological dynamics of the sexual abuse were dissociated in this case. The Court gave the father the right to discuss the best psychotherapeutic treatment for the daughter whom he denied he had sexually abused and failed to hold him responsible for breaking the restraining order. It was the same Court that prescribed the restraining order to protect the child against this father, because he was suspected of having sexually abused his daughter. This example shows how much more importance is given to the parental rights rather than to the child's rights.

This girl was referred to me after the street episode for a crisis intervention. She had developed posttraumatic symptoms which, as described by the mother, were the same emotional and behavioral reactions she had manifested at the time of the sexual abuse disclosure.

At her first therapy appointment, the girl was very reluctant to talk about the episode: *"I was coming back from school and suddenly I've found myself lying like this (she opens her arms looking to the ceiling with a bizarre gesture); when he (the father) heard M. (the au pair) calling my name he realized that it was me."* In her statement about the encounter, the girl is introducing a distorted perception through which she tells how helpless, surprised, and impotent she felt. The statement *"I've found myself lying like this"* depicts her internal sense of both mind and body paralysis.

A subsequent dialogue with the girl illustrated her need for dissociation. The girl talked about how she felt during this unexpected meeting with her father: *"I don't want to let this come out from my head"* (Therapist (T): So, what do you want?) *"I want to be happy"* (T: And what do you think you have to do to be happy?) *"I don't want this inside my head anymore."*

What this girl is apparently saying is that she doesn't want to talk about the stressful situation which is directly linked to her abusive father because this would certainly trigger the abusive memories. She decided to pretend that the encounter didn't exist anymore–and dissociate–in order to be happy. Her need for self-protection against these memories was also fueled by the legal system, which somehow had agreed with the father's need to avoid any sexual abuse related issues during her course of psychotherapy. The dissociation then maintains a survival condition, and the reinforcement of the myth that nothing happened strengthens the dissociative defenses (Goodwin, 1985). But if society deprives the last possible escape for the abused children (listen to them and believe their voices), much more pathology will be the only solution for the victim to cope with the unspeakable.

At the time period in which this is being prepared, the reunification process of a nine-year-old girl and her sexually abusive father was being decided. The Family Court ordered a first reunification process with the intervention of a Family Therapy team that had conducted only three interviews, after which the team concluded that the reunification had ended successfully. Therefore they had suggested that the Judge allow a visitation plan between the father and his daughter, stating that this could start at the waiting room of the girl's therapist office. The therapist agreed, but, at the time of the first meeting, and while the girl was inside her therapist's office, the girl had an explosion of rage followed by very regressive behaviors. No more meetings at the therapist's office were allowed, and the girl didn't want to come back to her former therapist after almost three years of a therapeutic relationship. Shortly after that first "re-unification" visitation by the father, the little girl had at least three other dissociative episodes, including self injuries, time loss, and dissociative fugues. These kinds of episodes weren't addressed as dissociative by the former therapist. In this case, it remains clear that there is a need to establish a link between the child's traumatization and her dissociative symptoms. This therapeutic process should be a priority to better understand when would be the appropriate moment to initiate a reunification process, and if so, under what conditions it should be done.

It is possible to hypothesize that all of the three girls had been dealing with trauma through the use of dissociative defenses even before the re-unification processes. The actions or even in-actions of the legal system described above might have been acting both as precipitating and/or perpetuating factors in regard to the child's trauma. In any case, it remains clear that a better understanding of the dissociative processes triggered by this kind of trauma are needed in order to reduce the damage to the child. Nevertheless, the willingness of the legal system to consider this knowledge in every decision-making process is out of a therapist's control.

In my opinion, these cases constitute extreme evidence of how much a child can be traumatized by a dysfunctional and abusive parental relationship. The societal denial of child sexual abuse has also been accompanied by the premise that sexual abuse doesn't harm, or at worse, does minimal harm to a child (Rind, Bauserman, & Tromovitch, 1998), which is not supported by the few empirical reliable data (Berliner, 1991; Dallam et al., 2001; Deblinger, McLeer, Atkins, Ralphe, & Foa, 1989; Kendall-Tackett, Meyer Williams, & Finkelhor, 1993; Mullen, Martin, Anderson, Romans, & Herbison, 1996; Roberts, O'Connor, Dunn, & Golding, 2004). Many times a child presenting as asymptomatic or having shown less symptoms specifically linked to the abuse has been used as evidence to minimize and even deny the traumatic effects of sexual abuse on children. Emphasis on both the traumatic dynamics and aftereffects of child sexual abuse should be always used as a way to counteract against these societal denial mechanisms. In addition the acknowledgement and recognition of dissociation and dissociative disorders in children due to sexual traumatization should be presented. Nevertheless, the large amount of research literature on adult dissociative disorders in contrast to the smaller amount of research on child dissociative disorders leads to the conclusion that a stronger body of research on dissociative disorders in childhood is still needed.

Dissociation in Argentina

Due to the important lack of research in Argentina, the literature on child sexual abuse that was utilized to understand the problem was mainly American and British. It was also American and British literature that introduced the concept of dissociation to Argentina. Today, the use of the term "dissociation" is widespread among professionals from many disciplines working in the field of child sexual abuse. Even a judge recently had written about how children cope with the reality of the sexual trauma by the extended use of dissociation (Rozanski, 2003).

Considering the main importance given to the psychoanalytical framework among the mental health professionals of this country, it is possible to hypothesize that both dissociation and dissociative disorders might still be resisted. Nevertheless, the obvious increase of papers related to dissociation presented during the last International Congress of Psychic Trauma and Traumatic Stress, celebrated in Buenos Aires every year since 2001, brings new winds of hope in this area.

Unfortunately, the lack of research in Argentina affects not only the field of trauma and sexual abuse. It is extended to many other fields of science, and reflects the deep financial, social and educative crisis of the country. Nevertheless, the efforts of many professionals who have been working in the field in very hard conditions counteract against these structural obstacles.

In the Concluding Comments of her brilliant Editorial to the special issue of the Journal of Trauma and Dissociation on "Dissociation in Culture," Lisa Butler (2004) states: *normative dissociative experiences are not incidental to daily life, but central to it–central not just in the sense that they are commonplace, but also in that they may be instrumental and integral to adaptive functioning"* (p. 8). It would be appropriate to ask what normative daily dissociation is made for. It is possible to assume that it serves the purpose to deal with an extremely stressful modern life, full of events, and goals to achieve, in societies that experience both small and huge actions of aggression and violence. If this is true it could certainly explain how much dissociation is "instrumental and integral to adaptive functioning" (Butler, p. 8), not only for individuals, but also for societies.

But following the continuum of dissociation, it is also appropriate to ask what makes "societal" dissociation pathological. Does this dissociation have the same function of coping with severe trauma as what may happen in childhood? If it is adequate to say that traumatized children use dissociation "to ignore, discount and forget critical experiences" (Friedrich, 2002, p. 53) and that serves "as a protective mechanism for the integrity of the self" (Ogawa, Sroufe, Weinfeld, Carlson, & Egeland as cited in Friedrich, 2002, p. 53) when facing catastrophic trauma, what integrity does societal pathological dissociation protect? All these questions move dissociation into the mainstream of daily life, and every human related discipline should attempt to answer them.

In this piece, I've been trying to show that, even if the concept of dissociation has been absent from the most important theoretical frameworks in the mental health field of my country, some way of dissociative functioning, both normative and pathological, could be found in the Argentine society along a period of time (military regime) or as a response to a particular event (childhood trauma).

The story of the children who had disappeared with their parents during the last military government in Argentina made it possible to assert that the way in which every society, as a whole, copes with its traumatic situations will also predict the successful or failed outcome of the intervention process with the victims of different types of trauma. This prediction can also include the length of time spent for both the recovery of the individual and society.

NOTES

1. *"On the floor was born a beautiful baby who was taken away a few hours later."*
2. *Desaparecidos* may be translated as "vanished." The word refers to the final product of a systematic action of persecution and capture of the people known or suspected as being opponents of the military government. Many times this action included also their relatives and friends.
3. During the military government, both the mothers and the grandparents of the desaparecidos used to meet in Plaza de Mayo, a big central square in front of the Government Palace in Buenos Aires, and with their weekly silent parades used to claim for their relatives to appear alive. They organized themselves in two separate organizations: Madres de Plaza de Mayo (Mothers of Plaza de Mayo) and Abuelas de Plaza de Mayo (Grandmothers of Plaza de Mayo). They are still actively involved in the finding of their grandchildren.

REFERENCES

Abuelas de Plaza de Mayo (Ed.) (1997). Restitución de Niños. Buenos Aires: Eudeba. On-line version www.conadi.jus.gov.ar

Baita, S. (2002). Impacto de los procedimientos legales en niños víctimas de abuso sexual. In G.L. Blanco (Ed.), *Bioética y Bioderecho. Cuestiones actuales.* (pp. 451-463). Buenos Aires: Editorial Universidad.

Baita, S. & Visir, P. (2004). Controversias de la revinculación en casos de abuso sexual y sus consecuencias para el psiquismo infantil. Unpublished paper.

Barach, P. (1991). Multiple Personality Disorder as an attachment disorder. *Dissociation,* 4, 117-123.

Baratta, A. (1995). La niñez como arqueología del futuro. In M.C. Bianchi (Ed.), *El Derecho y los Chicos.* (pp. 13-22). Buenos Aires: Espacio Editorial.

Berliner, L. (1991) The effects of sexual abuse on children. *Violence Update.* 1, 1-10.

Bringiotti, M.I. (1999). *Maltrato Infantil. Factores de riesgo para el maltrato físico en la población infantil que concurre a las escuelas dependientes del Gobierno de la Ciudad de Buenos Aires.* Madrid: Miño y Dávila Editores.

Butler, L. (2004). The dissociations of everyday life. *Journal of Trauma and Dissociation*. 5, 1-11.

Cazabat, E.H. (2002). Un breve recorrido a la traumática historia del estudio del trauma psicológico. *Revista de Psicotrauma para Iberoamérica*, 1, 38-41.

CONADEP. (1984). *Nunca Más. Informe de la Comisión Nacional sobre la Desaparición de Personas*. Buenos Aires: Eudeba.

CONADI (Comisión Nacional por el Derecho a la Identidad) (2004). *Biblioteca Digital por la Identidad*. www.conadi.jus.gov.ar/home_fl.html

Conte J.R. (1994). Child Sexual Abuse: Awareness and Backlash. *The Future of Children*. 4, 224-32.

Conte, L.J.de. (1997). La restitución, una respuesta identificante. In Abuelas de Plaza de Mayo (ed). *Restitución de Niños*. Buenos Aires: Eudeba. On-line version www.conadi.jus.gov.ar

Cook, A., Blaustein, M., Spinazzola, J. & van der Kolk, B. (2003). *Complex Trauma in Children and Adolescents*. National Child Traumatic Stress network. www.NCTS Net.org

Dallam, S.J., Gleaves, D.H., Cepeda-Benito, A., Silberg, J.L., Kraemer, H.C., & Spiegel, D. (2001) The effects of child sexual abuse: Comment on Rind, Tromovitch and Bauserman (1998). *Psychological Bulletin*. 127, 715-33.

Deblinger, E., McLeer, S.V., Atkins, M.S., Ralphe, D., & Foa, E. (1989). Post-traumatic stress in sexually abused, physically abused and nonabused children. *Child Abuse and Neglect*. 13, 403-408.

deMause, L. (1994). La evolución de la infancia. In L. deMause (ed). *Historia de la infancia*. (pp. 15-92). Madrid: Alianza Universidad.

Felitti, V.J., Anda, R.F., Nordenberg, D., Williamson, D.F., Spitz, A.M., & Edwards, V. et al. (1998). Relationship of childhood abuse and household dysfunction to many of the leading causes of death in adults: The adverse childhood experiences (ACS) study. *American Journal of Preventive Medicine*, 14, 245-258.

Figley, Ch.R. (2002). Origins of traumatology and prospects for the future, Part I. *Journal of Trauma Practice*. 1, 17-32.

Finkelhor, D. & Korbin, J. (1988). Child Abuse as an International Issue. *Child Abuse and Neglect*, 12, 3-23.

Friedrich, W. (2002). *Psychological Assessment of Sexually Abused Children and Their Families*. Thousand Oaks, CA: Sage Publications, Inc.

Ganduglia, A.H. (2002). Revinculación: una nueva oportunidad... ¿para quién? In J.R.Volnovich (ed) *Abuso sexual en la infancia*. (pp. 125-144). Buenos Aires: Editorial Lumen Humanitas.

Goodwin, J. (1985). Credibility problems in Multiple Personality patients and abused children. In R.P. Kluft (ed) *Childhood Antecedents of Multiple Personality* (pp. 2-15). Washington DC: American Psychiatric Press.

Grosman, C. & Mesterman, S. (1998). *Maltrato al menor. El lado oculto de la escena familiar*. Buenos Aires: Editorial Universidad.

Herman, J.L. (1992). *Trauma and recovery. The aftermath of violence–From domestic abuse to political terror*. New York: Basic Books.

INDEC (Instituto Nacional de Estadísticas y Censos) (2004) *Incidencia de la pobreza y la indigencia en el total de aglomerados urbanos y regiones estadísticas. Primer semestre 2004*.

ISSD Task Force on Children and Adolescents (2003). *Guidelines for the evaluation and treatment of dissociative symptoms in children and adolescents.* www.issd.org

Kempe, R.S. & Kempe, C.H. (1979). *Child abuse.* London: Open Books Publishing, Ltd.

Kendall-Tackett, K.A., Meyer Williams, L., & Finkelhor, D. (1993). Impact of sexual abuse on children: A review and synthesis of recent empirical studies. *Psychological Bulletin.* 113, 164-180.

Kluft, R.P. (ed). (1985). *Childhood antecedents of Multiple Personality.* Washington D.C.: American Psychiatric Press.

Lascaratos, J. & Poulakou-Rebelakou, E. (2000). Child sexual abuse: Historical cases in the Byzantine Empire (324-1453 A.D.). *Child Abuse and Neglect.* 24, 1085-90.

Lo Giudice, A. (1997). La Cajita. Subjetividad y Traumatismo. In Abuelas de Plaza de Mayo (ed). *Restitución de Niños.* Buenos Aires: Eudeba. On-line version www.conadi.jus.gov.ar

Makari, G.J. (1998). The seductions of history: Sexual trauma in Freud's theory and historiography. *International Journal of Psychoanalysis.* 79, 857-69.

Malacrea, M. (1998). *Trauma e riparazione. La cura nell'abuso sessuale all'infanzia.* Milano: Raffaello Cortina Editore.

Mullen, P.E., Martin, J.L., Anderson, J.C., Romans, S.E., & Herbison, G.P. (1996). The long term impact of the physical, emotional and sexual abuse of children: A community study. *Child Abuse and Neglect.* 20, 7-21.

Olafson, E., Corwin, D., & Summit, R. C. (1993) Modern history of child sexual abuse awareness: Cycles of discovery and suppression. *Child Abuse and Neglect* 17, 7-24.

Putnam, F.W. (1997). *Dissociation in children and adolescents. A developmental perspective.* New York: The Guilford Press.

Rind, B., Bauserman, R., & Tromovitch, P. (1998). A meta-analytical examination of assumed properties of child sexual abuse using college samples. *Psychological Bulletin.* 124, 22-53.

Roberts, R., O'Connor, D., Dunn, J., & Golding, J. (2004). The effects of child sexual abuse in later family life; mental health, parenting and adjustment of offspring. *Child Abuse and Neglect.* 28, 525-45.

Rozanski, C. A. (2003). *Abuso Sexual Infantil. ¿Denunciar o Silenciar?* Buenos Aires: Ediciones B.

Summit, R.C. (1988). Hidden victims, hidden pain: Society's avoidance of child sexual abuse. In G.E. Wyatt & G.J. Powell (Eds.), *Lasting effects of child sexual abuse.* (pp. 39-60). Newbury Park, CA: Sage Publications.

Terr, L. (1990). *Too scared to cry. Psychic Trauma in Childhood.* New York: Harper & Row.

Viar, J.P.M. & Lamberti, S. (2003). Algunas reflexiones acerca de la revinculación desde el ámbito jurídico. In S. Lamberti (Ed.), *Maltrato Infantil. Riesgos del compromiso profesional.* (pp. 153-168). Buenos Aires: Editorial Universidad.

Walker, L.E.A. (2002). Politics, psychology and the Battered Woman's Movement. *Journal of Trauma Practice.* 1, 81-102.

Dissociation in Australia

Francesca Collins

SUMMARY. There is growing interest in dissociative phenomena among Australian clinicians and researchers. This is in spite of a public mental health system that allocates services on the basis of diagnosis (predominantly depression and psychotic disorders) rather than need, and professional training programs that make only passing reference to the dissociative disorders. This piece provides an introduction to the Australian context, an overview of the status of dissociation and the dissociative disorders in Australia and a selective review of Australian dissociation research. Emphasis will be placed upon investigations into the correlates of normal dissociative phenomena and the nature and sequelae of peritraumatic dissociation. The concludes with an examination of the psychometric properties of the Dissociative Experiences Scale arising from Australian adult samples. *[Article copies available for a fee from The Haworth Document Delivery Service: 1-800-HAWORTH. E-mail address: <docdelivery@haworthpress.com> Website: <http://www.HaworthPress.com> © 2005 by The Haworth Press, Inc. All rights reserved.]*

KEYWORDS. Dissociation, dissociative disorders, normal dissociation, peritraumatic dissociation, Dissociative Experiences Scale, Australia

Francesca Collins, BA, BSc(Hons), PhD, is affiliated with the Faculty of Arts, Monash University, 900 Dandenong Road, Caulfield East, VIC, 3145, Australia (E-mail: frances.collins@arts.monash.edu.au).

[Haworth co-indexing entry note]: "Dissociation in Australia." Collins, Francesca. Co-published simultaneously in *Journal of Trauma Practice* (The Haworth Maltreatment & Trauma Press, an imprint of The Haworth Press, Inc.) Vol. 4, No. 1/2, 2005, pp. 55-79; and: *Trauma and Dissociation in a Cross-Cultural Perspective: Not Just a North American Phenomenon* (ed: George F. Rhoades, Jr., and Vedat Sar) The Haworth Maltreatment & Trauma Press, an imprint of The Haworth Press, Inc., 2005, pp. 55-79. Single or multiple copies of this article are available for a fee from The Haworth Document Delivery Service [1-800-HAWORTH, 9:00 a.m. - 5:00 p.m. (EST). E-mail address: docdelivery@haworthpress.com].

DISSOCIATION IN AUSTRALIA

The research and practice literature indicates a compartmentalisation of "trauma" and "dissociation" in Australia. Public and private investment in psychological trauma has grown enormously in last twenty years as evidenced by the establishment of the Australian Centre for Posttraumatic Mental Health, Australasian Society for Traumatic Stress Studies and the Victorian Foundation for Survivors of Torture. A concise, but thorough, review of the experience of trauma (including combat, sexual and physical trauma) and posttraumatic stress in Australia is provided by Rosenman (2002). However, the Australian trauma literature makes very little reference to dissociative processes or the dissociative disorders. The aim of this piece is to provide an overview of the status of dissociation in Australia. The context will be set by an introduction to the Australian public mental health system. This will be followed by a selective review of dissociation research activity including Dissociative Experiences Scale (DES) psychometrics.

THE AUSTRALIAN CONTEXT

Australia is a vast and empty land. To place this statement in context, Australia is almost as large in area as the United States (US) (excluding Alaska) and thirty-two times the size of the United Kingdom (UK). Whereas the population density of the US and the UK is around 29.5 and 245 person per km^2, respectively, the population density for Australia is a mere 2.5 persons per km^2 with about 85% of inhabitants living along the coast.

Aboriginal peoples have been the custodians of Australia for an estimated 40,000 years and have a profound spiritual and instrumental connection to "country." European Australians are relative new-comers to the land. The Dutch explorer Jansz discovered the land mass in 1606, dubbing it "New Holland"; however, it was not until 1788 that the first British colony was established in Sydney Cove. At the time of colonisation, the indigenous population was approximately 300,000; today, these numbers are close to 460,000 with Aboriginals and Torres Strait Islanders making up just over two percent of the Australian population.

Australian society is remarkable for its ethnic diversity with almost a quarter of the population having been born overseas. Australia has always had a substantial number of British-born citizens; however, shortly after World War Two, Australia became home to increasingly large numbers of Italian, Greek and Dutch immigrants. At the beginning of the twentieth-first century, almost three percent of the Australian population was of Asian descent (including Vietnamese, Chinese, Filipino, and Malaysian).

TRAUMA ON TERRA AUSTRALIS

The first 150 years following colonisation saw much mass trauma of natural and human origin. Significant, but unknown, numbers of Aborigines died in the years immediately following colonisation due to disease and conflict associated with European settlers. Other large-scale disasters during this period included ship wrecks, heatwaves, epidemics, and bush fires. In the last hundred years, Australians have witnessed major industrial accidents (e.g., the 1970 Westgate Bridge Collapse), shooting massacres (e.g., the 1996 Port Arthur Massacre), and transport accidents (e.g., the 1977 Granville Train Disaster). In the twenty-first century, Australians have fallen victim to terrorist activity in the United States (2001 September 11 Attacks) and Indonesia (the 2002 Bali Bombings); however, the main forms of large-scale trauma continue to be natural in origin–bush fires, floods, and heat waves.

Since the 1980s, the Australian public mental health system has embraced the concept of psychological trauma with state and federal governments investing large sums of money into diagnosis, treatment and research programs. Until very recently, however, dissociation and the dissociative disorders have received very little attention in Australian trauma literature and practice.

The Status of the Dissociative Disorders

In 1992, Australia adopted a co-ordinated national mental health system as outlined in the National Mental Health Plan 1992-1997 ("Plan"; Australian Health Ministers, 1992). The original Plan had four strategic aims: (1) to focus services on the diagnosis, treatment, and research of "serious mental illnesses"; (2) deinstitutionalisation involving the decommissioning of stand-alone psychiatric hospitals, which consumed half of the nation's mental health budget, and the development of community-based services; (3) the "mainstreaming" of mental health services into the general health system including the establishment of acute psychiatric inpatient wards in general hospitals with the goal of reducing stigma and improving service quality; and (4) the promotion of consumer and carer involvement in the mental health policy-making process. Each of these aims have been pursued with varying degrees of success. For example, by the end of the first Plan, Victoria (Australia's second most populous state) had closed all of its stand-alone psychiatric hospitals. At the time, this was promoted as an incredible success story for the Plan especially when compared to the relatively poor achievements in Western Australia. In the same year, Western Australia came under criticism for their slow implementation of the Plan. However, in 2004, Victoria faced a severe shortage of publicly funded psychiatric beds with 22 dedicated beds per 100,000 residents compared to 45 per 100,000 in Western Australian. Both figures are far below world standard; per 100,000 residents, Canada has 193 beds, New Zealand, 134, the US, 95, and the UK, 58 (Rosenman, 2002).

The Plan has also been criticised for allocating services based on an individual's diagnosis rather than their unique needs. This practice led to the privileging, within the system, of psychotic and mood disorder diagnoses over other complex clinical presentations (Brown, Middleton, Butler, & Driscoll, 1996; Meadows & Singh, 2003; Whiteford, Buckingham, & Mandersheid, 2002). Smith (2003) explains the situation:

> public psychiatry has become focused on psychosis, ending a century-long broader perspective . . . The concept of "serious mental illness" emerged, with a narrow definition of disorders meeting that criterion. It became the basis for determining access to public services and the type of staff employed . . . [However], lobbying by the [Consultation-Liaison] psychitry community . . . led to acknowledgement in the Second National Health Plan 1998 that some public mental health systems had erroneously equated severity with diagnosis rather than level of need and diasbility. (pp. 150-151)

Although some attempt was made to rectify this imbalance in resource allocation in the second (1998-2002) and third (2003-2008) National Mental Health Plans (Australian Health Ministers, 1998; 2003), the situation remains that access to acute hospital beds is effectively restricted to individuals deemed at immediate risk of harm to themselves and/or others, presenting as psychotic or severely depressed.

It should be noted that while the National Mental Health Plans (Australian Health Ministers, 1992; 1998; 2003) explicitly endorses the classification systems of the Diagnostic and Statistical Manual of Mental Disorders-IV and IV-TR (American Psychiatric Association, 1994;

2000) and the International Classification of Diseases, 10th edition (World Health Organisation, 1992), no reference is made in any of the Plans to the dissociative disorders. It is not surprising, then, that a basic knowledge of dissociation and the dissociative disorders is not a requirement of psychiatry and psychology training in Australia. And this "absence of such coverage has helped maintain the assumption that such disorders [are] either rare or non-existent" (Middleton, 1996, p. 43); "as in medicine in general, what's not considered or looked for, usually won't be found" (Middleton, 1996, p. 46).

As Brown, Middleton, Butler, and Driscoll (1996) point out, "while there is greater acceptance of dissociative disorders, they still prove difficult to recognise and diagnose, particularly where the prevailing clinical tradition gives them little emphasis, and they are not covered in depth any depth in psychiatric training" (p. 273).

An encouraging development is the establishment of the Royal Australian and New Zealand College of Psychiatrists, Special Interest Group on Psychological Trauma (Brown, 2000). Formed in 1996, the Group sponsored the 2000 World Conference of the ISTSS in Melbourne, Victoria, and a national lecture tour by dissociation scholar, Onno Van der Hart. The Group also plans to establish specialist postgraduate psychiatry training in psychological trauma.

In terms of the private mental health sector, the only dedicated hospital beds for sufferers of dissociative disorders are those in the Trauma and Dissociation Unit of the privately operated Belmont Hospital in Queensland. A small number of well-established dissociation-specific support organisations exist including the Dissociative Identity Society of South Australia, the New South Wales-based Merging All Parts and the nation-wide support group, Ritual Abuse Survivors and Supporters.

Research Directions

The 1990s saw the commencement of dissociation research in Australia. To date, the greatest amount of research has been conducted in relation to normal and peritraumatic dissociation; this research will be reviewed in the following section along with psychometric data for the DES administered to Australian non-clinical samples. This research emphasis on dissociation as a normal response to both everyday and extraordinary events can be seen as reflecting the Australian mental health community's reticence regarding the dissociative disorders. However, this picture is changing. Emerging areas of research activity include the forensic implications of dissociation, the neuropsychology of Dissociative

Identity Disorder (DID) and the relationship between dissociation and alexithymia. Selected studies are briefly presented here.

Criminal responsibility. A legal scholar, McSherry has tackled the question of dissociative states and legal responsibility under Australian law (1998; 2004). Her work has focused upon the status under Australian law, of the "fleeting mental state" of "psychological blow" automatism; she notes that "there is some suggestion that automatism resulting from dissociation is now beginning to be raised as a matter of course in Australia, along with other defences such as provocation and/or self defence" (McSherry, 1998, p. 174). Under Australian law, an individual experiencing dissociation-related automatism at the time of the crime would be considered sane, but unable to fully control their actions. In contrast, the same person would, under Canadian law, be considered insane and unable to control their actions. The legal status of dissociation-related automatism clearly has huge implication for the defendant who successfully brings the defence of automatism. In Australia, the defendant would be acquitted; in Canada, the individual may be detained indefinitely in a secure psychiatric ward. This legal definition of dissociation-related automatism is at odds with accepted psychological definitions in that an individual experiencing dissociation-related automatism can still perform goal-directed and purposeful behaviours (McSherry, 2001). McSherry does not offer a final solution to this dilemma but foresees its importance increasing as legal defences develop.

Juvenile offenders. Preliminary work has commenced investigating the rate and severity of dissociation in juvenile prison populations. Walker (2002) administered the Adolescent Dissociative Experiences Scale (A-DES; Armstrong, Putnam, & Carlson, 1997) to 58 young males aged 16 to 18; participants were incarcerated juvenile offenders and 29 were drawn from the general population. The offender group reported significantly higher A-DES scores (mean = 3.0) than the general population group (mean = 1.58). The authors of the A-DES state that scores greater than 4 are indicative of a pathological level of dissociation. Two members of the general population group scored above 4 while eight members of the offender group scored above 4.

EEG coherence. Led by Joseph Ciorciari, the Swinburne University of Technology Centre for Neuropsychology has begun investigating EEG coherence (a measure of cortical connectivity) between host and alters in individuals diagnosed with DID. In one of their first studies (Hopper, Ciorciari, Johnson, Spensley, Sergejew, & Stough, 2002) the team compared EEG coherence in DID individuals and professional actors who acted as if they were DID. Results revealed significant EEG coherence among genuine DID hosts and alters but not among acted-DID "hosts" and "alters." "The professional actors were not able to simulate the coherence patterns of the alter personalities indicating that EEG coherence, at least in the present study is not able to be simulated or faked from information relating to age and sex" (Hopper et al., 2002, p. 84).

Alexithymia. Clayton (2004) has investigated the relationship between dissociation and the five dimensions of alexithymia: difficulty analysing, identifying, verbalising, emotionalising, and fantasising emotions. In a university population, the author found that somatoform dissociation is predictive of alexithymia, especially in young males.

NORMAL DISSOCIATION

In this section, Australian research pertaining to normal dissociation will be reviewed including investigations into antecedents and correlates. Peritraumatic dissociation has been included in a separate section although it can be a seen as a normal response to abnormally stressful or arousing situations.

That dissociation is a normal psychological process has been accepted by most authorities involved in the investigation of dissociative phenomena. In fact, the Diagnostic and Statistical Manual of Mental Disorders (4th Ed.), Text Revision *(DSM-IV-TR)* states explicitly that "dissociation should not be considered inherently pathological and often does not lead to significant distress, impairment, or help-seeking behavior" (APA, 2000, p. 477). Under the dimensional conceptualisation, dissociation may be viewed as a normal process that can lead to psychopathology under certain conditions.

At the "normal" end of the dissociative continuum are the phenomena of mild, transient depersonalisation and derealisation and experiences of absorption and imaginative involvement (Bernstein & Putnam, 1986; Bowers, 1994; Frischholtz Braun, Sachs, Schwartz, Lewis, Schaeffer et al., 1991; Irwin, 1999a; Norton et al., 1990; Putnam, 1989; Sapp & Evanow, 1998; Sterlini & Bryant, 2002; Waller et al., 1996). Normal dissociative phenomena are useful for dealing with a vast range of unpleasant experiences from simple boredom to chronic abuse. Dissociation, however, can also be employed as a defense against the cognitions and affects associated with overwhelming, albeit pleasurable, experiences.

Antecedents of Normal Dissociation

The most prolific Australian investigator of dissociation in non-clinical populations is Dr. Harvey Irwin (1994; 1995; 1996; 1997; 1998a; 1998b; 1998c; 1999a; 1999b; 2000). He stated that "traumatized children differ in the extent to which their social environment promotes a healthy resolution of the experiences of trauma" (Irwin, 1996, p. 701), therefore, all traumatised children should not be expected to develop dissociative tendencies in adulthood as a result of this trauma. Similarly, Putnam (1997) noted that other "non-trauma-related factors, such as disturbed family environments, make important contributions to pathological dissociation" (p. 63). In particular, Putnam points to inconsistent parenting, where a child's behaviour is sometimes positively reinforced, sometimes punished by the parent, as being associated with dissociation in adulthood. Merckelbach and Muris (2001), in a review of the literature regarding the traumagenesis of adult dissociation, found that the relationship between childhood abuse and adult dissociation appears to be modulated by the effects of family environment. Walker (2002) suggests that "it is likely that the [dissociative] psychopathology arises in a repeatedly abused child within a dysfunctional family which fails to protect the child and in which there are prohibitions against the child being able to disclose the abuse" (p. 59). Walker's views echo those of Putnam (1995) who stated that significant others also play an important role in the development of dissociative tendencies; he suggested that the generalisation of dissociative defences may be encouraged by the failure of significant others to provide adequate nurturance and reassurance.

In an investigation of the impact of family environment in the experience of dissociation in adulthood, Irwin (1996) found that, in an Australian non-clinical adult sample ($N = 239$), although dissociative tendencies in adulthood were predicted by physical and sexual abuse and family-related loss, the effects of these events were mediated by the perceived availability of childhood emotional support. Irwin (1996) concluded from these findings that perceived emotional support in childhood plays a mediating role in the relationship between childhood trauma and the development of dissociative tendencies in adulthood.

Unresolved Grief and Guilt

Irwin (1998c) also investigated the possible role of unresolved feelings of grief, shame and guilt in mediating the relationship between childhood trauma and dissociative tendencies in adulthood.

Irwin (1994) proposed that dissociation in non-clinical populations may only be indirectly, if at all, related to childhood trauma and more directly related to unresolved feelings of loss resulting from childhood trauma. Specifically, he hypothesised that the strength of feelings of unresolved guilt would influence an individual's reliance upon dissociation as a coping strategy.

Irwin (1994) investigated the possibility of this relationship in an Australian sample of non-clinical adults ($N = 121$). He did not inquire directly about childhood trauma, rather, he inquired about feelings of grief on the grounds that "traumatic memories may be difficult to tap, but associated emotions may be relatively more accessible to observation" (Irwin, 1994, p. 86). Multiple regression analysis revealed that as much as 54% of variance in level of dissociation was accounted for by gender and unresolved grief. Irwin (1994) interpreted these results as suggestive of the mediating role of grief in the relationship between childhood trauma and dissociative tendencies in adulthood.

In regard to shame and guilt, Irwin (1998c) hypothesised that if childhood trauma leads to feelings of shame and guilt, lack of resolution of these affects may, in turn, lead to a reliance on dissociative coping strategies in later life. According to the literature (for a review, see Irwin, 1998c), shame and guilt differ in that shame is related to one's negative evaluation of oneself while guilt relates to one's negative evaluation of one's own behaviour. In an Australian sample of non-clinical adults ($N = 103$), Irwin found that as much as 32% of variance in level of dissociation was accounted for by age and feelings of shame and grief. Irwin (1998c) interpreted these results as suggestive of their mediating role in the relationship between childhood trauma and adult dissociation.

Schumaker (as cited in Dorahy, Schumaker, Krishnamurthy, & Kumar, 1997) has stated that "adaptive dissociation regulates mental health, so that stimuli aversive to psychological well-being are filtered out before integrating with conscious experience. . . . Individuals who have adaptive dissociative processes operating effectively will be less troubled by transient guilt than individuals with more inefficient dissociative functioning" (p. 968). That is, a tendency toward high levels of guilt reflects a high level of "adaptive" dissociation. By this argument, Irwin's findings may reflect an association between guilt and maladaptive, rather than adaptive, use of dissociation.

Dorahy et al. (1997) in a later (although earlier published) study, further investigated Irwin's (1998c) findings regarding dissociation and guilt. The authors administered trait measures of dissociation and guilt to an Australian adult non-clinical population ($N = 259$) and found that trait guilt was predictive of dissociation, providing support for Irwin's (1998c) findings.

Dorahy et al. (1997) integrated their findings with those of attachment theorists (e.g., Liotti, 1992) who stated that the on-going effects of childhood trauma may be ameliorated to some extent by stable and supportive attachment experiences. Dorahy et al. (1997) noted that guilt arising from trauma during childhood cannot be redressed or ameliorated by the child's own actions or by the support of an attachment figure because "an interpersonal transgression did not create the feeling" (Dorahy et al., 1997, p. 970). But, because the child was not responsible for the guilt-producing event, they are unable to reduce the feelings of guilt by use of dissociation.

Correlates of Normal Dissociation

The correlates of dissociation in non-clinical populations have not been widely investigated, however, a small number of reliably associated variables have emerged in Australian research, namely, age, the use of emotion-focused coping strategies, and external locus of control.

Emotion-Focused Coping

According to Folkman and Lazarus' cognitive appraisal model of coping (Folkman, 1984), coping involves a *conscious* effort to reduce stress. Within this model, coping strategies can be broadly categorised as either *problem-focused*–attempts to manage or alter the problem causing the stress–or *emotion-focused*–attempts to regulate emotional responses to the stressful situation. By virtue of its spontaneous and unconscious nature, dissociation cannot be considered a conscious attempt to reduce stress. However, some dissociative responses to stressful situations resemble emotion-focused coping responses such as attempts to avoid registering the stressful event, attempts to suppress upsetting emotions and attempts to psychologically remove oneself from the stressful situation. Given this, one would expect the use of emotion-focused coping strategies to be associated with the tendency to experience dissociative phenomena.

That dissociation is automatic and effortless is central to the notion of dissociation. Harvey and Bryant (2002) explicitly endorse acute dissociation as a coping mechanism and further note that "inherent in the notion of dissociative response is the premise that many cognitive responses to trauma are automatic and effortless" (p. 895). Such responses include emotional distancing, imaginative involvement, absorption, avoidance, depersonalisation, derealisation and alterations of identity.

In a sample of Australian adults (N = 130), Collins and Ffrench (1998) found DES scores to be correlated with scores on the Escape-avoidance (r = .47, p < .05) and Distancing (r = .21, p < .05) sub-scales of the Ways of Coping Questionnaire (Folkman & Lazarus, 1988). In a later study, again involving Australian adults (N = 161), Collins (2004a) found correlations between DES scores and Escape-avoidance (r = .37, p < .01) and Distancing (r = .4, p < .01) coping. The magnitude of the correlations increases along with increases in DES scores (Collins, 2004a).

In attempting to explain this relationship between dissociation and emotion-focused coping, Collins (2004a; Collins & Ffrench, 1998) suggested that the automatic nature of dissociative phenomena may reflect a qualitative shift in the way in which emotion-focused coping strategies are performed. Strentz and Auerbach (1988) noted that escape-avoidance-type emotion-focused coping strategies are most useful in the early stages of prolonged trauma. It is plausible, then, that with repeated use, emotion-focused coping strategies may transform from being consciously produced behaviours to the effortless, automatic processes that characterise dissociation (Collins, 2004a). Conversely, the use of emotion-focused coping strategies may represent the con- scious production of automatic dissociative states.

External Locus of Control

In addition to a general preference for one approach or the other, the decision to employ a particular coping strategy is also affected by one's perceptions of personal control over the stressful situation. In this regard, control beliefs can be seen as "pre-existing notions about reality that serve as a perceptual lens . . . [determining] how things are in a given [situation]" (Folkman, 1984, pp. 840-841).

Locus of control (LOC) refers to an individual's beliefs regarding sources of control in life. Levenson (1972) proposed a multi-dimensional conceptualisation of LOC that differentiated between the degree to which individuals believe that they are in control of their fate (Internal), the degree to which they believe their fate is subject to the forces of chance (Chance), and the degree to which they believe their fate is contingent upon the actions of powerful others (Powerful Others). The strength of an individual's orientation to each of the three dimensions is measured via Levenson's Multidimensional Locus of Control Scale (LLC; Levenson, 1972).

Where an individual perceives a stressful situation to be beyond their control, they are more likely to utilise emotion-focused coping strategies; where the individual believes there exists an opportunity to alter the situation or the problem causing it, problem-focused coping strategies will be preferred. It is not surprising, then, that researchers have found individuals demonstrating a predominantly External locus of control orientation (both Chance and Powerful Others) more likely to employ emotion-focused, rather than problem-focused coping strategies, given that a perceived lack of control is integral to their cognitive schema.

Collins and Ffrench (1998) hypothesised that the constructs of locus of control and dissociation would be related based upon their shared relationship with emotion-focused coping. They tested this hypothesis in an Australian adult sample ($N = 130$) and found that DES scores were positively correlated with Chance ($r = .26$) and Powerful Others LOC ($r = .21$) orientations and negatively correlated with Internal LOC orientation ($r = -.22$). In a later replication of this study (N = 161), Collins (2004a) found positive correlations between DES scores and Chance ($r = .26$, p < .01) and Powerful Others LOC ($r = .17$, p < .05) orientations. Once again, the magnitude of the correlations increases along with increases in DES scores (Collins, 2004a).

PERITRAUMATIC DISSOCIATION

Peritraumatic dissociation refers to dissociative phenomena experienced in anticipation of, during and immediately after a subjectively traumatic event. Investigations into the psychological effects of emergency service work have proven a rich source of information regarding peritraumatic dissociation (Barnes, 2000; Hershiser & Quarantelli, 1976; Marmar, Weiss, Metzler, Delucchi, Best, & Wentworth, 1999; Paton, Smith & Stephens, 1998; Strentz & Auerbach, 1988; Taylor & Frazer, 1982; Werner, Bates, Bell, Murdoch, & Robinson, 1992). Findings arising from such investigations indicate that peritraumatic dissociation is often associated with emergency situations that have personal meaning to the individual. For example, dissociation may occur where the emergency victims are known to the worker or are similar in some way (e.g., age and gender) to the worker or to people close to them. In such cases, the personal or emotional impact of the event can be overwhelming and the accompanying thoughts and feelings unacceptable and, consequently, dissociated (Marmar et al., 1999).

Although emergency service workers are trained to deal with worst case scenarios and are exposed during training to the gruesome and terrifying situations that may be encountered in the course of their work,

> no amount of training, can prepare emergency responders for the trauma of dismembered bodies, the screams of injured children, knowing that people may be trapped in a burning building, or having to deal with distressed people who suspect family members may be trapped. Such experiences are often so extreme that the ability to cope with them is overwhelmed. (Barnes, 2000, p. 60)

In many cases, peritraumatic dissociation is the only coping strategy available.

Sequelae of Peritraumatic Dissociation

There is some research evidence suggesting that individuals who experience peritraumatic dissociation are at greater risk of going on to develop Posttraumatic Stress Disorder (PTSD; Bremner & Brett, 1997; Marmar et al., 1996, Marmar et al., 1999; Marshall, Orlando, Jaycox, Foy, & Belzberg, 2002; Morgan et al., 2001; Shalev et al., 1996).

The apparent causal relationship between peritraumatic dissociation and ongoing posttraumatic stress has been questioned by Australian researchers Harvey and Bryant (2002), who pointed out, "peritraumatic" dissociation may be experienced in relation to a non-traumatic event and that in such cases, this "peritraumatic" dissociation did not place the individual at risk for continued "post-trauma" dissociation or other psychopathology. Harvey and Bryant (2002) noted that "there are reasons to question the notion that dissociation is necessarily linked to maladaptive outcomes. For example, novice skydivers display elevated levels of dissociation during their skydive, even though they do not develop a subsequent psychological disorder" (p. 894).

Panasetis and Bryant (2003) noted that peritraumatic dissociative responses may not lead to ongoing psychopathology, however, "persistent dissociation may impede access to and resolution of traumatic memories and associated affect, and this may contribute to ongoing psychopathology" (p. 563).

In a study involving 53 Australian victims of motor vehicle accidents and non-sexual assaults, Panasetis and Bryant (2003) found that ongoing posttraumatic psychopathology was more strongly associated with persistent, as opposed to peritraumatic, dissociation in victims of car accidents and non-sexual assaults (Panasetis & Bryant, 2003, p. 563). The authors concluded that "peritraumatic dissociation does not necessarily serve a maladaptive function following a traumatic experience" (p. 565).

Peritraumatic Dissociation and Coping

The widespread use of dissociative/emotion-focused coping strategies in response to acute trauma has been established in the Australian research literature examining the psychological effects of emergency service work (Evans, Coman, Stanley, & Burrows, 1993; Raphael, Singh, Bradbury, & Lambert, 1983-84; Taylor & Frazer, 1982; Werner et al., 1992). Two of the most commonly reported peritraumatic coping strategies in this population are the compartmentalisation of emotional material and imaginative involvement.

Compartmentalisation allows the individual to switch off from, or avoid consciously registering, the signs and symptoms of stress (Werner et al., 1992). For example, McFarlane and Raphael (1984) describe a Victoria fire-fighter attending the 1983 Ash Wednesday fires, who reported "switching off" from his fear and driving a truck down an avenue of burning trees, admitting afterwards that he would not have done so had he thought about it at the time. Similarly, Raphael et al. (1983-84) report the suppression of feelings of fear and dread in rescue workers attending to the victims of the 1977 Granville bridge collapse in suburban Sydney; these workers felt unable to abandon their duties despite the threat of gas leaks and the further collapse of the bridge onto the area in which they were working. Workers engaged in the recovery, handling, and identification of the dead after natural and human-made disasters have described suspending affective ties to the victims by avoiding looking at their faces, narrowly focusing concentration onto a small aspect of their work and generally ignoring the bodies (Hershiser & Quarantelli, 1976; Werner et al., 1992). The value of compartmentalisation of emotional material in the acute stages of a disaster has been noted by Taylor and Frazer (1980) who found that, among body-handlers during the 1979 Mt. Erebus aircrash in Antarctica, such strategies were employed by the most efficient workers, and enabled them to carry out their duties emotionally unencumbered.

A further peritraumatic dissociative/emotion-focused coping strategy is imaginative involvement. Imaginative involvement is the process whereby an individual withdraws into a self-induced trance state, accompanied by alterations in the individual's sense of self. Imaginative involvement serves the function of automatising certain behaviours and allows for the escape from unpleasant or unacceptable situations.

Examples of the peritraumatic use of imaginative involvement have been reported by Taylor and Frazer (1982). In their study examining the stress associated with body handling and victim identification following an air-crash in Antarctica, Taylor and Frazer (1982) found that 30% of the body recovery team engaged in imaginative involvement to help them cope with their gruesome task. The majority of this group imagined that the bodies were mere objects while others imagined them to be pieces of frozen or roasted meat, plane cargo, waxworks, or scientific specimens. This spontaneous use of imaginative involvement allowed these workers to distance themselves from the victims' plight and enabled them to function effectively within their professional roles. In addition, this group reported experiencing significantly lower levels of stress during this period than those workers who did not engage in imaginative involvement (Taylor & Frazer, 1982).

"Peritraumatic" Dissociation During Positive Events

Cameron (1963) recognised the role of dissociation during positive events such as abrupt changes in one's surroundings experienced during overseas travel. Transient feelings of derealisation are not uncommon both during travel and on arrival back home. Nearly thirty years later, Spiegel and Cardena (1991) picked up this thread stating that "whether trauma is a necessary and sufficient condition or a mere incidental correlate of [dissociation] is far from clear" (p. 368).

Pica and Beere (1995) sought to determine whether trauma is central to the experience of dissociation in an investigation of dissociative phenomena experienced during non-traumatic, subjectively positive events. Such events included last minute sporting victories, intense sexual encounters, performing in front of an audience and receiving good news. According to Beere's (1995a; 1995b; 1996; Beere & Pica, 1995) perceptual theory, dissociation occurs in the face of intense stimulation which need not be subjectively traumatic or unpleasant; it is the overwhelming or "captivating" nature of the stimulus that triggers dissociative reactions. In this study, both low and high dissociators reported experiencing dissociative phenomena during positive events leading the authors to conclude that (1) an individual does not need to be highly dissociative to experience dissociation during positive events and (2) trauma is not necessary for the experience of dissociation.

Further evidence of peritraumatic dissociation during positive events comes from Sterlini and Bryant (2002). In their investigation of dissociation in 100 Australian novice sky-divers, they found that, during their first skydive, about a third of the participants experienced distortions of time and derealisation while a quarter felt as though they were "on auto-pilot."

A recent sporting incident involving Australian tennis player Mark Philippoussis provides an illustration of the experience, and function, of peritraumatic dissociation during an undoubtedly positive, yet extremely painful, event. The 2003 final of the Davis Cup (a prestigious international tournament in which teams play for their country) was contested by Australia and Spain in Melbourne, Australia. Prior to Philippoussis' match, Australia led 2-1 in the "best of five" final. Apart from the obvious pressure on him to secure the championship by winning his match, Philippoussis also felt the pressure of playing for his country, on home-soil, in front of his father and his home-town crowd.

Philippoussis had taken the lead in the match by two sets to love before suffering a suspected torn pectoral muscle. In intense pain, he lost the next two sets badly bringing the score to two sets all. After the match, Philippoussis reported that at this point "There was no way I was going to pull out. I just kept telling myself to take it one point at a time, that's all I could do. I mean, this is the Davis Cup and you leave your heart out there" (Pearce, 2003, online). Philippoussis' painful experience was well corroborated; in addition to his own reports, data regarding his level of pain were available from a number of sources: the team chiropractor ("A normal match, he would have pulled out. Absolutely"), his team-mates ("I thought he was done, done like a dinner, to be honest"), the team coach ("I will be honest; I didn't see how he could turn that around"), and a sports journalist ("He was almost shrieking with the pain").

Philippoussis went on to play for another 33 minutes, winning the fifth and deciding set and securing the Davis Cup for Australia. In the obligatory post-match interview, Philippoussis described feeling "numb" during this final set; "It felt like I wasn't playing . . . I was sort of watching from the side. I didn't know what was going on, but, thank God, the shots were going in" (Pearce, 2003, online).

Hyperarousal and Uncontrollability

Collins and Jones (2002) proposed that, in non-clinical adult populations, hyperarousal and uncontrollability are the key features of "peritraumatic" dissociation. That is, it is not the traumatic or negative character of an event that provokes the dissociative reaction, rather, it is its highly arousing nature and perceived uncontrollability. By this argument, the "trauma" provoking the "peritraumatic" dissociative response may be either a negative or positive event. If this is so, under conditions that are highly arousing (e.g., psychologically, sensorially, physiologically) and where there is no apparent opportunity for control over the arousal, all individuals should experience "peritraumatic" dissociation regardless of whether they experience the situation as positive or negative and regardless of whether they are low or high dissociators. Based on this assumption, Collins (2004b) predicted that in non-clinical adult populations, all individuals, both low and high dissociators, would experience dissociative phenomena under conditions that are highly arousing and uncontrollable such as riding a roller-coaster.

Collins (2004a) tested this assumption in a non-clinical sample of Australian adult visitors of a Melbourne amusement park (N = 37). All participants completed the DES, rode on the park's rollercoaster, and then completed semi-structured interviews regarding their experience of the ride.

Phenomenological analysis revealed that 33 (90%) of the 37 participants experienced one or more dissociative phenomenon during the ride. The dissociative phenomena reported fall into the categories of derealisation, depersonalisation and time distortions. The most frequently experienced dissociative phenomenon was time distortion, which was reported by 70% of all participants. Around half of all participants (46%) reported experiences of derealisation while a relatively small number (14%) reported depersonalisation.

Time distortion. The most frequently reported dissociative experience was time distortion, being reported by 70% of all participants. Time distortion took three main forms: time speeding up which was reported by 35% of all participants; time slowing down, reported by 11% of participants; and time standing still or an absence of time which was reported by 27% of participants. The variety of perceptions of time distortion was illustrated by the following statement,

> 'No concept of time really. Um, I guess when the ride starts you sort of, there's a bit of a journey ahead of you. And when it's finished, it sort of feels like, um, it feels like only a couple of seconds has gone past. But while you're on the ride, you don't have any concept of time at all.' (Collins, 2004a, p. 208)

Depersonalisation. A small number of participants (two low and three high dissociators) reported depersonalisation experiences as illustrated by the following statement: "Your body just feels, you didn't feel as if you were actually in your own body 'cause you, you're thinking in your own head, so you weren't worried about your body" (Collins, 2004a, p. 207).

Derealisation. Almost half of all participants reported derealisation experiences. Derealisation phenomena took many forms including the experience of dream-like or surreal states, sensory (i.e., vision and hearing) loss, narrowed focus or attention, and a sense of being in one's own little world or the absence of the "outside world" "[Time] felt like it was standing still because I felt like I wasn't actually–you know, I was there but I wasn't so kind of . . . Well it was kind of like in my own little world; I mean I was in another . . . I was in a world within a world" (Collins, 2004a, p. 206).

THE DISSOCIATIVE EXPERIENCES SCALE

Australian samples have produced psychometric data for the DES, similar to those found in other Western societies (Collins, 2004a). Mean and standard deviations for Australian adult populations are shown in Table 1.

As can be seen, Australian samples produce DES scores comparable to those obtained by van IJzendoorn and Schuengel (1996) who, in their extensive meta-analysis of studies involving the DES, derived a mean DES score of 11.57 (*SD* = 10.63) from 7 studies involving 1458 non-clinical adults.

In terms of the reliability, the internal consistency coefficient obtained by Collins (2004a), .93 (N = 162), was the same as that obtained by van IJzendoorn and Schuengel (1996).

Factor Analysis

Since its publication in 1986, a good deal has been written about the factor structure of the DES, much of it conflicting and some of it leading to important advances in the assessment of dissociative pathology (Waller et al., 1996). The main point of contention has been the number of factors that best describe DES data in clinical and non-clinical populations. I shall restrict my review of the factor analytic literature to that pertaining to non-clinical populations.

TABLE 1. DES mean and standard deviation scores for Australian non-clinical samples.

Collins & Ffrench (1998)	17.51 (13.25)	130
Irwin (1998c)	12.01 (7.47)	103
Irwin (1998b)	10.32 (6.91)	92
Irwin (1998a)	12.39 (9.85)	106
Collins (2004a)	11.37 (10.20)	162

Factor analyses of DES scores in non-clinical populations have been conducted by a number of authors in an effort to clarify the underlying constructs of the DES producing solutions ranging from one to four factors, depending on technique used (Bernstein, Ellason, Ross, & Vanderlinden, 2001; Holtgraves & Stockdale, 1997; Modestin et al., 2002; Ray, June, Turaj, & Lundy, 1992; Ross, Ellason, & Anderson, 1995; Sanders & Green, 1994; Waller et al., 1996; Wolfradt, 1997; see Carlson & Putnam, 1993, for a review of early factor analytic studies and Wright & Loftus,1999, for a review of later studies). Waller (1995) has observed, however, that the distributions for individual DES items are positively skewed in both clinical and non-clinical populations, thus distorting the Pearson's correlations on which factor analyses are based, and possibly, resulting in the emergence of spurious factors.

With the aforementioned in mind, Collins (2004a) conducted a principal components analysis (PCA) using DES data from an Australian, non-clinical population (N = 335) which yielded four factors with eigenvalues greater than 1.0. All 28 DES items loaded on the first factor with loadings ranging from .52 to .81. This first factor had an eigenvalue of 13.51 and accounted for 48.25% of variance in DES scores. Factors 2, 3, and 4 accounted for a further 7.1%, 4.7%, and 4.1% of the variance, respectively. Given that all items loaded strongly on the first factor, a single factor solution can be accepted.

To establish whether the skewness and kurtosis of the DES score distribution affected the solution, the analysis was repeated on DES data to which a square root transformation had been applied. This second PCA also yielded four factors with eigenvalues greater than 1.0. Once again, all 28 DES items loaded on the first factor with loadings ranging from .53 to .79. This first factor had an eigenvalue of 12.67 and accounted for 45.22% of variance in the scores. Factors 2, 3, and 4 accounted for a further 6.2%, 4.9%, and 4.1% of the variance, respectively. Given that a single factor solution accounting for a almost half of the variance has been arrived at using both transformed and untransformed data, it is accepted in the present work that in non-clinical adult populations, the DES measures dissociation as a unidimensional construct.

Internet-Based Administration

In a study involving 335 Australian adults, Collins and Jones (2004) investigated the psychometric equivalence of traditional pen and paper (PP) and Internet-based versions of the DES. The DES demonstrated excellent internal consistency for both the PP and online groups with Cronbach's alphas of .95 and .96 produced by the PP and online samples, respectively.

The online responders reported higher levels of dissociation than did the PP responders. However, the overall pattern of online responses was found to mirror that found by Collins and Ffrench (1998) among PP responders. Collins and Ffrench (1998), in a PP investigation of the relationship between dissociation, coping strategies and locus of control orientation in non-clinical populations, found that the tendency to dissociate was positively related to external locus of control and the use of emotion-focused coping strategies. In the present study, in addition to reporting higher DES scores than their PP counterparts, the online responders reported higher external locus of control scores and higher emotion-focused coping scores than did the PP responders.

This finding suggests that differences in mean scores reflect differences in the dissociative tendencies of the two groups rather than instability in the online mea sures.

CONCLUSION

The last decade of the twentieth century saw a blossoming of interest in dissociation and the dissociative disorders among Australian practitioners and researchers. At the beginning of the twenty-first century, there is still some resistance in the public mental health sector to dissociative phenomena, however, this situation is poised for change as the growing community of dissociation researchers begins to convey their findings to their clinical colleagues.

REFERENCES

American Psychiatric Association (1994). *Diagnostic and statistical manual of mental disorders-fourth edition.* Washington, DC: Author.
American Psychiatric Association (2000). *Diagnostic and statistical manual of mental disorders-fourth edition, text revision.* Washington, DC: Author.

Armstrong, J., Putnam, F. W., & Carlson, E. B. (1997). Adolescent Dissociative Experiences Scale. In F. W. Putnam, *Dissociation in children and adolescents* (pp. 357-360), New York, NY: The Guilford Press.

Australian Health Ministers (1992). National Mental Health Plan 1992-1997. Canberra, ACT: Commonwealth Department of Health and Family Services.

Australian Health Ministers (1998). Second National Mental Health Plan 1998-2002 Canberra, ACT: Commonwealth Department of Health and Family Services.

Australian Health Ministers (2003). National Mental Health Plan 2003-2008. Canberra, ACT: Commonwealth Department of Health and Family Services.

Barnes, P. H. (2000). The experience of traumatic stress among urban firefighters. *Australian Journal of Emergency Management, Summer*, 59-64.

Beere, D. (1995a). Loss of "background": A perceptual theory of dissociation. *Dissociation: Progress in the Dissociative Disorders, 8*, 165-174.

Beere, D. (1995b). Dissociative reactions and characteristics of trauma: Preliminary tests of a perceptual theory of dissociation. *Dissociation: Progress in the Dissociative Disorders, 8*, 175-202.

Beere, D. (1996a). Switching part 1: An investigation using experimental phenomenology. *Dissociation: Progress in the Dissociative Disorders, 9*, 48-59.

Beere, D., & Pica, M. (1995). The predisposition to dissociate: The temperamental traits of flexibility/rigidity, daily rhythm, emotionality and interactional speed. *Dissociation: Progress in the Dissociative Disorders, 8*, 236-240.

Bernstein, E. M., & Putnam, F. W. (1986) Development, reliability, and validity of a dissociation scale. *The Journal of Nervous and Mental Disease, 174*, 727-735.

Bernstein, I. H., Ellason, J. W., Ross, C. A., & Vanderlinden, J. (2001). On the dimensionalities of the Dissociative Experiences Scale (DES) and the Dissociation Questionnaire (DIS-Q). *Journal of Trauma and Dissociation, 2*, 103-123.

Bowers, K. S. (1994). Dissociated control, imagination, and the phenomenology of dissociation. In D. Spiegel (Ed.), *Dissociation: Culture, mind, and body* (pp. 21-38), Washington, DC: American Psychiatric Press.

Bremner, J. D., & Brett, E. (1997). Trauma-related dissociative states and long-term psychopathology in Posttraumatic Stress Disorder. *Journal of Traumatic Stress, 19*, 37-49.

Brown, P. (2000). The Special Interest Group on Psychological Trauma: A progress report. *Australasian Psychiatry, 8*, 153-154.

Brown, P., Middleton, W., Butler, J., & Driscoll, H. (1996). Society, trauma, and dissociation. *Australasian Psychiatry, 4*, 272-275.

Cameron, N. (1963). *Personality development and psychopathology*. Boston, MA: Houghton Mifflin.

Carlson, E. B., & Putnam, F. W. (1993). An update on the Dissociative Experiences Scale. *Dissociation: Progress in the Dissociative Disorders, 6*, 16-27.

Clayton, K. (2004). The interrelatedness of disconnection: The relationship between dissociative tendencies and alexithymia. *Journal of Trauma and Dissociation, 5*, 77-101.

Collins, F. E. (2004a). *Dissociation, coping and control: A cognitive model of dissociation in non-clinical populations*. Unpublished doctoral dissertation, Monash University, Melbourne, Australia.

Collins, F. E. (2004b). 'Peritraumatic' dissociation during positive events: A response to hyperarousal and perceived lack of control. *Proceedings of the 39th Australian Psychological Society Annual Conference*, 52-56.

Collins, F. E., & Ffrench, C. H. (1998). Dissociation, coping strategies and locus of control in a non-clinical population: Clinical implications. *Australian Journal of Clinical and Experimental Hypnosis, 26,* 113-126.

Collins, F. E., & Jones, K. V. (2002). Dissociation under highly arousing and uncontrollable conditions: Responses to riding a roller-coaster. *Under the Southern Cross: Proceedings of the 23rd Stress and Anxiety Research Society Conference, Melbourne, Australia,* 9-13.

Collins, F. E., & Jones, K. V. (2004). Investigating dissociation online: Validation of a Web-based version of the Dissociative Experiences Scale. *Journal of Trauma and Dissociation, 5,* 133-147.

Dorahy, M. J., Schumaker, J. H., Krishnamurthy, B., & Kumar, P. (1997). Religious ritual and dissociation in India and Australia. *The Journal of Psychology,* 131, 471-476.

Evans, B. J., Coman, G. J., Stanley, R. O., & Burrows, G. D. (1993). Police officers' coping strategies: An Australian police survey. *Stress Medicine, 9,* 237-246.

Folkman, S. (1984). Personal control and stress and coping processes: A theoretical analysis. *Journal of Personality and Social Psychology, 46,* 839-852.

Folkman, S., & Lazarus, R. S. (1988). *Ways of Coping Questionnaire.* Palo Alto, CA: Mind Garden.

Frischholtz, E. J., Braun, B. G., Sachs, R. G., Schwartz, D. R., Lewis, J., & Schaeffer, D. et al. (1991). Construct validity of the Dissociative Experiences Scale (DES): 1. The relationship between the DES and other self-report measures of the DES. *Dissociation: Progress in the Dissociative Disorders, 4,* 185-188.

Harvey, A. G., & Bryant, R. (2002). Acute Stress Disorder: A synthesis and critique. *Psychological Bulletin, 128,* 886-902.

Hershiser, M. R., & Quarantelli, E. L. (1976). The handling of the dead in a disaster. *Omega, 7,* 195-208.

Holtgraves, T., & Stockdale, G. (1997). The assessment of dissociative experiences in a non-clinical population: Reliability, validity, and factor structure of the Dissociative Experiences Scale. *Personality & Individual Differences, 22,* 699-706.

Hopper, A., Ciorciari, J., Johnson, G., Spensley, J., Sergejew, A., & Stough, C. (2002). EEG coherence and Dissociative Identity Disorder: Comparing EEG coherence in DID hosts, alters, controls and acted alters. *Journal of Trauma and Dissociation, 3,* 75-88.

Irwin, H. J. (1994). Affective predictors of dissociation: I. The case of unresolved grief. *Dissociation: Progress in the Dissociative Disorders, 7,* 86-91.

Irwin, H. J. (1995). Affective predictors of dissociation: III. Affect balance. *Journal of Psychology, 129,* 463-467.

Irwin, H. J. (1996). Traumatic childhood events, perceived availability of emotional support, and the development of dissociative tendencies. *Child Abuse and Neglect, 20,* 701-701.

Irwin, H. J. (1997). Dissociative tendencies as a marker of parapsychological phenomena: Constructive observations with reference to Michelson and Ray's Handbook of Dissociation. *Journal of the American Society for Psychical Research, 91,* 133-141.

Irwin, H. J. (1998a). Dissociative tendencies and the sitting duck: Are self-reports of dissociation and victimization symptomatic of neuroticism? *Journal of Clinical Psychology, 54*, 1005-1015.

Irwin, H. J. (1998b). Attitudinal predictors of dissociation: Hostility and powerlessness. *Journal of Psychology, 132*, 389-400

Irwin, H. (1998c). *Affective predictors of dissociaiton II: Shame and guilt. Journal of Clinical Psychology, 54*, 237-245.

Irwin, H. J. (1999a). Pathological and nonpathological dissociation: The relevance of childhood trauma. *Journal of Psychology, 133*, 157-164.

Irwin, H. J. (1999b). Violent and nonviolent revictimization of women abused in childhood. *Journal of Interpersonal Violence, 14*, 1095-1110.

Irwin, H. J. (2000). The disembodied self: An empirical study of dissociation and the out-of-body experience. *Journal of Parapsychology, 64*, 261-277.

Levenson, H. (1972). Distinction within the concept of Internal-External control: Development of a new scale. *Proceedings of the 80th Annual Convention of the American Psychological Association*, 261-262.

Liotti, G. (1992). Disorganized/disoriented attachment in the etiology of the dissociative disorders. *Dissociation: Progress in the Dissociative Disorders, 5*, 196-204.

Marmar, C. R., Weiss, D. S., Metzler, T. J., & Delucchi, K. (1996). Characteristics of emergency services personnel related to peritraumatic dissociation during critical incident exposure. *American Journal of Psychiatry, 153*, 94-102.

Marmar, C. R., Weiss, D. S., Metzler, T. J., Delucchi, K. L., Best, S. R., & Wentworth, K. A. (1999). Longitudinal course and predictors of continuing distress following critical incident exposure in emergency services personnel. *The Journal of Nervous and Mental Diseases, 187*, 15-22.

Marshall, G. N., Orlando, M., Jaycox, L. H., Foy, D. W., & Belzberg, H. (2002). Development and validation of a modified version of the Peritraumatic Dissociative Experiences Questionnaire. *Psychological Assessment, 14*, 123-134.

McFarlane, A. C., & Raphael, B. (1984). Ash Wednesday: The effects of a fire. *Australian and New Zealand Journal of Psychiatry, 18*, 341-351.

McSherry, B. (1998). Getting away with murder? Dissociative states and criminal responsibility. *International Journal of Law and Psychiatry, 21*, 163-176.

McSherry, B. (2001). Expert testimony and the effects of mental impairment: Reviving the ultimate issue rule. *Law and Psychiatry, 24*, 13-21.

McSherry, B. (2004). Criminal responsibility, "fleeting" states of mental impairment, and the power of self-control. *Law and Psychiatry, 27*, 445-457.

Meadows, G., & Singh, B. (2003). "Victoria on the move": Mental health services in a decade of transition 1992-2002. *Australasian Psychiatry, 11*, 62-67.

Merckelbach, H., & Muris, P. (2001). The causal link between self-reported trauma and dissociation: A critical review. *Behaviour Research & Therapy, 39*, 245-254.

Middleton, W. (1996). Dichotomies, polarisations and dissociative processes. *Psychotherapy in Australia, 3*, 43-47.

Modestin, J., Lotscher, K., & Erni, T. (2002). Dissociative experiences and their correlates in young non-patients. *Psychology and Psychotherapy: Theory, Research and Practice, 75*, 53-64.

Morgan, C. A., Hazlett, G., Wang, S., Richardson, E. G., Schnurr, P., & Southwick, S. (2001). Symptoms of dissociation in humans experiencing acute, uncontrollable stress: A prospective investigation. *The American Journal Psychiatry, 158*, 1239-1247.

Norton, G. R., Ross, C. A., & Novotny, M. F. (1990). Factors that predict scores on the Dissociative Experiences Scale. *Journal of Clinical Psychology, 46*, 273-277.

Panasetis, P., & Bryant, R. A. (2003). Peritraumatic versus persistent dissocaition in Acute Stress Disorder. *Journal of Traumatic Stress*, 16, 563-566.

Paton, D., Smith, L. M., & Stephens, C. (1998). Work-related psychological trauma: A social psychological and organisational approach to understanding response and recovery. *The Australasian Journal of Disaster and Trauma Studies, 1*.

Pearce, L. (2003, December 1). Winged Scud stands tall. *The Age*. Retrieved December 1, 2003, from http://www.theage.com.au/

Pica, M., & Beere, D. (1995). Dissociation during positive situations. *Dissociation: Progress in the Dissociative Disorders, 8*, 241-246.

Putnam, F. W. (1989). Pierre Janet and modern views of dissociation. *Journal of Traumatic Stress, 2*, 413-429.

Putnam, F. W. (1995). Development of dissociative disorders. In D. Cicchetti & D. J. Cohen (Eds.), *Risk, disorder, and adaptation* (pp. 581-608). New York, NY: John Wiley and Sons.

Putnam, F. W. (1997). *Dissociation in children and adolescents: A developmental perspective*. New York, NY: The Guilford Press.

Raphael, B., Singh, B., Bradbury, L., & Lambert, F. (1983-84). Who helps the helpers? The effects of disaster on the rescue workers. *Omega, 14*, 9-20.

Ray, W. J., June, K., Turaj, K., & Lundy, R. (1992). Dissociative experiences in a college age population: A factor analytic study of two dissociation scales. *Personality & Individual Differences, 13*, 417-424.

Rosenman, S. (2002). Trauma and posttraumatic stress disorder in Australia: Findings in the population sample of the Australia National Survey of Mental Heath and Wellbeing. *Australian and New Zealand Journal of Psychiatry*, 36, 515-520.

Ross, C. A., Ellason, J. W., & Anderson, G. (1995). A factor analysis of the Dissociative Experiences Scale (DES) in Dissociative Identity Disorder. *Dissociation: Progress in the Dissociative Disorders, 8*, 229-235.

Sanders, B., & Green, J. A. (1994). The factor structure of the Dissociative Experiences Scale in college students. *Dissociation: Progress in the Dissociative Disorders, 7*, 23-27.

Sapp, M., & Evanow, M. (1998). Hypnotizability: Absorption and dissociation. *Australian Journal of Clinical Hypnotherapy & Hypnosis, 19*, v-xii.

Shalev, A. Y., Peri, T., Canetti, L., & Schreiber, S. (1996). Predictors of PTSD in injured trauma survivors: A prospective study. *American Journal of Psychiatry, 153*, 219-225.

Smith, G. C. (2003). The future of consultation-liasion psychiatry. *Austalian and New Zealand Journal of Psychiatry*, 37, 150-159.

Spiegel, D., & Cardeña, E. (1991). Disintegrated experience: The dissociative disorders revisited. *Journal of Abnormal Psychology, 100*, 366-378.

Sterlini, G. L., & Bryant, R. A. (2002). Hyperarousal and dissociation: A study of novice skydivers. *Behaviour Research & Therapy, 40*, 431-437.

Strentz, T., & Auerbach, S. M. (1988). Adjustment to the stress of simulated captivity: Effects of emotion-focused versus problem-focused preparation on hostages differing in locus of control. *Journal of Personality and Social Psychology, 55*, 652-660.

Taylor, A. J. W., & Frazer, A. G. (1980). Interim report on the effects on the recovery team after the Mt. Erebus disaster, November 1979. *New Zealand Medical Journal, 91*, 311-312.

Taylor, A. J. W., & Frazer, A. G. (1982). The stress of post-disaster body handling and victim identification work. *Journal of Human Stress, 8*, 4-12.

van IJzendoorn, M. H., & Schuengel, C. (1996). The measurement of dissociation in normal and clinical populations: Meta-analytic validation of the Dissociative Experiences Scale (DES). *Clinical Psychology Review, 16*, 365-382.

Walker, A. (2002). Dissociation in incarcerated juvenile male offenders: A pilot study in Australia. *Psychiatry, Psychology & the Law, 9*, 56-61.

Waller, N. G. (1995). The Dissociative Experiences Scale. In J. C. Conoley, J. C. Impara, & L. L. Murphy (Eds.), *The twelfth mental measurements yearbook*. Lincoln, NE: Buros Institute of Mental Measurement.

Waller, N., Putnam, F. W., & Carlson, E. B. (1996). Types of dissociation and dissociative types: A taxometric analysis of dissociative experiences. *Psychological Methods, 1*, 300-321.

Werner, H. R., Bates, G. W., Bell, R. C., Murdoch, P., & Robinson, R. (1992). Critical incident stress in Victorian emergency service volunteers: Characteristics of critical incidents, common stress responses and coping methods. *Australian Psychologist, 27*, 159-165.

Whiteford, H., Buckingham, B., & Mandersheid, R. (2002). Australia's National Mental Health Strategy. *British Journal of Psychiatry, 180*, 210-215.

Wolfradt, U. (1997). Dissociative experiences, trait anxiety and paranormal beliefs. *Personality & Individual Differences, 23*, 15-19.

World Health Organisation (1992). *ICD-10: The ICD-10 classification of mental and behavioural disorders: Clinical descriptions and diagnostic guidelines*. Geneva: Author.

Wright, D. B., & Loftus, E. F. (1999). Measuring dissociation: Comparison of alternative forms of the dissociative experiences scale. *American Journal of Psychology, 112*, 497-519.

Dissociative Experiences in the Peoples' Republic of China: An Empirical and Cross-Cultural Study

Stephanie Olen Kleindorfer

SUMMARY. This paper discusses the qualitative differences in dissociative experiences among normal college-age subjects in China and Japan. The paper first describes the process used to prepare the Mandarin version of the Dissociative Experiences Scale (DES). Baseline statistics comparing the two populations of interest are then presented. These results show fundamental differences across these two Asian cultures in terms of the mean DES scores obtained as well as the shape of the overall distribution of these scores. The results of a factor analysis of the DES responses corroborate both gender and cultural differences across the Japanese and Chinese data. Interestingly, the structure of the factors derived shows little relationship to factors from analyses of normal college-age subjects in North America. These contrasting results suggest that the DES can be a useful addition to other instruments and methods for exploring cross-cultural psychological differences, and that prior to

Stephanie Olen Kleindorfer, PsyD, is in Private Practice, Director, Center for Applied Psychology and Anthropology, and Founding Member, European Society for Trauma and Dissociation (ESTD).

Address correspondence to: Mme. Stephanie O. Kleindorfer, PsyD, 8, rue de l'Odéon, Paris, 75006, France (E-mail: drk@capaconsult.com).

[Haworth co-indexing entry note]: "Dissociative Experiences in the Peoples' Republic of China: An Empirical and Cross-Cultural Study." Kleindorfer, Stephanie Olen. Co-published simultaneously in *Journal of Trauma Practice* (The Haworth Maltreatment & Trauma Press, an imprint of The Haworth Press, Inc.) Vol. 4, No. 1/2, 2005, pp. 81-94; and: *Trauma and Dissociation in a Cross-Cultural Perspective: Not Just a North American Phenomenon* (ed: George F. Rhoades, Jr., and Vedat Sar) The Haworth Maltreatment & Trauma Press, an imprint of The Haworth Press, Inc., 2005, pp. 81-94. Single or multiple copies of this article are available for a fee from The Haworth Document Delivery Service [1-800-HAWORTH, 9:00 a.m. - 5:00 p.m. (EST). E-mail address: docdelivery@haworthpress.com].

clinical use baseline DES norms for each culture need to be established.
[Article copies available for a fee from The Haworth Document Delivery Service: 1-800-HAWORTH. E-mail address: <docdelivery@haworthpress.com> Website: <http://www.HaworthPress.com> © 2005 by The Haworth Press, Inc. All rights reserved.]

KEYWORDS. Dissociation, China, Japan, dissociation and gender

In the summer of 1994, when I embarked on this study of dissociative experiences in the Peoples' Republic of China, there were few, if any, empirical studies on the phenomenal psychology of the Chinese and no reported studies on dissociation or dissociative disorders. The field of cross-cultural psychology did, however, describe aspects and elements of Chinese mental and physical health and pathology. The movement of "Ch'i," for instance, could become blocked or imbalanced by the relationship of "yin-yang" in the body. "Hseih-ch'i," a free-floating energy force could invade the body causing "Hseih-ping," a possession illness. (Gaw, 1993, pp. 589-592). The practice of Qi-gong, a recent phenomenon based upon the ancient Chinese martial art and exercise regimen of Tai chi ch'uan, could lead to a syndrome known as Qi-gong psychotic reaction. This syndrome is described in the DSM-IV (American Psychiatric Association, 1994) as "an acute, time-limited episode characterized by dissociative, paranoid, or other psychotic or non-psychotic symptoms." Instances of Qi-gong psychotic reactions are commonly treated by psychiatrists using forms of suggestion (personal communication, Y.T. Li, 2003). These fundamentally non-Western beliefs, together with the historical stresses associated with the Cultural Revolution (which reached its peak in the 1970s), prompted the author to wonder about the nature of adaptive dissociative responses in the normal Chinese population.

Dissociative experiences remain an unsettling prospect for most rationally minded Westerners who believe in the concept of an individual, willful, unified, conscious self that is based upon the development of a healthy primary narcissism and/or a secure attachment experience during childhood. However, dissociation is a biological, physiological, evolutionary psychic mechanism inherent to all *homo sapien sapiens* (modern humans), but different cultures may or may not conceptualize and construct the self in the same way. For example, dissociative experiences that are considered taboo or desirable may differ from culture to culture and one could well expect that the willingness to endorse such experiences would therefore also vary from one culture to another.

In order to investigate such culture-specific issues related to dissociation, this paper considers results from Japan and China based on the Dissociative Experiences Scale (DES, Carlson and Putnam, 1993). The DES is a 28-item self-report questionnaire that is based upon a North American construction of experiences that would be considered normal through pathological depending on item and percentage of time one endorsed having these experiences. Results of the DES scores of the Chinese subjects are compared with DES scores of Japanese subjects (another Asian country) and the extant North American data utilized to norm the instrument. The research null hypothesis was that the differences in mean DES score would be statistically insignificant in all comparisons between Asian cultures in non-clinical late adolescent populations, and in relationship to extant North American findings resulting from responses obtained on the Dissociative Experiences Scale.

The DES was originally developed to serve both as a clinical tool to help identify patients with dissociative pathology and as a research tool to provide a means of quantifying dissociative experiences (Carlson and Putnam, 1993, p.16). It asks subjects to report on the frequency of dissociative experiences in their daily life, described on a response scale from 0% (meaning "This never happens to you") to 100% (meaning "This always happens to you"). The resultant DES score is determined by taking the average of the scores of the 28 items on the instrument. While originally formatted along a 100 mm response scale for each item (the DES I), it was reformatted in 1993 to a response scale from 0 to 100 in increments of 10 (the DES II) without any significant differences reported in reliability, construct validity or the factor analytic structure and subscale reports (Carlson and Putnam, 1993, pp. 18-22).

According to Carlson and Putnam (1993), the 28 items that comprise the DES were developed from interviews with persons with the DSM-III diagnoses for the dissociative disorders and in consultation with experts in the diagnosis and treatment of the dissociative disorders. However, "Items were worded to be comprehensible to the widest possible range of individuals and to avoid implications of any social undesirability of the experiences" (Carlson and Putnam, 1993, p. 18). These requirements pose special difficulties in translating and using the DES that vary as much from the North American origins of the DES as do the Asian cultures of interest in this chapter. As Carlson and Putnam state:

> Some of the most important guidelines for translation are described by Brislin (Brislin, 1986). First, scale items should be

translated conceptually, not literally. This is to insure that collo-
quial expressions are not translated literally and that terms and
concepts unfamiliar in another culture do not appear in the translated items. Second, it is sometimes wise to eliminate items that do
not make sense in another culture or population. For example, in
translating the DES into Japanese, it was sensible to add "riding a
bicycle" to other modes of transportation listed in item one. Third,
it is important to include new items that represent experiences that
do occur in the second culture, but were not part of the cultural experience of those for whom the measure was originally developed
(A. Kleinman, personal communication, October 1991). Fourth, it
is crucial to perform a blind back translation of the translated measure so that the back translation can be compared and reconciled
with the original version. This provides a necessary check on the
accuracy of the translation. (Carlson and Putnam, 1993, pp. 21-22)

Translation can, and indeed should, be an ongoing process of the refinement of the accuracy, validity, and reliability of the multi-cultural
comparison of data resulting from the use of the instrument. For example, in the Ensink and Van Otterloo validation of the DES in the Netherlands, the authors used two versions of the DES–one which had been
previously validated and one which was substituted with nine "dummy
questions." The results of this small scale study (N = 80) indicated that
the questionnaire maintained good internal consistency and good criterion validity (Ensink and Van Otterloo, 1989).

It is not the purpose of this chapter to provide an exhaustive list of
studies using the DES-II. A review of other studies that have utilized a
translation of the DES-II has been completed by Kleindorfer (1998).
The essential point is that there is a broad and growing scope of the use
of this instrument internationally and when the DES-II, or any other instrument is used clinically in translation, there needs to be a norming of
that instrument based on a study of responses from samples of the normal population of that culture and language.

This chapter will focus on the development of the Mandarin DES, the
author's collaboration with Chinese colleagues in the generation and
collection of the data, the research design and the statistical approaches
utilized in the analysis of the data. Following this, summary statistics
will be presented, including a statistical comparison of the Chinese and
Japanese data. Thereafter, a factor analyses of the Chinese data will be
presented, with a comparison of those results with the factors derived
from the North American and Japanese populations. The discussion of

the results demonstrates statistical evidence of cultural differences in the underlying response structure of the DES for the Chinese, Japanese and North American populations studied. In conclusion, some particular features of Chinese culture are highlighted that may help explain these results.

METHOD

The Development of the Mandarin and Japanese Versions of the DES

During the spring of 1994, under the author's supervision and with the support of Dr. Wu, the English version of the DES was translated by three Chinese doctoral students at the University of Pennsylvania. Dr. Dong-Jun Wu, a native of Yancheng, was at the time a doctoral student at the University of Pennsylvania. Dr. Wu, with the author's assistance, then synthesized the Mandarin translations for best "fit of expression" and produced the first Mandarin DES and back translation. This Mandarin version was then refined by Professors Zhongheng Dai and Cun-Dao He of the Department of Psychology, East Shanghai Normal University, and by Professor Jiecheng Zhao of the Shanghai Institute of Mental Health. The final back translation was done with the assistance of Ms. Kate Fang of the University of Pennsylvania.

Professors Dai, He, and Zhao administered the DES to 125 hospitalized diagnosed schizophrenics (in accordance with the ICD-9 criteria) and 125 college students (ages 18-25 years old) from the East China Normal University. The author administered (coordinated by Dr. Wu) the DES to a group of 125 college students (ages 18-25 years old) from Yancheng Education Institute located in Jaingsu, a coastal province of China. All original data (i.e., original DES forms) were collected, coded, and analyzed by the author. The data included age, sex, date of administration and particular population sample–Yancheng college student, Shanghai college student, or hospitalized schizophrenic.

Data on the Japanese version of the DES were collected by Yuichi Hattori, MA, and shared with the author for independent analysis. The data provided was on two groups of Japanese university students at the Science University of Tokyo and Tokyo Home Economics University, collected in the early 1990s (N = 460 subjects).

There were three independent analyses conducted on the Chinese data from the three samples of late adolescent subjects from a city university, from a rural university, and from an adult clinical in-patient population of ICD-9 diagnosed schizophrenic patients. The central issue addressed was the comparison of DES scores of these three samples, calculating the overall mean score of each subject across all 28 questions in the DES as a measurement of his/her level of dissociation. The population means were tested to see if they were significantly different from one another. A principle components analysis and a factor analysis were also conducted to compare the covariance structures across the responses to the 28 questions, i.e., considering the score of each subject as a 28-dimensional observation.

The two population means of the Japanese Universities were also analyzed. A confounding variable of gender was noted as the Science University of Tokyo sample consisted of only female subjects. It was due to this confounding variable that no further statistical analysis was done on the covariance structures between the two Japanese university samples.

Based on the results of the comparison among different universities, the college students in each country were pooled and considered as a Chinese sample and a Japanese sample for the DES instrument. For these two samples, there are two issues of interest, potential cultural differences and potential gender differences. Of special interest in the norming of the Mandarin DES and in comparing its results to the Japanese and other cultures are differences, if any, in population means and population variances. Of further interest are the covariance (i.e., factor analytic) structures between genders within each culture and between the two cultures. We consider each of these issues in turn.

Norming of the Mandarin and Japanese DES

Standard t-tests for the means and F-tests for the variances of the two pooled populations were undertaken. Of special interest, given previous work in this area, are the distributions of the overall mean of each subject's response. A factor analysis of the correlation structure of the individual responses to the 28 questions in the DES was then conducted. This analysis then allowed further comparisons of both culture and gender according to the factor structure determined.

RESULTS

Norming of the Mandarin DES

Means and standard deviations were computed for the three Chinese populations noted above (Table 1). The resulting means for the Manda-

TABLE 1. Summary Statistics for Chinese and Japanese Populations

Chinese Populations			
	Mean DES Score	Standard Dev of DES Score	Number of Observations
Schizophrenics	9.27	11.79	122
University Students Yancheng University	21.54	9.42	117
University Students Shanghai University	18.75	10.05	124
Combined Chinese Student Populations	20.10	9.83	241
Japanese Populations			
Science University of Tokyo	9.80	9.47	345
Tokyo Homo Economics University	11.80	11.36	115
Combined Japanese Student Populations	10.41	10.00	460

rin DES scores were not inconsistent with the results from the existing North American studies on late adolescents: (Study 1 reporting a Mean = 23.8 (N: 259), and Study 2 reporting a Mean = 11.8 (N: 108)) and for diagnosed schizophrenics (Study 1 reporting a Mean = 17.7 (N: 61), and Study 2 reporting a Mean = 10.5 (N: 15)) from Carlson and Putnam (1993) (standard deviations for these studies are not currently available in the literature).

Concerning the Chinese data in Table 1, it is plain from these data that the clinical population of schizophrenics is quite different from the two student populations, with much smaller differences between the two student populations. In fact, using Tukey's Studentized Range (HSD), Kleindorfer (1998) formally tested these relationships and concluded that the two student populations were sufficiently similar, statistically, to allow them to be pooled. Thus, henceforth the data from the two university populations will be pooled and referred as the "Chinese data," as summarized in Table 1.

Norming of the Japanese DES

The statistical results for the Japanese subjects (N = 460) are also presented in Table 1. The pooled group of subjects generated a DES score of 10.41. It should be noted that while the two Japanese university populations exhibited mean DES scores that were not statistically different (at the p = .067 level), the variance in DES scores from these two university populations was statistically different. This significant difference may be related to the gender composition of the two universities as the Tokyo Home Economics University test subjects were only female and the Science University of Tokyo involved both male and female subjects.

Comparison of Chinese and Japanese Populations

Table 1 also summarizes the statistics contrasting Chinese and Japanese university pooled populations. There is a highly statistically significant difference (p-value < 0.0001) between the mean DES scores of the two university populations, with the Mean DES Score of the Japanese student population being 10.41 and that of the Chinese student population being 20.10.

Gender Differences

Table 2 provides statistics on the Chinese and Japanese populations by gender. In this case, the reader will note a striking difference between the Japanese and Chinese populations in terms of reports of dissociative experiences by gender. Both male and female subjects in the Chinese populations reported experiences on the DES scale that are not different at a statistically significant level, either in terms of the means or the variances of the gender-differentiated subjects. This contrasts with the Japanese data in which both the mean (p-value = .010) and variance (p-value = .0027) of DES scores are statistically different across gender.

Summarizing the Cultural Differences for Chinese and Japanese DES Responses

From Table 1, the reader will note that there is a highly significant difference in mean DES scores between the Chinese and Japanese university student populations (p < 0.0001). Actually, the distributions of responses from the Japanese and Chinese populations are even more different than these summary statistics would indicate. Figure 1 plots the histograms of responses for the Chinese and Japanese data, respectively. These histograms visually indicate the difference between the

TABLE 2. Statistics for Chinese and Japanese University Students by Gender

	Mean DES Score	Standard Dev of DES Score	Number of Observations
Chinese University Students			
Male Subjects	19.10	9.98	132
Female Subjects	20.95	9.58	109
Japanese University Students			
Male Subjects	9.41	9.12	285
Female Subjects	11.87	11.15	175

FIGURE 1. Histogram of Chinese and Japanese University Populations

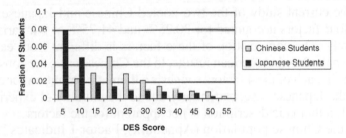

structures of the two data sets. In the Chinese data sets, a relatively symmetric distribution is seen, centered close to the Chinese mean of the DES scale (20.1). In the Japanese case, a very positively skewed distribution is seen, with the mode close to zero. These observations were found to be true regardless of whether the overall data sets or the gender-specific subsets of these data sets are considered.

An analysis of the Chinese schizophrenic population resulted in different means across gender and especially age. While the sample mean was 9.49, the mean for males was 10.0 and the mean for females was 8.90. This is relatively consistent with the lack of significance across gender in the normal population. However, there was a significant difference in mean scores across age: subjects age 35 and younger had a mean of 12.30, compared with a mean of 6.90 for subjects age 36 and older. A question for further study is whether this difference is an artifact of the tendency of dissociative experiences to decline with age or is associated with some idiosyncratic historical experience (e.g., the Cultural Revolution in China) of this age group.

Factor Analytic Structure and Comparisons Across Cultures

A factor analysis of non-clinical North American subjects (Carlson et al., 1991) yielded three categories of experiences which accounted for 40% of variance among item scores, giving rise to the following defined factors:

Factor 1: Absorption and Changeability
    DES Item Numbers: 12, 14, 15, 16, 17, 18, 20, 22, 23
Factor 2: Derealization and Depersonalization
    DES Item Numbers: 3, 4, 7, 11, 12, 13, 28
Factor 3: Amnestic Experience
    DES Item Numbers: 5, 6, 8

In the current study of the two pooled Chinese and Japanese populations, four factors accounted for 30.25% and 41.75% of the variance, respectively. The composition of these factors is different from each other and from the North American results. In the Chinese case, the constellation of items in each of the 4 factors suggests a thematic definition for each factor. In the Japanese case, particularly due to the plurality of experiences in factor 1, a thematic description is not apparent for the factors.

For the Chinese population (Appendix), Factor 1 indicates "Internal Absorption," Factor 2 "External Inattention," Factor 3 "Derealization/Depersonalization," and Factor 4 "Amnestic Experience." The mean DES scores for the items in Factor 1 are considerably higher than the mean item scores in Factors 2, 3, and 4. For instance, in Factor 1, items 14, 17 and 22 show means, respectively, of 55.60, 42.11 and 33.69, which are well over the mean scores of any of the items reported in Factors 2-4. These results suggest evidence of a significant cultural component that values dissociative internal absorption in normal Chinese experience. In addition, the study of the relatively high mean value of item 10 in Factor 2 revealed an interesting gender difference, i.e., males scored a mean of 30.68 while females scored a mean of 16.15.

DISCUSSION

The present study involved the translation of the DES into Mandarin, the norming of the translated DES for a normal PRC Chinese population, and the comparison of the translated scale to a clinical population.

In addition, the translated normed DES data was compared statistically with similar subject populations in Japan and North America. These results show fundamental differences across the Chinese and Japanese college-age populations studied in terms of the mean DES scores obtained as well as the shape of the overall distribution of these scores. The striking dissimilarities found between the Chinese and Japanese samples led to the speculation that gender differences may account for said differences. However, while the differences were striking across genders in the Japanese population, the same was not true for the Chinese population.

Factor analysis and component analysis was conducted to see whether the differences noted in the distribution of means of DES scores was the result of some fundamental differences in the structure of responses to particular items in the DES. The results further highlight the differences across cultures for the two populations of interest. Moreover, the factor analysis of the Japanese and Chinese data showed that the data was not structurally the same as those in North American studies. All of this leads to the central conclusion of this paper that the nature and intensity of the dissociative experiences evoked by the DES are different as a function of the culture and gender of the respondent, at least in Asia.

It should be noted that Ross, Keyes et al. (2003) collected data in Shanghai only months after the current study, utilizing the same translated version of the DES developed in Kleindorfer (1998) and used in this study. Their study involved 618 factory workers (mean age 41.8 yrs.) and resulted in a mean DES score of 2.6 (compared to the current study mean for the Chinese college-student sample of 20.10). Their analysis of 423 psychiatric in-patients resulted in a mean DES score of 4.1 (compared to the current study mean of 9.27). The contrasting results of the two studies illustrate the need for continued cross-cultural studies of the translation and utilization of the DES.

In conclusion, the words of Kirmayer seem appropriate: "the recognition of symptoms and syndromes is always selective and based on preconceived culturally shaped notions (of both patient and physician) as to what is deviant, pragmatically relevant, and worthy of medical attention" (Kirmayer, 1991, p. 26). The investigation of the phenomenology of experience and consciousness across cultures and individuals remains a richly fertile area of inquiry can lead us to whole new avenues of human understanding and potential.

REFERENCES

American Psychiatric Association (1994). *Diagnostic and statistical manual of mental disorders* (4th ed.). Washington, DC.

Brislin, R. (1986). The wording and translation of research instruments. In W.J. Lonner and J.W. Berry (Eds.), *Field methods in cross-cultural research* (pp. 137-164). Beverly Hills, CA: Sage.

Carlson, E. B. & Putnam, F. W. (1993). An update on the Dissociative Experiences Scale. *Dissociation, 6*, 16-27.

Carlson, E. B., Putnam, F. W., Ross, C. A., Anderson, G., Clark, P., & Torem, M. et al. (1991). Factor analysis of the Dissociative Experiences Scale: A multi-center study. In B. G. Braun and E. B. Carlson (Eds.), *Proceedings of the Eighth International Conference on Multiple Personality and Dissociative States*, Chicago: Rush.

Ensink, B. & Van Otterloo, D. (1989). A validation study of the DES in the Netherlands. *Dissociation, 2*, 221-223.

Gaw, A. C. (ed.) (1993). *Culture, Ethnicity and Mental Illness.* American Psychiatric Press, Washington, DC.

Kirmayer, L. J. (1991). The place of culture in psychiatric nosology: Taijin kyofusho and DSM-III-R. *Journal of Nervous and Mental Disease, 179*, 19-28.

Kleindorfer, S. O. (1998). *The Dissociative Experiences Scale: Gender and Cross-Cultural Considerations*, Doctoral Dissertation, Widener University, Institute for Graduate Clinical Psychology, UMI Dissertation Services, Ann Arbor, MI.

Ross, C. A., Keyes, B., Xiao, Z., Yan, H., Wang, H. Zhou, Z., Xu, Y., Cheng, J., & Zhang, Y. (2003). Trauma and dissociative disorders in China. Presentation at the ISSD 20th International Fall Conference, November 2-4, Chicago.

APPENDIX

Factor Analysis for Overall Chinese Student Population

Factor 1

Item Description	Mean	Value
14. Remembering/Reliving the past vividly	55.60	0.414
17. Absorption in a TV program or movie	42.11	0.404
18. Being so involved in a fantasy that it seems real	20.50	0.523
22. Feeling as though one were two different people	33.69	0.489
27. Hearing voices inside one's head	18.13	0.503

Factor 2

Item Description	Mean	Value
05. Finding unfamiliar things among one's belongings	10.42	0.690
06. Being addressed by a stranger as if he knows you	15.06	0.540
09. Forgetting important events in one's life	12.37	0.411

10. Being accused of lying but not thinking you lied   24.11   0.421

26. Finding one's writings, drawings, or notes without

     recalling having created them   12.57   0.424

Factor 3

Item Description	Mean	Value
12. Other people and objects don't seem real	19.42	0.613
13. Feeling as though one's body is not one's own	12.23	0.466
16. Being in a familiar environment but finding it strange	18.59	0.468
28. Looking at things and people as if through a fog	21.74	0.529

Factor 4

Item Description	Mean	Value
09. Forgetting important events in one's life	12.37	0.444
24. Confusing thinking about something and doing it	20.79	0.637
25. Finding out one has done things one can't remember	22.41	0.623

Factor Analysis for Overall Japanese Student Population

Factor 1

Item Description	Mean	Value
06. Being addressed by a stranger as if he knows you	08.00	0.488
07. Looking at your actions as if others are doing them	09.48	0.521
08. Not recognized by friends or family	02.89	0.561
10. Being accused of lying but not thinking they lied	07.00	0.401
11. Not recognizing one's own reflection in a mirror	07.28	0.519
12. Other people and objects don't seem real	11.72	0.483
13. Feeling as though one's body is not one's own	08.87	0.511
14. Remembering/reliving the past vividly	17.35	0.514
15. Being unsure if a remembered event happened or not	18.09	0.484
17. Absorption in a TV program or movie	23.65	0.420
18. Being so involved in a fantasy that it seems real	08.74	0.454
20. Thinking of nothing and not aware of time passing	18.89	0.529
21. Talking out loud to oneself when alone	10.67	0.562
22. Feeling as though one were two different people	16.61	0.536

Factor 2

Item Description	Mean	Value
22. Feeling as though one were two different people	16.61	0.563
23. Being able to do usually difficult things with ease	16.52	0.538

26. Finding one's writings, drawings, or notes without
recalling having created them 07.67 0.535
27. Hearing voices in one's head 07.44 0.647
28. Looking at things and people as if through a fog 06.61 0.505

Factor 3

Item Description	Mean	Value
01. Riding in a car/bus and not remembering	10.09	0.532
03. Being in a place but unaware of how one got there	03.15	0.684
04. Being dressed in clothes one can't recall putting on	00.98	0.445
09. Forgetting important events in one's life	08.87	0.487
12. Other people and objects don't seem real	11.72	0.572
13. Feeling as though one's body is not one's own	08.87	0.511

Factor 4

Item Description	Mean	Value
05. Finding unfamiliar things among one's belongings	01.76	0.480
24. Confusing thinking about something and doing it	20.07	0.524
25. Finding out one has done things one can't remember	12.17	0.637
26. Finding one's writings, drawings, or notes without recalling having created them	07.67	0.637
27. Hearing voices inside one's head	07.44	0.523

Experiences of Trauma and Dissociation in France

Jean-Michel Darves-Bornoz

SUMMARY. In France, trauma was identified as a cause of mental illness as early as the middle of the nineteenth century. Physical, sexual, or emotional abuse are the most frequent events. Interpersonal trauma, such as assault, abuse, confinement, or war, lead much more often to severe traumatic responses. In the aftermath of trauma, several traumatic syndromes exist. I discriminated especially *the dissociation and phobia traumatic syndromes, the reliving traumatic syndromes*, and *the narcissistic regression traumatic syndromes*. For us, posttraumatic clinics do not fundamentally differ from country to country. French mainstream psychotherapy still remains psychoanalysis. Maybe, the most significant research contribution in France lay in creating, many decades ago now, the first *medical Non-Governmental Organizations* as a therapeutic answer to mass trauma. *[Article copies available for a fee from The Haworth Document Delivery Service: 1-800-HAWORTH. E-mail address: <docdelivery@haworthpress.com> Website: <http://www.HaworthPress.com> © 2005 by The Haworth Press, Inc. All rights reserved.]*

Jean-Michel Darves-Bornoz, MD, PhD, is Head, Department of Psychiatry, General Hospital, Vendôme, France and Professor of Psychiatry, University of Kurdistan, Iraq.

Address correspondence to: Jean-Michel Darves-Bornoz, MD, PhD, 4 Faubourg Saint-Lubin, 41100–Vendôme, France (E-mail: darves-bornoz@wanadoo.fr).

The author wishes to thank Elaine Briggs for her consideration and help with this manuscript.

[Haworth co-indexing entry note]: "Experiences of Trauma and Dissociation in France." Darves-Bornoz, Jean-Michel. Co-published simultaneously in *Journal of Trauma Practice* (The Haworth Maltreatment & Trauma Press, an imprint of The Haworth Press, Inc.) Vol. 4, No. 1/2, 2005, pp. 95-111; and: *Trauma and Dissociation in a Cross-Cultural Perspective: Not Just a North American Phenomenon* (ed: George F. Rhoades, Jr., and Vedat Sar) The Haworth Maltreatment & Trauma Press, an imprint of The Haworth Press, Inc., 2005, pp. 95-111. Single or multiple copies of this article are available for a fee from The Haworth Document Delivery Service [1-800-HAWORTH, 9:00 a.m. - 5:00 p.m. (EST). E-mail address: docdelivery@haworthpress.com].

KEYWORDS. Human rights, France, survivors, trauma, traumatic syndromes, dissociation, conversion, somatization, phobias, reliving, narcissistic regression, borderline states, psychoanalysis, psycho- traumatology

Paul Briquet[1] stated as early as 1859 that he found determining causes of "hysteria" in certain events experienced by his patients. Even before, in 1857, Edouard-Adolphe Duchesne reported some traumatic illnesses in railway men that he named *"maladies des mécaniciens."*[2] Then, in France, trauma was identified as a cause of certain types of mental distress in the studies on railway accidents by Duchesne and de Martinet, and on several kinds of overwhelming private events in childhood or adulthood by Briquet.

At the same time, long-ignored scientific interest in the observation and theorization of the division of the mind was arising together with literary plays on interacting states of mind. This led to notions of the *double* in literature and *personnalité alternante* in psychopathology. Such ideas circulated loosely for some time before becoming organized in Jean-Martin Charcot and Pierre Janet's categorization of "traumatic hysteria."

The framework of knowledge accumulated over some decades in the nineteenth century in France became so impressive that even such an experienced doctor as Sigmund Freud visited Charcot's La Salpêtrière Hospital in Paris. In 1885, he had the opportunity to approach the field of trauma and dissociation in Paris, and even attended the very specialized activities on sexual crimes on children conducted by Brouardel, a professor in forensic medicine. Unfortunately, the followers of Charcot in La Salpêtrière left this stream of thinking and covered this knowledge over with a veil of so-called doubt and mistrust concerning the actual suffering of these patients.

However, other inspired clinicians revived the field. Among them were Alfred and Françoise Brauner, who went to Spain in 1936, and who imagined new techniques of psychiatric care for children in war conditions, including drawing techniques. They still remain a reference in France (Brauner, 1946). Such personalities maintained a creative stream of knowledge for trauma in some French circles.

A new wave of interest in France for mass trauma started in the early seventies with the foundation of Non-Governmental Organizations (NGO) such as *Médecins Sans Frontières* and afterwards *Médecins du Monde*. The founding doctors of these organizations wanted to speak out against human rights abuses around the world. One of them, Bernard Kouchner, once summarized their approach by saying: *"mankind's suffering belongs to all men."* Together with ideas for the respect of women's rights, and also fears of violent nationalist struggle reaching France in the 1980s, interest in trauma was definitely re-established in a significant sector of the French population.

TYPES OF TRAUMA

In order to appreciate the types of trauma that nowadays affect the French population, I present here, as an example, the description of my own outpatient department in the University Hospital in Tours. This consulting room was essentially oriented towards people exposed to traumatic events. More than half of them suffered from lasting *Post Traumatic Stress Disorder (PTSD)*.[3] We used the description of these patients for one of my resident student's master memoir. Its methodology was reported elsewhere (El Hage, Darves-Bornoz, Allilaire, & Gaillard, 2002).

All my outpatients older than sixteen were systematically approached for consent. They covered the whole range of ages from adolescence to elderly. The resulting sample over-represented women by five percent, but the mean ages of men and women did not appear significantly different.

Using the *Clinician-Administered PTSD Scale (CAPS)* developed by Blake and his colleagues (Blake et al., 1995) to assess *PTSD*, it was possible to gather which types of potentially traumatic events the patients experienced, through their rating of the exhaustive list of overwhelming incidents included in this instrument.

During the study, one hundred and sixteen subjects reporting one or several overwhelming incidents in their lives were interviewed. All together, these subjects had to face 491 potentially traumatic events, which meant an average of four to five experiences of that type for each person. This fact is crucial when thinking of treatment. Indeed, when such a person consults, it is not necessarily obvious which event was the key event in the process of traumatization. We ordered the overwhelming incidents reported by the patients, sometimes as witnesses, in four classes: physical, sexual or emotional abuse (37.5%), threat on health (31.9%), accidents (16.1%), disasters (10.8%), and war (or civil war) experiences (3.7%). The details of these events are shown in Table 1.

TABLE 1. Types of overwhelming events reported by French psychiatric out-patients (N = 116)

Overwhelming events	N = 491	
	n	%
Physical, sexual or emotional abuse	**184**	**37.5**
Physical assaults		
(physical maltreatment in childhood, assaults whether by the		
spouse, an acquaintance or a stranger, sometimes during a burglary)	54	11.0
Weapon assault		
(knife or sometimes firearms) seldom followed by a confinement	44	9.0
Sexual assaults		
(non-consensual sexual relations with the spouse, rape attempts or		
actual rapes, repeated or not, in childhood or adulthood; child		
abuse with sexual contact)	62	12.6
Severe emotional abuse or neglect	24	4.9
Threat on health	**157**	**31.9**
Illness or physical wound threatening life	30	6.1
Severe human suffering due to an illness	24	4.9
Witnessing a severe wound or personal damage	7	1.4
Sudden and violent death of one's nearest and dearest	28	5.7
Sudden and unexpected death of one's nearest and dearest	68	13.8
Accidents	**79**	**16.1**
Transport accident	50	10.2
Severe accident at work or in the home		
(with burn, cut, fall and then fracture, crush, or blast)	25	5.1
Exposure to dangerous toxic substance	4	0.8
Disasters	**53**	**10.8**
Natural disasters (earthquake, flood, storm)	23	4.7
Conflagration, explosion	30	6.1
War	**18**	**3.7**
Combat or exposure to a war zone	16	3.3
Captivity in a war (or civil war) context	2	0.4

THE DISSOCIATIVE RESPONSE TO TRAUMA

In our patients, these difficult experiences did not appear equally harmful for two main reasons. First, the repetition of certain incidents or their mix with other types of unfavourable contexts or chronic neglect deepened the traumatic wound as other authors have noted (Gold, 2000): it is not equivalent to undergo a car accident followed by immediate comfort from a warm family, and to experience the hard daily life of a prisoner of war for years subsequent to war combat; it is not equivalent to be raped once at twenty-five by a stranger, and repeatedly from five to ten by one's father (Darves-Bornoz, 1998a,b). Second, events by themselves do not equally overwhelm subjects: in our observations, experiences with an interpersonal dimension, like assault, abuse, confinement or war, lead much more often to severe traumatic responses whether in the traumatic reliving field, or in the traumatic withdrawal and numbing field. In order to fit the broadest range of traumatic syndromes, our clinical outcome studies were then undertaken among one of these groups, rape survivors, where subjects seldom remain non-traumatized (Darves-Bornoz, Lépine, Choquet, Berger, Degiovanni, & Gaillard, 1998). However, we must not forget that any type of overwhelming experience can lead, though more sporadically, to the same extensive clinics in some subjects.

In previous writings (e.g., Darves-Bornoz, Pierre, Berger, Lansac, Degiovanni, & Gaillard, 1997), I stated that in the aftermath of trauma, several traumatic syndromes exist. I discriminated especially three types of syndromes, distinct in their semiotics and independent in their outcome, whose occurrence follows each other: *the dissociation and phobia traumatic syndromes, the reliving traumatic syndromes,* and *the narcissistic regression traumatic syndromes.* Their onsets, in general, were hardly or not at all delayed from each other.

The patients let us know, often loudly, their traumatic reliving symptoms, but in many ways, the two other types of syndromes preoccupied us much more, especially as far as children and adolescents were concerned, because of the major psychic development disorders they induced in them (Darves-Bornoz, Berger, Degiovanni, Soutoul, & Gaillard, 1994c; Darves-Bornoz, Degiovanni, Berger, & Soutoul, 1995; Darves-Bornoz, 1995).

The *dissociation and phobia traumatic syndromes* represented the subject's defence mechanisms during the traumatic experience, and afterwards their attempt at processing, on the one hand, an identity wound by fragmenting the memories and the mind, and on the other hand, a traumatic reliving of trauma by avoiding the world. When using the term of dissociation, we meant a soma-psyche as well as purely intrapsyche splitting.

The intrapsychic dissociations included disorders such as psychogenic amnesias (related to the traumatic event or not), depersonalisations (especially with out of the body experiences), derealizations (for instance, feeling of watching one's own life like a movie), identity fragmentations (at worst, feeling one is two different persons), and automations (especially in fugues). To different degrees, they gave an answer to the subject's psychic pain when unprepared for the emergence of a representation of the world which was contradictory with the one he thought appropriate until that event.

The European psychiatric tradition used to speak of conversions when speaking of soma-psyche dissociation, for example non-epileptic seizures or anaesthesia. For us, these phenomena, as well as purely intra-psyche ones, also gave an answer to a pain, related in this case to the body, experienced before as safe and which was shown not to be so. These oppose the somatic reliving of the traumatic event as confirmed by daily physiological observations (Leroi, 2000).

Table 2 illustrates the close association of psychic dissociation, conversions and phobias to the experiencing of trauma. As for phobias, let us mention agoraphobia as the most specific, and social phobia as the least. Indeed, social phobia may result as much from the complication of a temperament, in other respects not very able to avoid adverse situations, as a traumatic consequence. Although the *reliving traumatic syndromes* had disappeared, we sometimes noticed that the only disorder which persisted was a psychogenetic amnesia or a panic disorder with agoraphobia. This clinical remark tallied with the current theorizations on panic attacks. Indeed, in order to understand the onset of the first attacks, the specialists needed to locate an environmental wound among the factors involved (Gorman, 2000).

The *dissociation and phobia traumatic syndromes* were the first traumatic syndromes occurring after the traumatic event. In some patients, they become recurrent. In that case, the clinical situation developed as if the experience of this defence during the traumatic event induced more frequent subsequent recourse to the same mechanisms in adverse events–but not necessarily traumatic–whereas other people would have reacted in a different way. Their persistency was shown to be a relevant alert sign for the dreaded long lasting *reliving traumatic syndromes* (Darves-Bornoz, 1996).

The clinics of the *reliving traumatic syndromes* consisted in reminiscences, nightmares or what we called trigger-associations which launched the reliving of the pain suffered in the traumatic experience or even the illusion of the traumatic experience itself (for example, a white car for someone who was assaulted in a white car). They formed the most specific and

TABLE 2. Definite psychiatric disorders (*) and their link to trauma experience *[in a six month outcome study of rape survivors]*

	Trauma experience:		
	if lasting at six months %	**if vanished** at six months %	**frequencies comparison** in lasting/vanishing groups p
Dissociation	84	38	< 0.0001
Conversions	75	42	< 0.01
Agoraphobia	70	20	< 0.0001
Specific phobia	56	25	< 0.02
Social phobia	49	29	ns
Panic disorder	18	0	< 0.03
Depressions	53	8	< 0.001
Gender identity disorder	41	4	< 0.001
Alcohol abuse	29	8	< 0.05
Drugs use	14	8	ns
Obsessional compulsive	12	0	ns
Generalized anxiety	7	17	ns
Psychotic or Bipolar	7	13	ns
Anorexia or Bulimia	20	8	ns

(*) Only the disorders occurring early and persistent in one form or another during the six months were taken into account in the table.

Reference. Darves-Bornoz, J.-M.(1997). Rape-related psychotraumatic syndromes. *European Journal Obstetrics & Gynaecology and Reproductive Biology, 71*, 59-65.

sensitive set of traumatic symptoms. Even though the American classification of mental disorders does not adopt such a cluster of symptoms as a sufficient criterion for diagnosing such *PTSD*, in practice when subjects suffered from painful traumatic reliving, these generally fulfilled the other clusters of symptoms required for this category, i.e., traumatic numbing or withdrawal, and traumatic hyper-arousal. In addition, the strength of the reliving was on a par with the strength of *PTSD* as a whole. The painful reliving was massive in physically or sexually assaulted subjects (Darves-Bornoz, Berger, Degiovanni, Lépine, Soutoul, Grateau, & Gaillard, 1994a). For the majority of rape survivors, the diagnosis was still present one year after the trauma (Darves-Bornoz, Pierre, Berger, Lansac, Degiovanni, & Gaillard, 1997) and is posed chronologically as one of the first therapeutic questions. Reliving occurred when the patient recalled an elementary sensory representation (for example, the image of the perpetrator's eyes), through reminiscences, nightmares, or trigger-associations. This proto-representation figured the whole trauma, and activated the emotion related to the traumatic experience. The traumatic reliving appeared to us then, as a disorder of the representation of the past.

In spite of its frequency in traumatized people–one in two–highlighting depression of the traumatized could lead to thinking that treating traumatized people is no more difficult than treating an isolated depression. It is not even of much use to qualify this as resistant depression. Let us mention, however, that the British professor of psychiatry Sir David Goldberg, after a whole life dedicated to the vulnerability factors in affective disorders, did not hesitate to present child abuse as the first etiological factor of depression (Goldberg, 1998).

In some cases or moments, the *narcissistic regression traumatic syndromes* came to light rather through psychic manifestations and, in others, rather through behavioural manifestations. At first, "the identity uncertainty" assumed the shape of a narcissistic depression (low self-esteem, shame, guiltiness, feelings of abandonment, emptiness or devitalisation) sometimes so severe that it could evoke melancholia if its traumatic aetiology had not been recognized. The identity disorder often became complicated afterwards, early on in some cases, especially in children and adolescents, by an impairing of the psychic development. Indeed, a peculiar "identity reconstruction" then appeared, including outbursts of paranoid omnipotence and acting. These features, well known in patients with a so-called borderline personality, were quite specific to the interpersonal character of trauma. They were infiltrated to such an extent by elements of dissociation, that the question arose as to whether the diagnoses of borderline personality and major dissociation states were redundant, as was suggested by another author (Sar, Yargic, & Tutkun, 1996). The impairing of relationships to other people and the world resulted from that interpersonal traumatic experience which promoted alienating identifications (in particular to the aggressor). In order to protect the psyche, the survivor paradoxically experiences masochism behaviours often described as "traumatophilia." The recurrence and severity of traumatic exposures increased the onsets of these *narcissistic regression traumatic syndromes*. In this manner, in Table 3, the narcissistic regression features were over-represented in incestuous rapes when compared to non-incestuous ones, especially in the fields of low self-esteem and feelings of abandonment, emptiness or devitalisation (Darves-Bornoz, 1998a,b). One must keep in mind that in the most severely traumatized, these syndromes were often the last ones to resist therapy long after any *reliving traumatic syndrome* had stopped.

TABLE 3. Link of narcissistic regression psychic and behavioral features (*) to event severity [in a six month outcome study of rape victims]

	Rapes	
	incestuous	non-incestuous
Low self-esteem	68%	37%
Recurrent fear of abandonment	64%	57%
Dissociative episodes	84%	60%
Affective disorder of the depressive type	49%	31%
Persistent feeling of emptiness	76%	56%
Idealization (versus devaluation) of one's nearest and dearest	28%	44%
Suicide attempts	33%	26%
Impulsive fugues	33%	21%
Rage leading to violence	54%	42%
At least five features out of the nine	58%	38%
Mean number of features	4.8	3.7

(*) Only the disorders occurring early and persistent under one form or another during the six months were taken into account in the table.

Reference. Darves-Bornoz, J.-M.(2000). Problématique féminine en psychiatrie. Paris : Masson, 270 pp.

They affected the subject's expectations and ideals for himself. As a consequence, we must not be surprised that they showed a more deleterious effect than the other types of traumatic syndromes on children and adolescents. In that way, the *narcissistic regression traumatic syndromes* could be seen as a failure of the representation of the future.

IS THERE A FRENCH SPECIFICITY IN CLINICS OR TREATMENTS?

As for the clinical expression of trauma in France, all the attempts to find major differences with other cultures or countries failed. For instance, many think that "Charcot's type of hysteria" disappeared in France a long time ago and remained present only in "Mediterranean countries." However, when working with a French department of neurology on supposed refractory epileptics recorded in video-EEG sessions,[4] we confirmed that some of them exhibited non-epileptic seizures, and that all of them had experienced severe trauma in their history. This finding showed once more that phenomena are discovered if they are looked for. Non-epileptic seizures exist in France as in the times of Charcot and as in other countries (Bowman & Coons, 2000). Our thesis lies in the idea that post-traumatic clinical manifestations do not fundamentally differ from country to country.

As for treatment, this is another story because, indeed, there is a French specificity for ways to treat traumatized people. In France, the mainstream psychotherapy still remains psychoanalysis. Actually, even though it seems strange to many colleagues elsewhere, some therapists in France even think that trauma could be a future for psychoanalysis. The example of American psychoanalysts such as Jean Goodwin could indeed show that such a statement does not arise from a new utopia.

Some psychoanalysts from the *Société Psychanalytique de Paris (SPP)*[5] in France became involved in the treatment of mass trauma survivors (Pérel Wilgowicz or Eva Weil); others approached the somatic expression of mental distress (with historical figures such as Joyce McDougall or Pierre Marty, and more recently Claude Smadja and Marilia Aisenstein). In my opinion, the main ability of psychoanalysis in these situations might lie in the actual reexperiencing of fragments of traumatic experiences in the sessions, but this time, in not alone and associative reexperiencing, instead of alone and dissociative reliving. As a matter of fact, the psychoanalytical therapies of borderline cases, well studied by the *SPP* members, differ radically from any spontaneous traumatic reliving. In my view, they allow the patient's psyche to internalise a new protective envelope which could be an image of his calming analyst. During an *SPP* seminar dedicated to that question in La Baule, France, in June 2003, Danielle Kaswin-Bonnefond nicely explored the personal effort to be made by the psychoanalyst with such patients around her report of a borderline case, and with Dolnald W. Winnicott as a permanent reference in her mind. Incidentally, Pierre Chauvel evoked in one of his case presentations the patient's expectation from the analyst, "of an ability to keep emotions as in a safe." Further, André Green, focusing on certain survivors whose development became too chaotic with so many traumatic exposures, stated that finally, one must consider them as if a "paranoia of destiny" preyed upon their lives. He would then incite the psychoanalyst to find new psychoanalytical therapies in these extreme cases.

When physicians do not believe in the usefulness of psychoanalysis, they then mainly centre their hopes on medication, mostly oriented, unfortunately, on unspecific diagnoses such as depression, or on the specific target of reliving. As a consequence, they leave aside all the other specific, but negative or regressive symptoms, such as numbing and narcissistic withdrawal. Such attitudes often disappoint the patients' expectations from a therapy: not only the vanishing of symptoms, albeit upsetting, but above all a restructuring of their internal world on new bases.

RESEARCH ON DISSOCIATIVE PHENOMENA AND TRAUMA

Pierre Janet noted that what was amazing in traumatic disorders lay in the coincidence of amnesia and hypermnesia. Many usual psychiatric symptoms seen in traumatic disorders, like psychogenetic memory disorders, can be referred to dissociation phenomena, and they are not infrequently identified as such in France, whether the traumatic cause is put forward or not. We are not surprised then, to observe interest in France on this topic whatever the point of view taken: today generally the point of view is psychoanalytical (studies on repression or splitting) even though the underlying phenomenon does not differ from Janet's (referred as to passive dissociation). Finally, one cannot say that French psychiatrists ignore the field of dissociation, rather they must be seen as processing them usually in a meta-psychological way.

There has been research on trauma and dissociation in France, but most, it is true, was not conducted in such a way as to allow publication in English language journals, because the interest for the current techniques of clinical epidemiologists, here, remained low. Nevertheless, certain French academicians do not ignore foreign scholars' research who have long since been attracted to this way of studying, whether from countries very close to France such as B.P.R. Gersons, O. van der Hart, S.O. Hoffmann, J.T.V.M. de Jong, J. Modestin, E. Nijenhuis, or U. Schnyder, or from further afield such as J. Chu, P. Fink, M.P. Koss, F.W. Putnam, D. Spiegel, or E. Witztum. So, one can say that French research has been in semi-captivity, although some knew what was going on abroad. This does not mean that the French researchers' findings were of no value for the development of the field. In several areas, studies have been extremely thorough: violence on women, mass trauma, disasters and terrorist attacks, psycho-somatic reactions, psychoanalytic meta-psychology, and some aspects of epidemiological clinics.

In the sphere of psychoanalysis, some refined the studies on meta-psychological concepts related to trauma even though this relation did not mobilize their interest much. For example, Claude Le Guen, studying repression, did not hesitate to state that research on this concept was over. The usefulness of meta-psychology in the understanding of eating disorders as a psychosomatic disorder continued to be explored by Philippe Jeammet. To my mind, indeed, Spitz's category of anaclitic depression, which is rarely lacking in the early history of a patient with anorexia, is in fact a trauma category.

As far as violence on women is concerned, one must not forget Eva Thomas's text entitled *Le viol du silence*. One could say this book is not research properly speaking, but everybody must be aware that her contribution went beyond the status of a narrative. Eva Thomas founded a survivors' association named *SOS Inceste*. Each year, they all meet for a *Research Meeting* and invite a guest to talk with them. I was that guest once, and I would like to say that I will never forget it. It was moving to see these people converging in Grenoble, France, from all over Europe, and to see how friendly they were toward those who tried to help. With emotion but accuracy, probably because they were the most lucid among these survivors, they all taught me a great deal, through our exchange of ideas: I proposed a theory which they echoed in their survivor feelings; I then suggested ways to get out of the trap, and they responded with brotherhood as a philosophy of existence. This is not the usual standardized research, but as theorization and communication of knowledge, it is definitely human research.

In this field, Catherine Bonnet's studies on sexually abused babies should also be mentioned. Gérard Lopez also stands as one of the first French male psychiatrists who expressed ideas on rape issuing from his consultations in the Hôtel-Dieu forensic centre in Paris. As far as perpetrators are concerned, great psychopathological work by Claude Balier and his pupils (Balier, 1996; Balier, Ciavaldini, & Girard-Khayat, 1996) must be noted, so much so that a French consensus conference was held in 2001 on the initiative of Jacques Fortineau, the president of the *Fédération Française de Psychiatrie*.

Mass trauma studies have mobilized much professional energy all over the world since World War II, and have spread to all kinds of collective violent conflicts (Albeck, 1981). Indeed, a theory has to be made on practitioners who respond to the exacerbation of community conflicts and violent ways of practicing politics by non-violent practices, and then work through mass trauma. This tendency was noticeable in the way the new South Africa processed the crimes of the past, or the way the mothers of the disappeared in Argentina quietly persisted. Now, the recommendation by the Iraqi branch of the NGO *Human*

Rights Watch to set up a *Truth Commission* for second rank citizens responsible for the past genocide crimes in Iraq is also planting some seeds of that nature. In France, Haydée Faimberg and Pérel Wilgowicz contributed greatly to the understanding of the alienating processes of intergenerational identifications in survivors and their offspring. In the nineteenth century, it was stated that Germany influenced Europe through the genius of its theoreticians, and France through the talent of its practitioners. Maybe this opinion still applies. Indeed, on the side of treatment, one can say that the French movement leading to the creation of the first *medical NGO* many decades ago now also represents a practical French answer to mass trauma in the sphere of therapeutics (Darves-Bornoz, Berger, Degiovanni, Soutoul, & Gaillard, 1994b).

As far as trauma through disasters or terrorist attacks is concerned, there has been a recent interest in two directions: early treatment and some aspects of epidemiological clinics. A network for early treatment of such traumas started to be established by the French government a decade ago. It consisted of one hundred psychiatrists, one responsible for each French administrative area, assisted by volunteers (nurses, psychologists, psychiatrists) and prepared for early interventions. Some of them had other experiences in the trauma field: for instance, Darves-Bornoz (assaults), Katz (firemen), and Vila (children). Until now, the assessment of its efficiency could not be made. Epidemiological studies of terrorists attacks have also been the subject of interesting publications (Jehel, Paterniti, Brunet, Duchet, & Guelfi, 2003).

In the sphere of psycho-somatic reactions, the French theoretical effort was important. The salient authors came from the *SPP*. Though they all refer somatization to some kind of trauma, their interest in the field, as mentioned above, lies in the will to understand the functioning of any subject rather than patients with definite disorders from a psychiatric point of view. Two different approaches to conceptualising these phenomena currently prevail. The first one, including Marty's followers (Smadja and Aisenstein), is centred on the category of "pensée opératoire," which is close to Sifneos's alexithymia, resulting from the loss of ability to associate and fantasize. The second one, represented by Joyce McDougall, who accomplished a part of her career in Paris and a part in New York, considers the psychosomatic phenomenon rather as a continuum of phenomena including slight daily manifestations, the so-called "hysterical conversions," up to severe illnesses with the reputation of comprising a strong psychosomatic component. She considers somatization as an archaic body language and a way to survive psychically for those who cannot find usual words for their trauma.

To my mind, any effort for theorizing trauma is useless if not founded on valid observations. I have therefore found it essential to lead clinical investigations using epidemiological techniques that are as modern as possible. Since the end of the eighties (Choquet, Darves-Bornoz, Ledoux, Manfredi, & Hassler, 1997; Darves-Bornoz, 1990; Darves-Bornoz, & Lempérière 1992; Lépine & Darves-Bornoz, 1993), we have tried to do so with Marie Choquet, Jean-Pierre Lépine, Thérèse Lempérière and Andrée Degiovanni, and now we are planning to combine other approaches with Hervé Le Louet. Our outcome studies of assault victims allowed us to discriminate early predictive factors of long lasting trauma. For instance, observing early and persistently a set of symptoms composed of low self esteem, permanent feelings of emptiness and fears unrelated to trauma such as agoraphobia, was found to be a strong predicting model of the persistency of *PTSD* one year later (Darves-Bornoz, 1998b). One could say this in another way: the more the narcissism or identity regress after the event, the longer the trauma will last. Moreover, we could also state that severity of trauma is on a par with the intensity of such psychic movements, including dissociation manifestations (Darves-Bornoz, 1996; Darves-Bornoz, Berger, Degiovanni, Gaillard, & Lépine, 1998b). For us, these findings fuel our opinion that narcissism or identity regressions subsequent to overwhelming incidents signal the most preoccupying change in traumatized populations.

CONCLUSIONS

In summary, in France, the subjects whose trauma refers to an interpersonal relationship with a third party in a sadistic position, suffer the most. They suffer without any doubt from traumatic reliving, but they also resort to intra-psyche or soma-psyche dissociations, and to phobic avoidances of the world in order to prevent the pain felt in their panics. At the same time, they transform, negatively or not, their identity and their narcissistic equilibrium.

A constituted trauma alters the usual activity of representing the past. In the *reliving traumatic syndromes*, the traumatic memory is reduced to a proto-representation–in our previous example, the sole image of the aggressor's eyes–and the pain felt in the whole overwhelming experience is attached entirely attached to this.

A constituted trauma alters the usual activity of representing the future. With the *narcissistic regression traumatic syndromes*, survivors wounded in their being aim at a neo-identity for the future implying new ways of thinking and behaving, for example in identifying with the aggressor, the lost object, or the damaged object.

The way in which the subject passes from the first register to the second is determined by the defences used during the overwhelming experience and combined what we called *dissociation and phobia traumatic syndromes*. Indeed, on one hand the phobic avoidance actualises the traumatic past again and again. Paradoxically, at the same time, the phobia carries its own projection into the future, the counter-phobic attitude of challenge. Thus, amnesia, and also conversion, through the fragmentation of the being, especially enable the past to be ignored. However, these dissociations also promote the emergence of neo-identities underpinned by new ideals and expectations for the future. With these jumps into the future, the survivor attempts to tune his being to the world as constituted after the trauma.

NOTES

1. In his *"Traité clinique et thérapeutique de l'hystérie."*
2. In a book entitled: *"Des chemins de fer et de leur influence sur la santé des mécaniciens et des chauffeurs."*
3. We will refer from here, as to PTSD, this psychotraumatic category within the current *American Psychiatric Association*'s classification of mental disorders.
4. During one week periods with a coupled electroencephalograph recording.
5. The French founding society of the *International Psychoanalytic Association*.

REFERENCES

Albeck, J.H. (1981). *Songs for the last survivor*. Boston: One-Generation-After.
Balier, C. (1996). *Psychanalyse des comportements sexuels violents*. Paris: Presses Universitaires de France.
Balier, C., Ciavaldini, A., & Girard-Khayat, M. (1996). *Rapport de Recherche sur les agresseurs sexuels*. Grenoble: [contrat financé par la Direction Générale de la Santé de France].
Blake, D.D., Weathers, F.W., Nagy, L.M., Kaloupek, D.G., Gusman, F.D., Charney, D.S., & Keane, T.M. (1995). The development of a Clinician-Administered PTSD scale. *Journal of Traumatic Stress, 8*, 75-90.
Bowman, E.S., & Coons, P.M. (2000). The differential diagnosis of epilepsy, pseudoseizures, dissociative identity disorder, and dissociative disorder not otherwise specified. *Bulletin of Menninger Clinic, 64*, 164-180.
Brauner, A. (1946). *Les répercussions psychiques de la guerre moderne sur l'enfance*. [Thèse de doctorat ès lettres]. Paris: Université de la Sorbonne.

Choquet, M., Darves-Bornoz, J.-M., Ledoux, S., Manfredi, R., & Hassler, C. (1997). Self-reported health and behavioral problems among adolescent victims of rape in France: Results of a cross-sectional survey. *Child Abuse & Neglect, 21*, 823-832.

Darves-Bornoz, J.-M., Lépine, J.-P., Choquet, M., Berger, C., Degiovanni, A., & Gaillard, P. (1998). Predictive factors of chronic post-traumatic stress disorder in rape victims. *European Psychiatry, 13*, 281-287.

Darves-Bornoz, J.-M. (1998a). *Dans le champ du traumatisme: paradigme et point singulier des violences sexuelles.* [Habilitation à Diriger des Recherches]. Tours: Université François-Rabelais.

Darves-Bornoz, J.-M. (1998b). *Specificities of incestuous rape in a French follow-up study.* Oral presentation to the 14th annual meeting of the *International Society for Traumatic Stress Studies.* Washington DC: 19-23 November 1998.

Darves-Bornoz, J.-M., Pierre, F., Berger, C., Lansac, J., Degiovanni, A., & Gaillard, P. (1997). *Mental disorders in a French follow-up study of rape victims.* Oral presentation, *New Research Program (oral/slide session)* of the 150th annual meeting of the *American Psychiatric Association.* San Diego: 17-22 May 1997.

Darves-Bornoz, J.-M. (1996). *Syndromes traumatiques du viol et de l'inceste.* [Thèse de doctorat de Sciences de la vie (Université Pierre et Marie Curie, Paris 6)]. Edition et présentation orale invitée comme *Rapport de Psychiatrie* de la 94ème session du *Congrès de Psychiatrie et de Neurologie de Langue Française.* Paris: Masson, 264 pp.

Darves-Bornoz, J.-M. (1995). *The trauma of rape in male victims.* Oral presentation to the 4th conference of the *European Society for Traumatic Stress Studies (ESTSS).* Paris: 7-12 May 1995.

Darves-Bornoz, J.-M., Degiovanni, A., Berger, C., Soutoul, J.-H. (1995). *Incestuous rape in adolescence.* Oral presentation at the 4th meeting of the *International Society for Adolescent Psychiatry (ISAP).* Athens: 5-8 July 1995.

Darves-Bornoz, J.-M., Berger, C., Degiovanni, A., Lépine, J.-P., Soutoul, J.-H., Grateau, M.-T., & Gaillard, P. (1994). *Les états de stress post-traumatiques chez les victimes de viol.* Oral presentation at the 7th meeting of the *Association of European Psychiatrists (AEP).* Copenhague: 18-22 September 1994.

Darves-Bornoz, J.-M., Berger, C., Degiovanni, A., Soutoul, J.-H., Gaillard, P. (1994). *Traiter les traumatismes psychiques: une urgence psychiatrique.* Présentation orale invitée au Colloque *La santé et les droits de l'homme.* Prague: May 1994.

Darves-Bornoz, J.-M., Berger, C., Degiovanni, A., Soutoul, J.-H., & Gaillard, P. (1994). Long term outcome of victims of rape in childhood or adolescence. Oral presentation, 13th international meeting of the *International Association for Child and Adolescent Psychiatry and Allied Professions (IACAPAP).* San Francisco: 24-28 July 1994.

Darves-Bornoz, J.-M., & Lempérière, T. (1992). *Sexual abuse in childhood and adolescence of schizophrenics-to-be.* Oral presentation at the 3rd meeting of the *International Society for Adolescent Psychiatry.* Chicago: 12-15 July 1992.

Darves-Bornoz, J.-M. (1990). *Recherche sur la sexualité des femmes schizophrènes.* [Mémoire de DEA]. Paris: Université Pierre et Marie Curie.

El Hage, W., Darves-Bornoz, J.-M., Allilaire, J.-F., & Gaillard, P. (2002) Posttraumatic somatoform dissociation in French Psychiatric outpatients. *Journal of Trauma and Dissociation, 3*, 59-74.

Gold, S.N. (2000). *Not trauma alone: Therapy for child abuse survivors in family and social context.* New York: Brunner-Routledge.

Goldberg, D. (1998). *The course of common mental disorders: Vulnerability, destabilization and restitution. Lecture, APA's Adolf Meyer Award.* 151st Annual Meeting of the *American Psychiatric Association.* Toronto: 30 May-4 June 1998.

Gorman, J.M. (2000). Neuroanatomical hypothesis of panic disorder, revised. *American Journal of Psychiatry, 157*, 493-505.

Jehel, L., Paterniti, S., Brunet, A., Duchet, C., & Guelfi, J.-D. (2003). Prediction of the occurrence and intensity of posttraumatic stress disorder in victims 32 months after bomb attack. *European Psychiatry, 18*, 172-6

Lépine, J.-P., & Darves-Bornoz, J.-M. (1993). Le traitement des états de stress posttraumatiques. *Acta Psychiatrica Belgica, 93*, 121-135.

Leroi, A.-M. (2000). De l'aspect organique à l'aspect psychologique des douleurs pelviennes. In: J.-M. Darves-Bornoz (Ed.), *Problématique féminine en psychiatrie* (pp. 46-51). Paris: Masson.

Sar, V., Yargic L.I., & Tutkun, H. (1996). Structured interview data on 35 cases of dissociative identity disorder in Turkey. *American Journal of Psychiatry, 153*, 1329-33.

The Concepts of Trauma and Dissociation in the German Language Area

Helga Matthess
Hanne Hummel
Arne Hofmann
Raimund Dörr

SUMMARY. In this article the development of research, training and therapy in the field of dissociation and psycho-traumatology in the German language area is summarized. In particular, the report describes the

Helga Matthess, MD, is Psychoanalyst and Specialist for Psychosomatic Medicine, Psychotraumatology Institute Europe, Board Member, Belgian Institute of Psychotraumatology and EMDR, and is affiliated with the Humanitarian Assistance Program (HAP-Europe and HHP), Germany.

Hanne Hummel, Dipl. Päd, is Psychotherapist, Psychotherapeutisches Institut im Park, Schaffhausen, Switzerland.

Arne Hofmann, MD, is Specialist for Psychosomatic and Internal Medicine, Director of the EMDR-Institute in Germany (University of Cologne), German national guideline commission on the treatment of PTSD, German guideline commission for the treatment of dissociative disorders, and Board Member, German speaking branch of the ISTSS (DeGPT).

Raimund Dörr, Dipl. Päd, is Psychotherapist, Psychotherapeutisches Institut im Park, Schaffhausen, Switzerland.

Address correspondence to: Helga Matthess, MD, Psychotraumatology Institute Europe, Grossenbaumer Allee 35 a D-47269 Duisburg, Germany (E-mail: Helga. Matthess@P-I-E.info).

[Haworth co-indexing entry note]: "The Concepts of Trauma and Dissociation in the German Language Area." Matthess et al. Co-published simultaneously in *Journal of Trauma Practice* (The Haworth Maltreatment & Trauma Press, an imprint of The Haworth Press, Inc.) Vol. 4, No. 1/2, 2005, pp. 113-132; and: *Trauma and Dissociation in a Cross-Cultural Perspective: Not Just a North American Phenomenon* (ed: George F. Rhoades, Jr., and Vedat Sar) The Haworth Maltreatment & Trauma Press, an imprint of The Haworth Press, Inc., 2005, pp. 113-132. Single or multiple copies of this article are available for a fee from The Haworth Document Delivery Service [1-800-HAWORTH, 9:00 a.m. - 5:00 p.m. (EST). E-mail address: docdelivery@haworthpress.com].

Available online at http://jtp.haworthpress.com
doi:10.1300/J189v04n01_08

possibilities of therapy and training in Germany and Switzerland. As an example, the curricula of the first two training courses are presented which have been a model for the development of general guidelines by the German language Society for Psycho-Traumatology. This training concept also is the base for the projects of training courses in Europe (i.e., Slovakia) and in Asia (i.e., China) by the German and the European Humanitarian Assistance Program (HHP & HAP-Europe). *[Article cop-*
ies available for a fee from The Haworth Document Delivery Service:
1-800-HAWORTH. E-mail address: <docdelivery@haworthpress.com> Web-
site: <http://www.HaworthPress.com> © 2005 by The Haworth Press, Inc. All
rights reserved.]

KEYWORDS. Dissociation, Germany, psycho-traumatology

Many well known researchers, psychiatrists and psychotherapists in the German language area have touched already very early upon the concept/concepts of trauma and dissociation. In addition to the case-report on the treatment of Anna O., the well known dissociative client of Josef Breuer, he published together with Sigmund Freud in "Studies on hysteria" (Freud & Breuer, 1895/1952), there are publications by military psychiatrists on so-called "war tremblers": soldiers who developed a dissociative movement disorder originating from traumatization in the trenches on the frontlines during World War I. At that time Hermann Oppenheim attributed this to an organic causing of the fight-reaction, but increasing knowledge about the psychogenesis led to a depreciating and unyielding attitude by the government and later by the National Socialist government and in the Second World War. At the beginning of the century there was already knowledge about dissociation and about dissociative identity disorders in the German-speaking psychiatry. Kraepelin spoke in 1915 about "strange mental disorders with different states of awareness that are changing several times." He discussed already different independent personalities in one client with separate memories. Also, the well-known psychiatrist Bleuler wrote in his textbook about alternating personalities with double awareness and amnesia for themselves. But this knowledge got lost in the following time, during the entire Nazi time all psychological symptoms were equated with lack of willpower or psychopathy, i.e., defects in character formation (Zimmermann, Hahne, Biesold, & Lanczik, 2004).

This attitude was weakened, but implicitly partly remained in Germany also after the end of World War II. Psychological traumatization was not perceived, and seldom named. If the psychological symptoms of Holocaust survivors persisted for more than a few months after their release from the concentration camps, it was hypothesized they must have had some other psychological problems in the time before, in addition to the traumatization by the Nazi regime.

Germany, as it seems now, has been dissociated for many decades from the knowledge about psychological traumatization, maybe also to protect itself from having to acknowledge that an entire nation is suffering from the consequences of both World Wars. It needed a long time to recover from this attitude and only in the late fifties different research results were accepted talking about "changing in the personality related to stressful situations." Especially the group around Venzlaff needs to be mentioned talking about the way the assessment changed over time in Germany (Venzlaff, 1958; Venzlaff, Dulz, & Sachsse, 2004).

Infrequently there were therapists who engaged in the subject of trauma; surely one of the pioneers was Hildegund Heinl, a Gestalt orthopedagogue with a humanistic training background, who engaged in somatoform dissociative symptoms from an early stage and found connections with war experiences.

But it was only in the beginning of the 80s that a major change in therapists' attitudes took place in the German language area, originating from new knowledge about the consequences of sexual violence (Sachsse, Venzlaff, & Dulz, 1997).

Initially, there were publications by psychoanalysts, e.g., Mathias Hirsch in Germany, or Ursula Wirtz in Switzerland, who occupied themselves with the changes in therapist attitude, setting, and therapy focus of incest victims.

In the time between 1990 and 1995 there were many different impulses: almost at the same time various organizations were founded by and for victims and for professionals, like Wildwasser, an organization of victims of sexual violence that offered social-educational and later also therapeutic support.

Other organizations concerning themselves with the interests of sexually traumatized children often were founded after the sexual molestation of children of a community had become known, e.g., Zartbitter in Cologne or Hobbit in Nordhorn.

At the same time, during the first and only European ISSD Conference, the German-speaking section of the ISSD was founded, and, at that same time, another small German association organizing an annual

ISSD Conference in Germany for 10 years. The latter association restricts itself to founding members, accepting no new members. The President has always been Michaela Huber, who published about dissociative disorders from an early stage and who, in the mid-nineties, wrote the first book entitled "Multiple personalities." This would remain the only book in the German language area for some years. Shortly thereafter, Michaela Huber offered a special 8 weekend course on dissociative disorders.

In addition the association "Vielfalt" (German translation of multiplicity) was founded in Bremen, that dedicated itself primarily to the task of translating into German all American literature not yet translated in the first half of the nineties.

Almost at the same time there were two more initiatives in the trauma field: the first one coming from the feminist domain, with the exemplary names of Ingrid Olbricht and Luise Reddeman. Luise Reddeman, drawing from her far-reaching experience as head of a clinic, soon started a 4-part training course on the treatment of trauma disorders, including stabilization techniques using imagination, and hypnotherapeutic techniques for trauma confrontation.

The second initiative was the training course for the EMDR-method which was established by Arne Hofmann and the German EMDR-Institute. In 1994 Arne Hofmann established as first therapist in Germany a special trauma unit in a clinic. His unit had the first explicit treatment program for patients with dissociative disorders in Germany.

Unlike in the United States, there were no different organizations built for traumatherapy in general (like ISTSS), and for the specific study of dissociative disorders (like ISSD)

Because the German association organizing the ISSD Conferences under the leadership of Michaela Huber had decided to include only the 7 founding members required by German law and advised all other interested persons to join the ISSD International in America, the German ISSD conferences could not be organized without the efforts of Tina Overkamp who is leading the German office and also publishes a newsletter that she sends via e-mail that includes summaries of important papers, announcements of conferences and sometimes a review about the ISSD-world and the DISSOC-discussion group.

Most trauma oriented colleagues organized themselves either in the largest trauma-association in Germany, the EMDRIA (with more than 700 members), or in the German speaking Society for Psychotraumatology, DeGPT (with about 250 members), which is closely connected to the ISTSS.

Also the division between organizations from a psychodynamic and behavior therapy background does not exist like in the American situation, where you find a fundamental cleavage between ISTSS and ISSD.

On the contrary: in Germany more psychodynamically trained psychotherapists than behavior therapists are members of the DeGPT.

This has to do with the fact that training in the trauma field originally came from psychodynamically oriented psychotherapists, and so far no "pure doctrine," to be distinguished from CBT on one side and analysis on the other side, has been developed.

Rather, a further integration took place with the general consensus that for the treatment of complex traumatized clients, more is needed than "pure" therapeutic behavior.

There is more than one reason for this: the "pure" behavioral researchers in Germany only discovered psychotraumatology at a late date, so the research on type I trauma, the most important research domain of CBT, was definitely less separated from the treatment of complex trauma than in other parts of the world. On the contrary: the search for the proper treatment of complex traumatized clients was and is the main reason why clinical working therapists in the German speaking area occupy themselves with psychotraumatology.

Besides the hypnotherapeutic and imaginative interventions, EMDR is taught in Germany as the main treatment method for trauma confrontation.

The attention of leading researchers in Germany, like Ulrich Sachsse, who gave courses on the treatment of complex traumatized clients together with Luise Reddemann, was drawn to EMDR from the beginning and they brought the method into psychodynamically-oriented therapy forms.

Arne Hofmann, as the leader of the German EMDR Institute, the Institute that offers by far the most EMDR trainings, puts a high value on integrating this method in both forms of therapy.

In addition to this, the leading psychodynamically-trained traumatherapists could accept without problems that the therapeutic procedures of the other schools were important.

So many times it is difficult to recognize, even for insiders in the German speaking area, what was the original training background of colleagues, because most of them are trained in more than one therapeutic approach and integrate much of what they learned in their treatments.

Moreover, some universities are offering research projects in the field of psychotraumatology: at the Medical University of Hannover, Ursula Gast is researching in the field of dissociation and psychotraumatology; furthermore, Friedhelm Lamprecht, together with Martin Sack and Wolfgang Lempa, are researching in teamwork in the field of complex-trauma as well as in the field of EMDR. At the University of Cologne the institute of Gottfried Fischer is working out a psycho-dynamic method for trauma-therapy, at the University of Mainz a team about Sven-Olaf Hoffmann and Ulrich Egle has built up a focal point in dissociative disorders, and Günther Seidler has built up a section of psychotraumatology in Heidelberg.

Even more colleagues from Germany, Austria and Switzerland could be mentioned. Just during the last three years, many efforts have started at many more universities and hospitals to establish focal points of psychotraumatology. Many of those persons concerned are organized in DeGPT, which organizes a congress once a year. Some of them also visit the congress of ISSD in Germany.

Up to the nineties there was no real tradition in therapy of traumatic disorders in Germany, so many ideas, impulses and enrichments came from other countries. Many American colleagues have organized semi-nars and courses in Germany, such as Richard Kluft, Cathrine Fine from ISSD, Bessel van der Kolk, and from the field of hypnotherapy John and Helen Watkins, Claire Frederics, Maggie Phillips, Phyllis Klaus, Carol Forgash, and even more.

Many of the last-mentioned have not been invited by the German ISSD, but they came to hypno-congresses like the Munich World Con-gress of Hypnotherapy and the first Ego-state World Congress in Bad Orb.

Of course there also was support by other countries. Vedat Sar from Turkey twice presented the main report at the ISSD-conference and also the Dutch colleagues like Suzette Boon and Ellert Nijenhuis made im-portant speeches at the yearly conferences of ISSD Germany. Felix Olthuis gave support in establishing one of the earliest in-patient trauma units in Bielefeld.

In the German language area and especially in Germany–different from America–the impulses in the field of trauma did not so much come from the treatment of the veterans who often are complexly trauma-tized, but have had traumatic experiences as adults only. Because of the different systems of insurance, more severely traumatized patients get treatment in the German language area, especially those who are caught up in the social net and who are legitimated by the national insurances to get psychotherapy. Unlike the Americans, they get significantly more therapeutic sessions, especially women who experienced sexual vio-lence during their childhood. Furthermore, these persons concerned have the possibility of getting national support by psychotherapeutic treatment, if they can prove physical and sexual violence during their childhood (state law for the financial compensation of victims of violence).

POSSIBILITIES OF TRAINING IN THE GERMAN LANGUAGE AREA

As mentioned above, in quite different fields initiatives of therapy and training in dissociative and complex traumatic disorders have developed since the middle of the nineties. There was no genuine separation of the different therapeutic schools. The training concentrated on physicians, psychologists and therapists of children and young persons.

The first seminars in the field of dissociation have been organized by Michaela Huber, who especially presented hypnotherapeutic techniques. She has been influenced by the developements of ISSD international. Further offers of training since the middle of the nineties came from Luise Reddemann who together with Ulrich Sachsse organized the first seminars as an analyst. The focal points were the imaginative and psychodynamic bases. Lutz Besser also was a trainer who soon after offered seminars in other German language areas like Switzerland and Austria.

Since 2002 there also is the possibility to participate in international ISSD-training offered by Helga Matthes.

An agreement developed in DeGPT to set up general guidelines for the treatment of traumatized people. Here, the integrative attitude came to everybody's aid just not to suggest a method of treatment for complexly traumatized patients, but to develop a curriculum to enable the therapists to treat differently traumatized patients. The acutely traumatized people belong to this group as well as the people traumatized during childhood, well-known for a long time by the health system for needing treatment. In the German language area there was no separation concerning the special needs of dissociative patients.

Before the detailed report about the curricula, here now is a short view of the special situation in Switzerland.

TRAUMA AND DISSOCIATION IN SWITZERLAND

In Switzerland, people also have experienced the increasing knowledge in this field: from the beginning of the scandal about the fact of sexual exploitation of women and children up to a range realized as traumatic. Trauma-specific methods had developed as well as a further theoretic progress in this field, so that this concept of dissociation gets more and more important. It seems that knowledge and possibility of training in the field of trauma and dissociation get to Switzerland with delay. In Europe most of the knowledge comes from the English language area which is supposed to bring a lot of news. But in our field of dissocation, the colleagues from the Netherlands and those who first were engaged in this subject surely belong to the avant garde. The new knowledge comes to Germany with delay, and from there with a further delay to Switzerland. Knowledge covers highly interesting ways, a fact that surely has to do with languages, but also with network.

But this delay in further knowledge is increasingly belonging to the past, because close connections between colleagues from Germany and the Netherlands have been established.

THE BEGINNING:
FIRST SEMINARS FOR PSYCHOTRAUMATOLOGY
AND TRAUMA-CENTRED PSYCHOTHERAPY

At the end of the eighties, trauma mainly was realized as a consequence of exploitation and violence towards women. When in 1987 the first radio- and TV-interviews concerning sexual violence and seminars for experts of various professional fields were given under the topic "Advisory and psychotherapeutic coping with severely traumatized people," there were very various reactions. On the one hand, many people depreciated and refused these informations and seminars. They accused outriders like Hanne Hummel of fouling her own nest, because they were convinced that in Switzerland there was no violence against women and children. People saying so must have a bad phantasy or just be promoting feministic propaganda.

That was one direction. On the other hand, there was great interest by various professional groups to deal with the topic thouroughly. During this time, in Switzerland there were established the first refuges for battered women and the first emergency phone numbers for raped women and girls. The topic of sexual violence was detabooed by and by.

Many colleages felt insecure, because they realized that there was a need of even more knowledge about the special psychodynamics in traumatic disorders and practical authority for advisory and psychotherapeutic coping with traumatized people, because their previous knowledge was limited.

At that time, seminars were addressed to psychotherapists, physicians, welfare workers, teachers, and educators as well as to lawyers and to the police. Besides that there was supervision for teams working in the field of support of victims.

The focal point of the seminars for psychotherapists at that time was a thourough introduction in psychotraumatology. Then, this field was in its infancy compared to the knowedge of today, the imparting of techniques of stabilization and the practice of resources as well as the screening technique for digestion of traumas which already were established.

Then for the first time, many (sexually) traumatized people could find somebody who believed the stories of their lives and who was willing to get involved in a treatment of their various detractions and disorders determined by traumas.

The names of women like Hanne Hummel were closely connected to the subject by numerous radio interviews and public relations for the special offer of the information centre. The more psychotherapists faced the fact that there was and is massive violence and even organized violence against children like prostitution of children and ritual violence in obscure circles, the more they were found by the persons concerned.

So, since the end of the eighties, they could experience even more the treatment of people with dissociative disorders like DID or DDNOS and could rapidly pass them on.

Noticeable were the irritation and insecurity, but also the fascination caused by parts of the workshops and reports about working with people with dissociative disorders. Some patients offered pictures for seminars drawn about the scenes of violence from the field of commercial violence against children and women. For a number of participants, these pictures were the first contact with these problems.

On the one hand, this confrontation caused insecurity and fears in the lecturer herself, connected with a loss of the illusion that such things did not exist in Switzerland and the idea that we are all living in a world where the cruelest violence is possible and does really exist.

On the other hand, many colleagues were fascinated by the idea to be able to even offer competent therapeutic help in severe disorders like these.

At that time, there was not much literature in the German language area. The well-known book "Sybil" by Flora Rheta Schreiber (1976) was one of the first books on this subject in the middle of the eighties.

Finally, in the middle of the nineties, specialist books were published on the subject, such as the specialist book "Multiple personalities" by Michaela Huber, also books by F. Putnam and R. Kluft et al., but also increasingly more reports from experience. These reports surely contributed to bringing this subject to the public.

CURRICULUM FOR PSYCHOTRAUMATOLOGY AND TRAUMA-CENTRED PSYCHOTHERAPY

In 1994 Hanne Hummel and Raimund Dörr founded the "Institute of Psychotherapy in the Park" in Schaffhausen, an institute offering psychotherapeutic treatment to people with traumatic disorders, that is to say with dissociative disorders as well. There the field of seminars for experienced psychotherapists also rated high.

In the course of time, the persons busy in seminars developed a basic agreement about knowledge and authorities which should be known to psychotherapists in their work with traumatized people. Furthermore, there was an increasing demand by patients for qualified psychotherapists with improved education on psychotherapy for traumatized people, Thus, the institute worked out an educative curriculum on trauma-centred psychotherapy, in cooperation with Lutz-Ulrich Besser, also an experienced colleague in this field from Germany. This curriculum is based on advanced training, i.e., it addresses psychotherapists having completed or at least partly completed their training.

Since the end of the nineties, this institute also organizes the training in the field of EMDR, which is to become part of the trauma education, in Switzerland. Since 2002, a modular curriculum has been established in Switzerland allowing qualified seminars in trauma-centred psychotherapy. In content, the meetings of this curriculum theoretically and practically are equivalent to the standards set by Arne Hofmann, Luise Reddemann, Michaela Huber and others, guided by the standards of the German Association of Psychotraumatology DeGPT.

At the same time, Helga Matthess developed a similar curriculum at the psychoanalytic institute in Sinzig, Germany.

One year later, in Berlin and Vienna similar curricula were offered in accordance with Helga Matthess, Hanne Hummel, Raimund Dörr and Lutz Besser as a forerunner of the later cooperatively developed training-program of DeGPT.

The participants of all recognized curricula need to meet the requirements of a completed training in psychotherapy on the master level as well as a psychotherapy licence.

The Swiss curriculum is to be presented as an example now. It contains the following subjects: general and special psychotraumatology, theory and practice of trauma-centred psychotherapy, installation of resources and methods of stabilization, methods of working on traumas and special aspects of therapy for traumatized people as well as supervision and self-experience. It is important to mention that trauma-training needs at least 2 trauma-confronting methods. These may either be hypnotherapeutic-imaginative methods, the EMDR- method which is mostly requested, or as a third method those from CBT. Every seminar listed in the curriculum may separately be attended. Every seminar has one subject. This is important, because we experienced that some colleagues already attended a single or several seminars concerning the subject psychotraumatology or trauma-centred psychotherapy in foreign countries. There is no obligation to attend the whole curriculum or complete it within a certain space of time.

The whole curriculum consists of ten weekend-seminars (see Box 1) which are offered within two years. If requested, there is the possibility of a final exam.

The weekend-seminars:

1. Introduction into psychotraumatology and therapy of psychotrauma
2. Methods of stabilization and mobilisation of resources 1
3. Methods of stabilization and mobilisation of resources 2
4. Installation of resources and trauma-exposition by the screening-method 1
5. Trauma-exposition and trauma-synthesis by the screening-method 2
6. Diagnostics and introduction into the treatment of dissociative disorders
7. EMDR introductary seminar (EMDR Level I)
8. EMDR advanced seminar (EMDR Level II)
9. Treatment of acute traumatizations
10. Seminar for special aspects and/or groups of patients

Seminar 10 provides the following choice of special subjects: (a) Psychotherapy of trauma in children. (b) Systemic aspects in therapy of psychotrauma. (c) Treatment of severe dissociative disorders. (d) Treatment of fear and phobias. (e) Trauma and processes of mourning.

The seminars may be attended separately; they are based one on the other–from theoretical aspects to practical aspects, from easy aspects to difficult aspects, from monotrauma to treatment of complex traumatizations and their consequences.

The practical part of the training needs the readiness and capability of attending exercises and self-experience on the part of clients, therapists, and observers. For a qualified exam the participant needs the certification of 40 lessons of supervision of casuistics and at least 5 sessions of 90 minutes of self-experience and coping with traumas. To pass the final exam, several casuistics have to be presented in the final colloquium.

The successful participants can be added to our list of qualified trauma-therapists on the Internet: *www.psychotraumtherapie.info*

For a complete outline of the curricular courses of the trauma-institute in Sinzig, Germany, which–besides the training in Switzerland–was the first curriculum of a nationally authorized institute in Germany, please contact the authors. Both curricula were important examples to establish guidelines for education in the German language area by DeGPT. The following is the final version:

Association for Psychotraumatology in the German language area (DeGPT)

Guidelines for an additional qualification "Special therapy of psychotrauma"

Preamble

In the last years, basic psychotrauma-knowledge has entered the educative curricula of psychological and medical therapists. Nevertheless, this knowledge is not sufficient for a qualified treatment of traumatized patients. That is why DeGPT recommends the following standards for qualification in special therapy of psychotrauma (DeGPT).

| A. | **Basic qualifications**
Qualification as a officially licensed medical or psychological psychotherapist | |

Qualification in Special Therapy of Psychotrauma (DeGPT)

	Curricular moduls/contents	**Std. (U)**
1.	**Theoretic basic knowledge** History of psychotraumatology, neurobiology, essentials of trauma-recollection, summary of trauma-specific methods of treatment, treatment with psychopharmaca, summary of the current research in psychotherapy in the field of trauma (metaanalyses etc.). Prevention of repeated victimization. Trauma-spezific diagnostics (at least 3 tests, interview and questionnaire), epidemiology and related disorders, spezific types of traumatizations (i.e., torture, sexual violence, problems of migration), relevant juristic basics, i.e., laws for support of victims (for Germany, i.e., OEG, GewSchG); possibilities of continuous seminars (guidelines, discussion of "Evidence-Based Medicine," specialized societies, professional journals),	20

2.	**Methods of stabilization and regulation of affect** Cognitive methods (diagnosis and altering of dysfunctional cognitions, working on feelings of guilt and shame (compare Ehlers, 1999), imaginative-hypnotherapeutic methods (compare Brom, Kleber, & Defares, 1989; Reddemann, 2001), or DBT-method (focal point interruption of intrusive phenomenons, self-injury and training in modulation of affect (compare Cloitre et al., 2002; Linehan, 1996a,b). At least one of the methods mentioned has to be trained and mastered practically, the presentation of the other two methods is sufficient. View at experimental protocols (in form of a manual, but up to now without a controlled randomized study).	20
3.	**Working on trauma (mainly related to non-komplex PTSD)** **Evidence-based method working on trauma** (Evidence-level 1a according to Cochrane) theoretically (models of disease, indication, contraindication, differential indication) and practically. **Methods:** *Actually* 1a-methods are cognitive *and* behavioural treatments or EMDR (compare Ehlers, 1999; Resick & Schniche, 1992) and various ways of exposure treatments (compare, e.g., Foa et al., 1991, compare Shapiro, 2001). One of these methods is to be taught in detail, a different one is to be introduced.	20
4.	**View on treatment of acute traumatizations and crisis management** Course and clinical features of acute traumatization, trauma-specific crisis management, support of natural recovering, prevention of retraumatization, reasonable acute interventions (evidence-based, documented approach, information on the effectiveness of various methods). Talking pattern in the acute situation, coping with phenomenons of acute stress disorder like dissociation. Diagnostics and treatment of acute stress disorders and multi-risk people (compare Bryant et al., 2000; Orner & Schnyder, 2003; Solomon et al., 1992). Cooperation with local organisations for support of victims.	10
5.	**Treatment of complex PTSD / Treatment of DESNOS** **Evidence-based methods** The concepts of treatment of complex PTSD are about to be developed at the time, although the research on this group of patients raises severe problems. So the findings in this field are equivalent to an evidence-degree level 2-3 according to Cochrane. The methods according to item 3, but especially according to item 2, can also be used within a general scheme of treatment of DESNOS. In the centre of this modul are graduated, well controllable methods of confrontation as well as the alteration of dysfunctional / disturbing affects and cognitions. Criterion is that the method is manualized, thoroughly described in detail and is clinically accepted. One of these methods is to be taught in detail, a different one is to be introduced. The contents of this modul are the special requirements in: • Therapeutic alliance: First of all the therapeutic alliance is especially emphasized and is considered to be the base. • Stabilization (compare 2) • Working on trauma and integration as well as • Information about the aftermath of severe interpersonel violence, especially in childhood (neuropsychology, development of relations, disorders in relationship as well as their effects on therapeutic relationship), and • View on the bases of dissociative disorders and methods of treatment	30

5. (cont.)	**At the time, the criterions are fulfilled by:** for example hypnotherapeutic methods, modified cognitive-behavioural methods, psychodynamic-imaginative methods, modified methods of depth psychology (compare: Mehrphasige integrative Traumatherapie, Butollo, 1998; Acceptance and Committment Therapy nach Hayes, Strosahl, & Wilson, 2002; van der Hart, Steele, Boon, & Brown, 1995; Mehrdimensionale Psychodynamische Traumatherapie, Fischer, 2000; Integrativ-psychodynamisch-kognitive Therapie, Horowitz, 1986; Phillips & Frederick, 2003; Psychodynamisch Imaginative Traumatherapie, Reddemann & Sachsse, 2000; Reddemann, 2001; Imagery Rescripting nach Smucker, Dancu, & Foa, 2002)	
6.	**Self-experience and psychohygienics** Subject-centred self-experience by of DeGPT authorized supervisors resp. by therapists qualified in therapy of psychotrauma named by institutes authorized for education.Psychohygienics for psychotherapists: self-diagnosis of secondary traumatisation and burnout, methods of self-protection for therapists (compare: Figley, 1995; Stamm, 2002).	10
7.	**Supervision** Supervision of own cases (if possible video-demonstrated) by qualified supervisors (among other things indication and scheme of treatment) in single-setting or groups (max. 6 participants in blocks of at least 4 U).	20
	Final colloquium Cooperative case-related discussion. For admission to the final colloquium six cases, supervised and demonstrated (short version), with different disorders (PTSD, complex traumatization, among other things trauma in childhood–at least 50 hours of treatment, and–if possible–acute traumatisation) are to be presented, 4 cases have to prove entire diagnostics (including at least three trauma-specific tests). The final colloquium bases on two of them.	
	Total hours (U)	140

The authors of the curriculum are aware that for qualified training of therapists treating dissociative disorders, it is necessary to even extend these bases. Certainly, it will also be necessary to impart the rapidly growing knowledge in the field of acute trauma. But the major demand will certainly be the imparting of therapeutic skills in treatment of trauma type 2.

SEMINARS IN GERMANY

Meanwhile, as the curriculum explained above, there is a number (now more than 15) of institutes specialized in the basic training according to DeGPT acknowledgement. The basic training in the treatment of traumatic disorders in general and dissociative disorders in particular is now established nationwide.

But, as mentioned above, there is a lack of experience in the treatment of patients with very severe disorders as well as patients with dissociative identity disorders.

That is why in the German language area there is still much support by qualified trauma-experts from all over the world.

Some of the most important and latest findings of the last years were taught by Ellert Nijenhuis, meanwhile offering seminars in Germany, who also offers seminars on Structural Dissociation of the personality in Switzerland, Norway, Sweden and Austria.

To invite authorized experts to seminars on dissociative disorders and complex trauma, the Psychotraumatology Institute Europe, PIE, has been founded by Ellert Nijenhuis and Helga Matthess. It is to initiate and support reseach in the field of dissociation and to invite experts beginning with Suzette Boon, Richard Kluft and Onno van der Hart, but also other colleagues like Janina Fisher, Pat Ogden, and Richard Chefetz are invited and they have promised to come.

IN THE FUTURE ALSO SPECIAL CURRICULA ON TREATMENT OF DISSOCIATIVE DISORDERS IN SWITZERLAND

In Switzerland there still is a lack of trainings in diagnosis and treatment of dissociative disorders. From the Internet there was only little result searching for trauma therapy and trainings in Switzerland–except for notes about our institute.

Of course there are single offers; particularly, colleagues from Germany are organizing workshops and lectures on various connections. Since 2002, Michaela Huber offers seminars in Switzerland in the institute in Schaffhausen and several Swiss colleagues have completed their training with her in Germany. In 2005, there was a structured offer of seminars on diagnosis and therapy of dissociative disorders on the scientific level of ISSD. A further series of seminars is planned by Ellert Nijenhuis.

There is a great demand for qualified seminars and they are very frequented. In Switzerland we have started to build up a network of therapists for patients with dissociative disorders. We are still far away from our own research in this field, but there seems to be a promising start.

Training standards are developed in cooperation with the German language Society of Psychotraumatology and the German language section of ISSD.

POSSIBILITIES OF TREATMENT
OF COMPLEX-TRAUMATIZED
AND DISSOCIATIVE PATIENTS IN GERMANY

In Germany, the treatment of choice for dissociative patients certainly is ambulatory therapy. Meanwhile, there is a great number of authorized and well trained therapists which is due to the education by Luise Reddemann and Michaela Huber, but also to the nationwide network of EMDR-supervisors who cover besides the training in the EMDR-method also the whole field of stabilization techniques. In the meantime, Arne Hofmann's second part of EMDR-training refers to the treatment of DESNOS-patients and in his institute he regularly offers seminars on EMDR and dissociative disorders.

The demand for seminars is great, particularly by established psychotherapists in the German language area, because contrary to most other European and American insurances the national German insurances are paying for quite a number of psychotherapeutic sessions. The insurances are paying for different numbers of sessions according to the various methods. Applications by experts are necessary. For behaviour therapy there are from 80 up to 100 sessions; psychodynamic therapists can get 80-120 sessions, psychoanalysts even more.

Many in-patient therapies in Germany are done in general psychiatric hospitals which are general clinics not yet well prepared to offer a good treatment in aftermath-disorders of trauma. But in the meantime, there is quite a number of specialized institutions known to most of the ambulant-working therapists who offer treatment to dissociative patients in particular. The period of treatment is quite various: some specialized hospitals offer an interval treatment, especially for those patients living in a region without a sufficient number of trauma-therapists. The in-patient treatment lasts about 3-4 months and may be continued after 6 months or 1 year, if required. Another concept is to hospitalize a patient immediately for stabilization and to dismiss him for ambulant therapy as soon as possible. In Switzerland, special units for the treatment of traumatized patients are not yet developed.

An important possibility to secure a long-time therapy in Germany is the law of reimbursement for victims. In case of acknowledgement of mental, sexual, and physical violence in childhood it secures the reimbursement of costs of treatment at public expense. Originally, this law has been installed for victims of the Second World War, who, at the time, had no public support and who suffered from physical and mental injury. Ten years ago, this law was extended to the victims of sexual and physical violence in childhood, who mostly suffer from a dissociative disorder. In Switzerland, a comparative law supports people being victims of a crime. Of course, criminal offences like sexual violence are also included.

The German language area surely still is a "developing country" with regard to diagnostics, therapy, and research in the field of dissociative disorders, but there are many promising signs for increasing development.

Here, the ISSD Europe will surely be very helpful. Maybe in the foreseeable future it might be possible to organize a European conference of ISSD.

DEVELOPMENTS IN THE FIELD OF TRAUMA BY MEANS OF THE GERMAN HUMANITARIAN ASSISTANCE-PROGRAM (HHP), (AMERICAN ORGANIZATION: HAP–HUMANITARIAN ASSISTANCE PROGRAM)

There is a European pendant to the American organization: Humanitarian Assistance Program (HAP). The purpose of the program is to organize free trauma-curricula including the basic knowledge about dissociative disorders in countries where professional training is not possible because of financial problems.

On the whole, the training follows the curricular training suggested by DeGPT as practiced by the Swiss institute as well as by the institute in Sinzig. The main components are three seminars. The first one offers diagnostics, methods of stabilization, and hypnotherapy, especially the screen-technique; the second one offers an increased knowledge of the first one and also an EMDR-level 1. The third seminar mainly concerns dissociative and complex disorders including the EMDR-level 2, extended by Arne Hofmann for DESNOS-treatments.

The training gets completed by supervisions between and after the seminars.

Up to now, the HHP, the German branch of HAP-Europe, has organized and completed two complete training curricula. The first training has been organized by Arne Hofmann and Helga Matthess in cooperation with Qian Mingyi and Fang Xin at the Psychological Institute of Peking University. Fifty Chinese colleagues attended the training; most of them had finished a basic therapeutic training by the German-Chinese Society of Psychotherapy. The Chinese colleagues come from all regions of China: from the north down to the south provinces, most of them are university lecturers and psychotherapy trainers. Before the next training program is started some Chinese participants of the first training program are attending further intensive training in order to give part of the seminars and lectures by themselves. Some colleagues are considering coming to Europe for some time in order to continue their training.

Meanwhile, the Chinese colleagues have founded a working group on psychotrauma within their Union of Psychologists. A special organisation for psychotraumatology according to the model of the German DeGPT is to be founded soon. Similar to the German language countries, no differentiation of various therapy methods is to be made at the moment. The Chinese colleagues still are in their infancy on diagnostics and treatment of dissociative disorders, although they have to treat a lot of dissociative patients already. The DES meanwhile is translated into the Chinese language. An important element of the training seminars is an introduction to the treatment of dissociative disorders. Further guidelines of treatment are worked out with the Chinese colleagues attending the seminars on a trainer qualification offered by HAP.

There was a parallel development in Slovakia. Here, about 40 participants completed the basic training of 3 years in the sense of a trauma curriculum. Two colleagues, Andrea Sevcikova and Daniel Ralaus, additionally qualified by further seminars in Germany in order to lead supervisions independently in their own countries. Colleagues from the Netherlands, Belgium, and Germany are about to complete their training. A training series with Helga Matthess, especially concerning dissociative disorders, is planned. An independent trauma organization was founded in 2005.

The Humanitarian Assistance Program is planning a training curriculum for colleagues in Thailand in autumn, which will be attended by therapists from the other adjoining countries like Indonesia and Sri Lanka suffering from the high tide disaster.

Further projects are planned, but not yet about to be concretely realized.

REFERENCES

Brom, D., Kleber, R. J., & Defares, P. B. (1989). Brief psychotherapy for Posttraumatic Stress Disorders. *Journal of Consulting and Clinical Psychology, 57,* 607-612.

Bryant, R. A. & Harvey, A. G. (2000). *Acute stress disorder: A handbook of theory, assessment, and treatment.* Washington, DC, US: American Psychological Association.

Butollo, W., Krüsmann, M., & Hagl, M. (1998). *Leben nach dem Trauma,* München: Pfeiffer.

Cloitre, M., Koenen, K. C., Cohen, L. R., & Han, H. (2002). Skills training in affective and interpersonal regulation followed by exposure: A phase-based treatment for PTSD related to childhood abuse. *Journal of Consulting and Clinical Psychology*, 70, 1067-1074.

Ehlers, A. (1999). *Posttraumatische Belastungsstörungen*, Göttingen: Hogrefe.

Figley, C. R. (1995). *Compassion fatigue: Coping with Secondary Traumatic Stress Disorder in those who treat the traumatized*. New York: Brunner Mazel

Fischer, G. (2000). *MPTT Mehrdimensionale Psychodynamische Traumatherapie*, Asanger-Verlag, Heidelberg.

Foa, E. B., Rothbaum, B. O., Riggs, D. S., & Murdock. T. B. (1991). Treatment of posttraumatic stress disorder in rape victims: Comparison between cognitive-behavioral procedures and counselling. *Journal of Consulting and Clinical Psychology*, 59, 715-723.

Freud, S. (1895, 1952). *Studien über Hysterie*, London: Imago

Hayes, S. C., Strosahl, K. D., & Wilson, K. G. (2002). Acceptance and commitment therapy: An experiential approach to behavior change. *Cognitive & Behavioral Practice, Vol 9*, pp. 164-166.

Horowitz M. J. (1986). *Stress Response Syndromes*, Northvale: Jason Aronson.

Kraepelin, E. (1909, 1915). *Psychiatrie, Ein Lehrbuch für Studierende und Ärzte*. Leipzig: Barth.

Linehan, M. M. (1993a). *Cognitive-behavioral treatment of Borderline Personality-Disorder*, New York: The Guilford Press.

Linehan, M. M. (1996a). *Dialektisch-Behaviorale Therapie der Borderline-Persönlichkeitsstörung*, CIP-Medien.

Linehan, M. M. (1993b). *Skills training manual for treating borderline personality disorder*. New York: The Guilford Press.

Linehan, M. M. (1996b). *Trainingsmanual zur Dialektisch-Behavioralen Therapie der Borderline-Persönlichkeitsstörung*, CIP-Medien.

Orner, R. & Schnyder, U. (2003). *Reconstructing early intervention after trauma*. Oxford, New York: Oxford University Press.

Phillips, M. & Frederick, C. (2003). *Handbuch der Hypnotherapie bei Posttraumatischen und dissoziativen Störungen*, Heidelberg: Carl Auer.

Phillips, M. & Frederick, C. (1995). *Healing the divided self*, New York, London: Norton

Priebe, S., Nowak, M., & Schmiedebach, H.-P. (2002). Trauma und Psyche in der deutschen Psychiatrie seit 1889, *Psychiat Prax*, 29, 2-9.

Reddemann., L. & Sachsse, U. (2000). Traumazentrierte imaginative Therapie. In Egle, U. T., Hoffmann, S. O. und Joraschky, P. (Hrsg.). *Sexueller Missbrauch, Misshandlung, Vernachlässigung. Erkennung und Therapie psychischer und psychosomatischer Folgen früher Traumatisierungen*. Stuttgart: Schattauer.

Reddemann, L. (2001). *Imagniation als heilsame Kraft*. München: Pfeiffer.

Resick, P., & Schnicke, M. (1992). Cognitive processing therapy for sexual assault victims, *J Consult Clin Psychol*, 60, 748-756.

Sachsse, U., Venzlaff, U., & Dulz, B. (1997). 100 Jahre Traumaätiologie, *Persönlichkeitsstörungen*, 1, 4-14.

Schreiber, F. L. (1976). *Sybil*, München: Scherz.

Shapiro, F. (2001). *Eye movement desensitization and reprocessing: Basic principles, protocols, and procedures*, New York, NY, US: Guilford Press.

Smucker, M., Dancu, C., & Foa, B. (2002). Imagery rescripting: A new treatment for survivors of childhood sexual abuse suffering from posttraumatic stress. In: Leahy, Robert L. (Ed); Dowd, E. Thomas (Ed); *Clinical advances in cognitive psychotherapy: Theory and application*. New York, NY, US: Springer, pp. 294-310.

Solomon, S. D., Gerrity, E. T., & Muff, A. M. (1992). Efficacy of treatments for posttraumatic stress disorder. *Journal of the American Medical Association, 268*, 633-638.

Stamm, B. H. (2002). *Sekundäre Traumastörungen*, Paderborn: Junfermann.

Stamm, B. H. (1999). *Secondary Traumatic Stress: Self-Care Issues for Clinicians, Researchers and Educators*, Lutherville, MD: Sidran Press.

Van der Hart, O., Steele, K., Boon, S., & Brown, P. (1995). Die Behandlung traumatischer Erinnerungen: Synthese, Bewusstwerdung und Integration; Hypnose und Dissoziation: Milton Erickson Gesellschaft (Ed): *Hypnose und Kognition*.

Van der Hart, O., Steele, K., Boon, S., & Brown, P. (1993). The treatment of traumatic memory: Synthesis, realization, integration, *Dissociation, 6*, 162-180.

Venzlaff, U. (1958). *Die psychoreaktiven Störungen nach entschädigungspflichtiger Ereignissen*. Berlin, Göttingen, Heidelberg: Springer.

Venzlaff, U., Dulz, B., & Sachsse, U. (2004). Zur Geschichte der Psychotraumatologie. In U.Sachsse (Ed.), *Traumazentrierte Psychotherapie*, Stuttgart, Schattauer.

Zimmermann, P., Hahne, H.-H., Biesold, K.-H., & Lanczik, M. (2004). Psychogene Störungen bei deutschen Soldaten des Ersten und Zweiten Weltkrieges, *Fortsch Neurol Psychiat*, pp. 101-112.

Trauma and Dissociation in Paradise (Hawaii)

George F. Rhoades, Jr.

SUMMARY. This chapter will introduce the types of traumas experienced in Hawaii historically and in the present day. The three different cultural groups that present for treatment of trauma and dissociation were noted as the indigenous Hawaiians, individuals that have been in Hawaii for multiple generations, but who are from different countries or the Continental U.S., and transplanted peoples that are in Hawaii for a prescribed period of time, i.e., U.S. military and contract employees/workers. The six essential components of working with the different Hawaiian cultures were presented as: (1) Determine the primary and/or mixture of cultural background of your patient; (2) If an immigrant to Hawaii, ascertain the generational status of the patient, i.e., first generation, second generation immigrant; (3) Determine how traditional was the cultural upbringing of the patient; (4) Determine how traditional the patient is in regards to their cultural background; (5) Determine how functional the patient is within their cultural context; and (6) Determine how functional the patient is within the overall cultural context where they have chosen to live. The elements of Hawaiian culture that related to the diagnosis

---

George F. Rhoades, Jr., PhD, is Director, Ola Hou Clinic, 98-1247 Kaahumanu Street, Suite 223, Aiea, HI, 96701 (E-mail: rhoades@pdchawaii.com).

The author would like to thank Mr. Leon Siu for his review of this chapter for historical accuracy.

[Haworth co-indexing entry note]: "Trauma and Dissociation in Paradise (Hawaii)." Rhoades, George F., Jr. Co-published simultaneously in *Journal of Trauma Practice* (The Haworth Maltreatment & Trauma Press, an imprint of The Haworth Press, Inc.) Vol. 4, No. 1/2, 2005, pp. 133-145; and: *Trauma and Dissociation in a Cross-Cultural Perspective: Not Just a North American Phenomenon* (ed: George F. Rhoades, Jr., and Vedat Sar) The Haworth Maltreatment & Trauma Press, an imprint of The Haworth Press, Inc., 2005, pp. 133-145. Single or multiple copies of this article are available for a fee from The Haworth Document Delivery Service [1-800-HAWORTH, 9:00 a.m. - 5:00 p.m. (EST). E-mail address: docdelivery@haworthpress.com].

and treatment of dissociative disorders were presented and illustrated with case examples. *[Article copies available for a fee from The Haworth Document Delivery Service: 1-800-HAWORTH. E-mail address: <docdelivery @ haworthpress.com> Website: <http://www.HaworthPress.com> © 2005 by The Haworth Press, Inc. All rights reserved.]*

KEYWORDS. Trauma, dissociation, Hawaii, Cross-Cultural Therapy, Noho, Possession Trance Disorder, Culture-Bound Syndromes, Akualele

Hawaii, formerly called the Sandwich Islands was "discovered" on January 18, 1778 (Daws, 1968) and described as "the world's most isolated land mass," by the British explorer Captain James Cook (Stone, 2003). The first discoverers were probably Polynesian from the Marquesas Islands before A.D. 400. Polynesians from Tahiti began to voyage to Hawaii in A.D. 1200, *Kahuna Nui* (high priest) and *Ali'i Nui* (high royalty) Pa'ao came to conquer and set up a new social and religious order with an oppressive taboo system in A.D. 1300. There was much warfare and bloodshed between Hawaiian Chiefs, until 1795 when King Kamehameha I conquered and unified[1] all the Hawaiian Islands into the Hawaiian Kingdom. Peace ensued and Kamehameha traded and parlayed with European, American and Oriental nations. In 1819, Kamehameha II abandoned the taboo system and welcomed Christianity into the realm. Within 25 years, the spread of Christianity transformed Hawaii from a pagan nation into "the most Christian nation on earth" (Kikawa, 1994). In 1840 King Kamehameha III changed Hawaii from an absolute monarchy into a constitutional monarchy and Hawaii soon became a modern, progressive, full participant in the family of nations. In 1893, Caucasian foreign businessmen and United States (U.S.) Marines illegally overthrew Queen Lili'uokalani and the government of the Hawaiian Kingdom. Hawaii subsequently became a U.S. Territory and eventually a U.S. State in 1959 (Kikawa, 1994).

The Hawaiian Islands has been described as the "Melting Pot" of the nations (Akana, 1992) or even an "International Nidus" (Raymond, Chung, & Wood, 1991). Raymond, Chung, and Wood (1991), speaking from the perspective of prevention research, saw Hawaii as being,

a natural nidus for international activity for the Asia and Pacific regions. Its year-round favorable climate, multilingual and multicultural citizenry, and a geographical location add to its desirability as a place for international exchange of knowledge. Its stable demography and ethnic mix likewise contribute to its value as a focus for behavior-oriented epidemiologic studies. Hawaii's ecological and cultural background is similar to that of many regions of the Pacific rim. (p. 528)

The centrality of Hawaii has made it an ideal location for prevention research studies, but also for the study of trauma and dissociation throughout the Pacific Rim Countries. Trauma has been defined as,

> The result of a painful event, physical or mental, causing immediate damage to the body or shock to the mind. Psychological traumas include emotional shocks that have an enduring effect on the personality, such as rejection, divorce, combat experiences, civilian catastrophes, and racial or religious discrimination. (Corsini, 1999, p. 1019)

Dissociation has been defined as "an unconscious process in which one or more parts of mental functioning become split off from others and appear to operate outside of consciousness" (Corsini, 1999, p. 288). The two concepts may be seen as inter-related as the experiencing of a trauma often leads to dissociation as a coping mechanism. In contrast the person that has dissociated parts of their emotional pain and even experiences in life has often experienced trauma in their lives. The different dissociative disorders (American Psychiatric Association, APA, 2000) are present within the patient population in Hawaii, expressed through the culture of the individual/group.

This chapter will introduce the types of traumas experienced in Hawaii historically and in the present day. The different cultural groups that present for treatment of trauma and dissociation will be noted. The elements of Hawaiian culture that relate to the diagnosis and treatment of dissociative disorders will be presented and illustrated with case examples.

TRAUMA IN HAWAII

It is difficult to realize that a land that is regarded and referred to as "paradise" could have traumatic events. Historically, the Hawaiian people went through a time of trauma subsequent to the arrival of Pa'ao in 1300 A.D. The Kapu system made clear distinctions between the Ali'i

(Chiefs) and the commoners. Those conquered in battle were considered kauwa (untouchables/slaves) and were utilized in human sacrifices (Pukui, Haertig & Lee, 1972b). The breaking of a kapu could lead to severe punishments such as the losing of an eye or even death. The kapu system even extended to the eating patterns of men and women. Only men were allowed to eat certain foods such as pork, bananas, coconuts and the sea turtle. The penalty was death for a woman that was clearly caught eating these forbidden foods (Malo,[2] 1951; Kikawa, 1994). The kapu system and the Hawaiian gods were overthrown by Ka'ahu-manu, the high chiefess and a widow of King Kamehameha in 1819 (Pukui, Haertig & Lee, 1972b).

The loss of the Hawaiian Kingdom in 1893 has caused a trauma among the Hawaiian people in the loss of their monarchy, their nation, their lands and for many their identity and "birthright had been stolen" (Fuchs, 1961, p. 3). There are a number of sovereignty movements in Hawaii at the present time, with a desire to restore the Hawaiian Kingdom in some form. The likelihood of a restoration of a Hawaiian nation, however, diminishes as each year passes and the importance of Hawaii as a strategic military location for the U.S. increases. Sovereignty members are hopeful and for the sake of justice work diligently for the restoration of the Hawaiian Kingdom as an independent nation. Either way, there remains the underlying problems of unresolved injustice, injury loss, and disassociation.

The four types of natural disasters in Hawaii are earthquakes, tsunamis, hurricanes, and volcanic eruptions. The earthquakes are often part of the volcanic activity which has mainly affected the island of Hawaii in recent history. The lava flows have destroyed entire housing developments and even threatened the city of Hilo in the past. Historically, 46 fatalities were recorded in a tsunami of 1819. Two tsunamis hit the island of Hawaii in1946 and 1960, resulting in damage to the city of Hilo and 83 and 61 deaths, respectively (Stone, 2003). Eight hurricanes have threatened the Hawaiian Islands between 1950 and 2000. Two hurricanes were noteworthy in their traumatic impact on Hawaii, the first being Hurricane Iwa which occurred in 1982 resulting in one death and 234 million dollars of property damage. Hurricane Iniki concluded in 1992 with eight deaths and 1 billion, 900 million dollars of property damage (Hawaii Government, 2000).

Violence is seemingly prevalent in all societies, including murder, rape, domestic violence and child abuse. Chemtob and Carlson (2004) studied the effects of domestic violence on 25 children and their mothers in Honolulu, Hawaii. The psychological measures utilized revealed (two years after the violence) that 40% of the children and 50% of the mothers had Posttraumatic Stress Disorder (PTSD). The variables that determined the disorder in the mothers was not found related to the development of the disorder in the children. Sadly, 91% of the mothers with PTSD had not obtained psychiatric services for their children, even though 92% of the mothers had themselves sought services. In regards to child abuse (including physical, sexual, psychological abuse and neglect) in Hawaii, the number of reported cases accepted for investigation rose from 1,079 (499 confirmed) in 1973 to 7,318 (3,744 confirmed) in 2002 (Hawaii Government, 2003).

The central location of Hawaii in the Pacific Basin has led to the establishment of multiple military bases and the placement of many servicemen and servicewomen and their families in Hawaii. The presence of a major military Hospital (Tripler Army Medical Center) and Veteran's Administration facilities has attracted many PTSD patients that served in the Vietnam Conflict, both Gulf Wars, and the present volatile deployments in Afghanistan and Iraq. The veterans of these traumatic tours of duty are often seen in private practice, along with their families.

CULTURAL GROUPS IN HAWAII

It is due to the fact of Hawaii being a "melting pot" that there are diverse cultural groups with corresponding needs in the treatment of trauma and dissociation. The first group is the indigenous Hawaiians themselves. The second group is those that have been in Hawaii for multiple generations, but who are from different countries or the Continental U.S. The third group is transplanted peoples that are in Hawaii for a prescribed period of time, i.e., U.S. military and contract employees/workers. There are multiple levels within these three groups depending on the generation of the individual/family (1st, 2nd generation Chinese) and the determination of how traditional the person's adherence to their ancestral heritage is. Rhoades (1999) noted six essential components of working with the different Hawaiian cultures, principles that are practical with essentially all cultures.

1. *Determine the primary and/or mixture of cultural background of your patient.* A standard aspect of an intake interview is to determine the racial/ethnic/cultural background of a patient. Should the patient be multi-cultural in upbringing, the patient is asked for a

breakdown of this mixture. The patient is then asked for the cultural mix of each individual parent. Be aware that culture and ethicnicity are not necessarily the same. A person may be Caucasian and have been raised in China, thereby having the traditional cultural upbringing of a Chinese person.

2. *If an immigrant to Hawaii, ascertain the generational status of the patient, i.e., first generation, second generation immigrant.* The generation of the patient in Hawaii is very important in regards to the Asian person. A general rule of thumb is that the more generations removed from the original country (i.e., Japan, Philippines, etc.) the less traditional is the patient's cultural heritage that is practiced. This principle can easily be thwarted as the first generation parents may choose to "let go" of their culture to better fit in with the Americans.

3. *Determine how traditional the cultural upbringing of the patient was.* A more critical question for your client is how traditional was the parenting practices of the patient's parents. One's parents may be many generations removed from the country of origin and yet treasure or go back to those countries' traditions.

4. *Determine how traditional the patient is in regards to their cultural background.* A patient may be raised by a traditional parents and choose to not be traditional in his/her belief structure or practice. In contrast, a person may choose to recapture his past cultural heritage regardless of his familial upbringing.

5. *Determine how functional the patient is within their cultural context.* The question here is whether the patient's dissociative behavior fits within their cultural context. A female patient of the current author was taught to read the melted wax candles and "manifest" a spiritual entity in the Philippines. This possession trance disorder was considered quite normal within the context of her spiritualist, Filipino cultural upbringing.

6. *Determine how functional the patient is within the overall cultural context where they have chosen to live.* The patient mentioned above moved to Hawaii and continued to "manifest." This behavior was no longer appropriate for her new cultural environment, i.e., the professional work environment in Hawaii and the patient sought psychological treatment.

The challenge for each therapist is to provide psychological treatment for their patients/clients that are within the context of and respect for their culture and to do no harm. This challenge is difficult to be accomplished without knowledge of the patient's background and how they apply this cultural fiber in every day living. This chapter will focus now on the Hawaiian cultural aspects that relate to the treatment of trauma and dissociation in Hawaiians.

HAWAIIAN CULTURE AND DISSOCIATION

The Hawaiian word "noho" refers to sit, to dwell or dwelling place. In old Hawaii, the "Hawaiian believed he could be *noho* by good spirits or bad; possession could be total or partial, but always temporary; spirits could possess spontaneously or by invitation" (Pukui, Haertig & Lee, 1972a). A spontaneous *noho* or possession could occur when a kahu (master), functioning as a spirit master would send a spirit to possess a person without holding a séance ritual. The possession could be by a family *aumakua* (ancestor-god) or a spirit of the dead. The possessing spirits, single or multiple were seen as either beneficial or harmful, but were not regarded as demons or devils. Pukui, Haertig, and Lee (1972a) gave the following case of a 17-year-old girl, in a rural, largely Hawaiian community after World War II,

> She was looking in a mirror and talking, and it was as if she were two persons talking. She would say "I don't want my hair combed that way. I want it this way." Then she went on combing her hair, and then she said, "I'm going to slap your face." And with that she'd slap her own face. Then she said, "You slapped my face. I'm going to slap yours, too." And then she would slap her face on the other side.

> Later, her father told me, "Poor Lucy. She and her sister, Luella [names disguised] were twins. When they were still very young, Luella died. Lucy was very sick. About two years later–Lucy was three or so then–she made me mad and I told her I felt like chopping off her head. A few days later we noticed she was acting like two persons, herself and her twin sister." (pp. 160-161)

The Hawaiian teenager would be seen as having a *noho*, partially due to unresolved grief and the obvious trauma by the father's violent threat at a tender age. Another historical case from the 1940s was related by Pukui (Pukui, Haertig & Lee, 1972a),

This happened in Kalihi [town on Oahu] and was told to me by a *haole* ["foreigner," "who-do-not-breathe," typically seen as Caucasian] Mormon elder . . . He was called in when a young woman began screaming and crying and tearing her clothing. He believed she was possessed, so he called for the spirit to come out, just about as it is described in the Bible. The woman became calm, for only a few minutes. Then she became even wilder. The elder thought this must be possession by many spirits and he didn't feel he could handle this. So he sent for an old Hawaiian who was also a Mormon elder. He came and prayed over the woman. Then he asked, "Where are you from?" And the woman answered "From Molokai." "Why did you come?" asked the elder. "Because she turned down a marriage proposal from one of our family." "We?" inquired the elder, "How many are you?" "Nineteen" came the answer.

And then the elder commanded each spirit, one by one, to come out. And to each one he said, "Now go back to where you came from. Leave the girl alone." After this the girl was calm and normal. (p. 161)

This *noho* was the result of a rejected marriage proposal and this possession was seen as bad as the spirits were sent for the detriment of the young woman. The resolution/removal of the spirits in this case showed a mixture of Hawaiian and Mormon beliefs. The Hawaiians viewed spirit possession as temporary, that the spirits would eventually leave on their own. The pain and concern caused by the spirits led to the development of exorcism rites to "speed their departure." These rituals were described as,

First the family prayed over the one who was noho. Then someone asked the spirit "Who are you? Where are you from? Who sent you?" And then this family member would command the spirit to leave by saying "Ho'i no 'ai I kou kahu." That means "go back and destroy your keeper."

Then it was wise to get the ohana (family clan) together for ho'oponopono ["to set to right," Hawaiian conflict resolution] to find and correct the wrongs or the bad behavior that allowed the spirit to take possession. (Pukui, Haertig & Lee, 1972a, p. 162)

Should a person be unable to talk, the one experiencing *noho*, the exorcism could be done by using *ti* leaves or white *tapa* (cloth made out of tree bark) in a ritual called kuehu (shaking out),

> The family senior or the *kahuna* [*kahu* = master/expert, *na* = present or continuing] made the possessed one lie down with his feet toward the house doorway. Then he struck him lightly with the *ti* from head to feet. The he shook the leaves in the doorway, just as you might shake out a dust cloth. This was to shake the possessing spirit out of the house. Then *ti* leaves were spread under the sleeping mat to keep the spirit from coming back. (Pukui, Haertig & Lee, 1972a, p. 163)

One patient that the current author treated came from a long line of *kahunas* [Commonly seen as Hawaiian Priests/Priestesses, were actually known as a present or continuing "Master" of an area such as medicine or, in this case, spirits] presented with many different spirits, mostly of Hawaiian origin. One spirit that troubled the patient identified itself as an Egyptian god. This puzzled the current author until research with Hawaiian authorities revealed one oral tradition of the Hawaiians as originally migrating from Egypt.

The Hawaiians were also able to distinguish between a true possession (*noho*) and a pseudo-possession (*ho'onohonoho*). The reasons for a *ho'onohonoho* given were to impress or frighten, or as an alibi for behavior that was socially disapproved. There was also a distinction of *noho* from physical illness and a lasting state of insanity (*pupule*).

A person could also experience a dissociative state when their "grief work" was incomplete. Pukui, Haertig, and Lee (1972a) cite the following example,

> Anytime she drinks and gets mad and upset, she goes off into a trance, and then she speaks Hawaiian. But when she is herself she can hardly speak Hawaiian at all. She starts off by wailing and *oli*-ing [chanting] and then she talks in Hawaiian. I think she is possessed by her mother or grandmother [both dead]. After it's all over, she doesn't remember a thing. I don't know enough Hawaiian to know what she is saying, but one of the neighbors heard her and said that she was speaking pure, very old Hawaiian. (p. 165)

The authors noted that the Hawaiian language was spoken by the patient's mother and grandmother when the patient was a child. The assumption being that the language was still known by an unconscious part of the person, not expressed until a time of *noho*, caused by incomplete grief work.

Noho may be seen as a culture-bound syndrome or a possession trance disorder as described in the *Diagnostic and Statistical Manual of Mental Disorders-Fourth Edition-Text Revision, (DSM-IV-TR, APA)*. Culture-bound syndromes (cbs) are defined as,

> recurrent, locality-specific patterns of aberrant behavior and troubling experience that may or may not be linked to a particular DSM-IV diagnostic category. Many of these patterns are indigenously considered to be 'illnesses,' or at least afflictions, and most have local names. (p. 898)

The Possession Trance Disorder (APA, 2000) is a single or episodic replacement of a person's personal identity with a new identity. This new identity is attributed to the influence of a spirit, deity, power or another person. This influence is indicated by either culturally determined or stereotyped behaviors, or a sense that the person is controlled by the possessing agent. The person also has full or partial amnesia for the event. The possession trance disorder causes significant distress in important areas of functioning such as social and occupational and is not seen as a normal part of the collective culture or religious practice. The Hawaiian trance possession as noted in previous examples can be quite detrimental to the person, but in come cases a possession was meant to be and seen as beneficial. This is often seen in the possessions of an *aumakua*, meant to help a troubled or ill person. Another example of a "mild, helpful possession" called *ho'oulu ia* was inspiration given by one's aumakua in an artistic endeavor (Pukui, Haertig, & Lee, 1972a, p. 80).

Hearing voices and seeing visions may be seen as culturally normal for a Hawaiian (Pukui, Haertig, & Lee, 1972a, pp. 11-12). There are several criteria to determine if a voice or vision is true (culturally normal) or wrong. First, if a person is in a group and he/she is the only person that hears a voice or sees a vision, and nobody else even senses it, then the voice or vision is false. Second, should the person be alone when he/she experiences the voice or vision, then two tests are applied. First, if no one else can understand the voice or vision, then it is false. Second, a true vision or voice must not bring any harm.

A Hawaiian may also talk about a sign (*ho'ailona*) or a revelation (*ho'ike*). The current author was at a Hawaiian internment ceremony when a "whirlwind" of air came around the mourners. The absence of wind before and after this incident was acknowledged by all in attendance. The mourners all had seen and felt a *ho'ailona*, but (Pukui, Haertig, & Lee, 1972a, p. 80) the resulting *ho'ike* depended on the individual. Many felt that the spirit of the deceased had made his presence known in a positive manner, while others felt that it was a display of power that was ominous.

A sign of unfinished grief may be the dead returning in Hawaiian dreams. This is seen as quite natural and a motivation to complete the healing process. The dreams may last for years, produce no anxiety, having mild emotion resulting in a "healing sadness" (Pukui, Haertig, & Lee, 1972b, p.189). The dreams may be seen as pathological by the Hawaiian when "the dead appear in recurring dreams that continue over a long period, and when the dreams arouse intense emotion and marked anxiety" (p. 189).

The Hawaiian Fire Ball or *Akualele* was seen as a "flying god" that was sent on a destructive errand (Pukui, Haertig, & Lee, 1972a, p. 25). It may also be seen as a vision or sign leading to dissociative symptoms. Grant (1996) described the creation of a fire ball,

> First they made a *pulolo* or bundle which had the vining *awa* root and fingernails of a dead person inside. As those things are put into the bundle, the *kahuna* continually prays. This must all be done in one action. Then the *kahuna* takes one deep breath to say the prayer. They must pray with one deep breath, chanting, chanting for it to fly. When the chanter finally drops out of breath, the bundle catches on fire and flies off to kill the person it has been directed against. You can see the light of the *akualele* for miles. (p. 97)

The current author consulted on a case wherein a 17-year-old Hawaiian girl "broke-up" with her Hawaiian boyfriend. The mother of the boyfriend made a curse on the teenage girl and sent an *akualele*, Hawaiian fireball, to the girl. The teenager saw the fireball in the sky and became acutely psychotic and was taken to a hospital emergency room with severely combative behaviors. The mother of the girl approached the ex-boyfriend's mother and apologized on behalf of her daughter. The daughter became well within the hour of the apology. It is of interest that the daughter did not know that her mother had approached and apologized for the scorning of the teenage boy. Medical records revealed that the teenager had the equivalent of one mixed drink in her system, not enough to account for her rapid onset of aggressive, psychotic behavior or her sudden return to sanity. This episode of *noho* was seen as generated by the sight of the *akualele*.

A final note is for the professional to be willing to work with a patient's *ho'ola*, i.e., healer or minister that practices healing. The Hawaiian patient that is traditional in their cultural practices has a strong reliance on prayer and consultation with their kahuna or kahu. The modern day interpretation of the two titles would be the Hawaiian priest (continuing master of traditional religious practices) or the Christian pastor, respectively.

CONCLUSION

The types of historical trauma experienced in Hawaii were the past wars, *kapu* system, natural disasters and even the Hawaiian's loss of their "birth right." The present traumas of natural disasters, violence in the home, and violence in the *aina* (land) can produce traumatic responses and dissociative disorders. The treatment of the disorders must be conducted within the culture of the patient for the maximum benefit.

NOTES

1. The Island of Kauai was never militarily conquered, but added to the kingdom via a treaty.
2. David Malo's *Hawaiian Antiquities (Moolelo Hawaii)* was translated from the Hawaiian Language by Dr. Nathaniel B. Emerson in 1898.

REFERENCES

Akana, A. (1992). *Light upon the mist: A reflection of wisdom for the future generations of native Hawaiians*. Edited by E. M. DeFries. Honolulu: Mahina Productions.
American Psychiatric Association (2000). *Diagnostic and statistical manual of mental disorders-text revision (4th ed.)*. Washington, DC: Author.
Chemtob, C. M. & Carlson, J. G. (2004). Psychological effects of domestic violence on children and their mothers. *International Journal of Stress Management*, 11 (3), 209-226.
Corsini, R. J. (1999). *The dictionary of psychology*. Philadelphia: Brunner/Mazel.
Daws, G. (1968). *Shoal of time: A history of the Hawaiian Islands*. Honolulu: University of Hawaii Press.
Fuchs, L. H. (1961). *Hawaii Pono: An ethnic and political history*. Honolulu: Bess Press.

Grant, G. (1996). *Obake files: Ghostly encounters in supernatural Hawai'i*. Honolulu: Mutual Publishing

Hawaii Government (2000). Major hurricanes: 1950 to 2000. *The State of Hawaii data book 2000*. Retrieved February 21, 2005 from http://www.hawaii.gov/dbedt/

Hawaii Government (2003). Child abuse and neglect reports: 1973-2002. *The State of Hawaii data book 2003*. Retrieved February 21, 2005 from http://www.hawaii.gov/dbedt/

Kikawa, D. I. (1994). *Perpetuated in righteousness: The journey of the Hawaiian people from Eden (Kalana i Hauola) to the present time (4th ed.)*. Kea'au: Aloha Ke Akua Publishing.

Malo, D. (1951). *Hawaiian Antiquities (Moolelo Hawaii)*. Honolulu: Bishop Museum

Pukui, M. K., Haertig, E. W., & Lee, C. A. (1972a). *Nana I Ke Kumu (Look to the source) (Vol. 1)*. Honolulu: Hui Hanai.

Pukui, M. K., Haertig, E. W., & Lee, C. A. (1972b). *Nana I Ke Kumu (Look to the source) (Vol. 2)*. Honolulu: Hui Hanai.

Raymond, J. S., Chung, C. S., & Wood, D. W. (1991). Asia-Pacific prevention research: Challenges, opportunities, and implementation. *American Psychologist*, 46 (5), 528-531.

Rhoades, G. F. Jr. (1999). *Cross-cultural presentation of Dissociative Identity Disorder in British, Hawaiian & American Clients*. Paper presented at the 15th annual meeting of the International Society for the Study of Dissociation, Miami, Florida.

Stone, S. C. S. (2003). *Yesterday in Hawaii: A voyage through time*. Waipahu: Island Heritage Publishing.

"Djinnati," A Possession State in Baloochistan, Iran

Mohsen Kianpoor
George F. Rhoades, Jr.

SUMMARY. The consideration of culture-bound syndromes is important for both the practitioner and the academician in the treatment and
study of the psychopathology in a given region of the world. The mental
health professional would as a result be better able understand normal
behavior patterns of that culture and to communicate with patients and
"local healers" of that culture in a nonjudgmental manner. This piece
presented a study of *Djinnati,* a culture-bound syndrome and possession
trance disorder, found in Baluchistan of Iran and Pakistan. The main
characteristics of ten observed cases of Djinnati are presented, including
episodes of impaired consciousness followed by agitation, restlessness,
hallucination and incoherent speech. The episode/attack is seen as a possession wherein the patient introduced herself as a discrete identity or

Mohsen Kianpoor, MD, is affiliated with the Zahedan University of Medical Sciences.

George F. Rhoades, Jr., PhD, is Director of Ola Hou Clinic.

Address correspondence to: George F. Rhoades, Jr., PhD, Ola Hou Clinic, 1247
Kaahumanu St., Suite 223, Aiea, HI 96701 (E-mail: rhoades@pdchawaii.com).

The authors thank Dr. N. M Bakhshani, for his encouragement on this subject and
his guidance in each step for defining the condition, and to Dr. S.A.R. Sadjadi, their cooperative colleague.

[Haworth co-indexing entry note]: "'Djinnati,' A Possession State in Baloochistan, Iran." Kianpoor,
Mohsen and George F. Rhoades, Jr.. Co-published simultaneously in *Journal of Trauma Practice* (The
Haworth Maltreatment & Trauma Press, an imprint of The Haworth Press, Inc.) Vol. 4, No. 1/2, 2005,
pp. 147-155; and: *Trauma and Dissociation in a Cross-Cultural Perspective: Not Just a North American Phenomenon* (ed: George F. Rhoades, Jr., and Vedat Sar) The Haworth Maltreatment & Trauma Press, an imprint
of The Haworth Press, Inc., 2005, pp. 147-155. Single or multiple copies of this article are available for a fee
from The Haworth Document Delivery Service [1-800-HAWORTH, 9:00 a.m. - 5:00 p.m. (EST). E-mail address: docdelivery@haworthpress.com].

entity known as "Djin." The psychopathology of the Djinnati culture-bound syndrome was discussed in the light of Socio-cultural, Communication, and Dissociation/psychoanalytic theories. The authors conclude that Dissociation theory is most effective of the three in explaining the psychopathology of Djinnati syndrome in Iran. *[Article copies available for a fee from The Haworth Document Delivery Service: 1-800-HAWORTH. E-mail address: <docdelivery@haworthpress.com> Website: <http://www. HaworthPress.com> © 2005 by The Haworth Press, Inc. All rights reserved.]*

KEYWORDS. Possession, dissociation, Djinnati, culture-bound syndrome, local healer, multiple personality, dissociative identity disorder, patriarchal

The identification and understanding of "Cultural Bound Syndromes" may be one of the most important tasks of academicians and therapists involved in cross-cultural studies. This understanding may allow for better understanding of normal, patient, and local/cultural "healer" behavior in a given culture, promoting nonjudgmental communication of persons, and an efficacious therapeutic space or stance. A culture-bound syndrome may be defined as,

> recurrent, locality-specific patterns of aberrant behavior and troubling experience that may or may not be linked to a particular DSM-IV diagnostic category. Many of these patterns are indigenously considered to be 'illnesses,' or at least afflictions, and most have local names. (American Psychiatric Society [APA], DSM-IV-TR, 2000, p. 898)

Many of the culture-bound syndromes may be seen as falling into the category of the dissociative disorders. Examples of such culture-bound dissociative disorders are Amok, Ataque de Nervios, "Falling-Out," Latah, Nervios, Pibloktoq, Qi-gong, Shin-Byung, Spell, Susto and Zar (Rhoades, 2003; APA, 2000). In addition, a dissociative state may be identified as a dissociative trance disorder which also involved a possession or trance state (APA, 2000). A possession trance is defined as a single or episodic alteration in the state of consciousness characterized by the replacement of customary sense of personal identity by a new identity. This is attributed to the influence of a spirit, power, deity, or other person, as evidenced by one (or more) of the following: (a) stereotyped and culturally determined behaviors or movements that are experienced as being controlled by the possessing agent; (b) full or partial amnesia for the event (p. 747).

Possession states are seen as widespread (Table 1) and are culturally accepted in about 90% of the world's populations (Pereira, 1995). Scientifically trained observers have reported different presentations of possession states from different regions such as Sibery (Korolenko, 2001), India (Shanmugan, 1981), Singapore (Kua, 1986), Egypt (Nelson, 1971), New Guinea (Salisbury, 1968), Ceylon (Obeysekere, 1970) and South America (Pineros, 1998). In northeast Africa and the Middle East, including the south of Iran, a prevalent presentation of possession syndrome is known as "Zar" (Sa-edi, 1975; Grisaru, 1997).

Possession states (Table 1) have been found in regions of the world where European and American psychiatric belief systems have not re-

TABLE 1. Some possession states known all around the world

Possession State	Location	Characteristics
Brief dissociative stupor (Alexander, 1997)	India	altered consciousness, change of voice, psychomotor agitation
Dybbuk (Billu, 1989)	Israel	hysterical symptoms involving spirits of the dead
Kizil kootalak (Korolenko, 2001)	Sibery	possession by the spirit of fertility
Madness attacks (Pineros, 1998)	Colombia	conversive disorder with dissociative features (ataques de locura)
Oolamachak (Korolenko, 2001)	Sibery	depression with lethal exit (imbalance of inner & outer spirits)
Orak (Korolenko, 2001)	Sibery	moving in of the spirit of suicides
Yi-Ping (Gaw, 1998)	China	loss of control
Zar (Sa-edi, 1975)	Africa Middle East	involuntary movements, mutism, incomprehensible language

placed older, ritualistic patterns of belief (Allison, 1985). These possession states/culture-bound syndromes may also be prevalent in Western
societies due to the migration of people from these regions of the world
and the tendency of modern cultures to be more multi-cultural and
multi-racial. It is important for therapists to both know and understand
the culture-bound syndromes in the region of the world where they are
treating patients. It is also essential for therapists to know the lay terms
of regional psychological and physical conditions and to have the
matching scientific/psychiatric terms for effective communication with
colleagues.

Several studies in eastern societies (Das, 1991; Adityanjee, 1989;
Saxena, 1989) have noted that the ICD-10 (International Statistical
Classification of Diseases and Related Health Problems-Tenth Revision; World Health Organization [WHO], 1992) criteria for trance and
possession disorders, were more satisfactory than the DSM III-R (APA,
1987) classification system. The DSM-IV (APA, 1994) classifica-
tion/diagnostic system was seen as more similar to the ICD-10, due to
the suggested set of diagnostic criteria for "Dissociative trance disorder" (Kaplan, 1998). It is hoped that this diagnostic trend by psychiatry
academicians will continue to be followed in the area of possession
trance disorders and culture-bound syndromes.

CLINICAL PRESENTATION

Djinnati or Djinnoki is a term used widely by the Balooches (indigenous people living in Baloochistan) for a possession state, commonly seen in rural areas and typically managed by local healers.
This clinical presentation is an effort to better define the culture-
bound syndrome of Djinnati. It is based on a number of sources: the
observation of ten patients from the Sistan and Baloochistan provinces of Iran; the observation of a therapeutic session for extruding
(exorcising) the Djin (the entity which had captured the patient) by a
local healer (the priest named "Molla" in the region); and an interview with two local healers.

The subjects/patients were nine females and one male. The age range
was between ages 16 and 32, with the majority between ages 18 and 23.
Six of the "possessed" women were married and had been married at
very young ages (age 13-16). Eight of the patients lived in the rural area
and all of them were illiterate or primarily lettered. Their main com-
plaint was episodes of impaired consciousness and unresponsiveness to

external stimuli, confirmed by their family members. The patients were completely amnesic about the "attacks." Other common symptoms reported by relatives of the patients were: psychomotor agitation with a serious urge for escape, often accompanied by screaming; behaviors suggesting visual or auditory hallucination, e.g., looking scared and self talking; speaking in a changed voice, accent or even language; and a change in identity. The new identity was strange both to the patients and their relatives. It was typically of the opposite gender, and presented itself as an existing Djin, complete with a different name and address if asked. Eight patients were possessed by only one Djin, which presented itself in all of the attacks for those patients. Two of the patients were reportedly captured by multiple Djins, all of which presented themselves in each attack. The attacks lasted from a few minutes to a few hours, and had sudden onset and termination, sometimes culminating in a state of sleep. One of the patients had a positive history of psychiatric disorders and was previously diagnosed as having "Bipolar mood disorder." The other nine patients had no history of medical or psychiatric problems.

The common cultural belief was that the problem was not a psychiatric disorder, but a kind of spell which would be best treated by religious men, i.e., the local therapist/healer called "mulla." During a hypnotic-like process, utilizing spiritual words, the mulla would command and commonly threaten the Djin to leave the patient. The effect of the suggestive process was usually temporary and the condition had a high tendency for recurrence.

CASE EXAMPLE

Sheila is a 24-year-old married female who was brought to the clinic from Karachi of Pakistan by her brother (who translated his sister's Urdu language into English, as the patient did not speak Persian or English). She presented with the chief complaints of irritability, apprehension, impaired concentration and memory, restlessness, fearfulness and episodes of impaired consciousness and change of identity. The problems had developed gradually six months after her obligatory marriage at age13 to an age 40 wealthy widower. The husband had lost his previous wife in a serious car accident, surviving the accident along with his 10-year-old-son and eight-year-old daughter. The patient reported that her husband had a very ugly burn scar on the right side of his face as a result of the accident.

The attacks, as her brother explained, would start with a trance state after staring for a while. Then the patient would exhibit escape-like behavior, accompanied by screaming. The family would not leave her alone during these attacks and would prevent her from physically hurting herself. The patient would calm down after approximately three to five minutes and would begin to speak in a different voice in fluent English. During the attacks, the patient would introduce herself as a female Djin named Flora. Flora noted that she lived in England, but liked Sheila and her beautiful features and so would sometimes capture Sheila's body. Sheila, possessed by the Djin called Flora, behaved and spoke in a dis-inhibited way with the family, especially the son and daughter of her husband. The attacks would last up to one hour. The family would usually take the patient to the local healers to "push out" the Djin.

Sheila presented as a tall, beautiful, and polite lady who was born to a rural farming family in Saravan, a city and a region in Iran, next to the border of Pakistan. She was only allowed to attend primary school and, similar to other girls in the region, was compelled to marry at a very young age. She was the third child of the family of three girls and four boys, with no family history of psychiatric or medical disorders. There was no apparent psychotic or frank thought disorder evident in her mental status exam and she presented as very cooperative and reliable. She had no memory of the attacks or of Flora, but was aware that there are many episodes of amnesia when she didn't know what had happened.

DISCUSSION

Due to apparent impairments in consciousness, identity, and memory found in the cases studied, "Djinnati" would seem to be a dissociative condition as defined in the diagnostic category of "Trance and possession disorders" in ICD-10 or "Dissociative trance disorder" in DSM-IV.

Similar to other Dissociative conditions, a possession state may be seen as both a part of normative experience in one culture (e.g., religious experience), and symptomatic of disordered personality organization in other cultures (Pereira, 1995). There are at least three different perspectives for understanding the underlying psychopathological basis of possession disorders (Pereira, 1995).

Socio-cultural theories suppose that spirit possession is a culturally sanctioned, heavily institutionalized phenomenon, and that children were exposed to it from an early age, with an expectation that they may experience possession at a later date (Pereira,1995). It has also been argued that polytheism and belief in reincarnation and spirits may be related to the possession syndrome, whereas high social approval of deliberate role-playing may foster multiple personality disorder as a diagnosis (Varma, 1981). It has been reported that pathological spirit possession, especially in South Asia, has a similar etiology to multiple personality disorder in North America (Castillo,1994b) and we can consider both of them as variants in the same spectrum with obvious similarities. The differing presentations of the two disorders seem to be mostly due to culture differences. This perspective can lead to a better understanding of the effect of cultural beliefs on presenting psychiatric signs and symptoms. A strong religious belief about the presence of "Djin" in the region supports the socio-cultural theory in the Sistan and Baloochistan provinces.

Communication theory views possession as a form of communication, exhibited by those oppressed groups who are unable to communicate in another way. In many societies, the persons most affected are women and the poor. It has been proposed that possession and exorcism arise together when there is an oppressive social structure or a loss of trust in social institutions, or in conditions where protest is dangerous or unacceptable and there is a seeming inability to resolve social conflicts (Pereira,1995). In Iran and especially in deprived regions like Baloochistan, communication skills are not employed well in social relationships and young people have not learned those skills for application in later life. Children in these societies are taught to hide their feelings and not to express their emotional and even basic needs. Communication theory would also seem to be appropriate in explaining the development of Djinnati syndrome in these areas of Iran. The majority of the cases being from rural areas and occurring among illiterate women would also support this point of view.

One model of dissociative theory maintains that possession is explained as a return of repressed conflict or desires, where the *Id* wishes to overwhelm the *Ego* in a state of dissociation following a major psychological trauma. In this model, relief from *intrapsychic* tension is a primary gain, and attention and sympathy are secondary gains (Pereira, 1995). This psychoanalytic formulation may explain well the presence of Djinnati predominantly in young women who have married at early ages (ages 13-16). It is the senior author's belief that marriage at these early ages (especially with the intense pressure of the father) is a major psychological trauma (which may even be construed as a form of sexual abuse). Such abuse/trauma may be seen as probable precipitating factor(s) for dissociative conditions such as Djinnati. The predominant extended patriarchal family in these areas may also potentially expose both women and children to more serious psychological traumas. It may be, with respect to the religious beliefs and cultural restrictions noted, that possession by a "Djin" would be an acceptable means (by employing dissociative mechanisms) or applicable defense mechanism for relief from intrapsychic tension for the person's *Ego*.

The socio-cultural, communication and, dissociation theoretical models could well be applied to better understand Djinnati in the Baloochistan society. The dissociation theory would seem, however, to be the most relevant to understanding the prevalence of Djinnati in Baloochistan. This theory seems more applicable among the young illiterate women, living in rural areas with strong religious beliefs, with a history of unwanted marriage at early ages, in addition to the special interpersonal relationships (and thus, pressures) of extended patriarchal families. More research and longitudinal studies are needed to develop a more comprehensive knowledge in the epidemiology, etiology, diagnosis, and management of the possession state of Djinnati.

REFERENCES

Adityanjee, R.G.S. & Kandelwel, S.K. (1989) Current status of Multiple Personality Disorder in India. *American Journal of Psychiatry*. 146(12): 1607-10.

Alexander, P.J., Joseph, S., & Das, A. (1997). Limited utility of ICD-10 and DSM-IV classification of Dissociative and Conversion Disorder in India. *Acta Psychiatrica Scandinavia*. March; 95(3): 177-82. (abst)

Allison, R.B. (1985). The Possession Syndrome on trial. *American Journal of Forensic Psychiatry*. 6(1): 46-56.

American Psychiatric Association (1987). *Diagnostic and statistical manual of mental disorders-revised (3rd ed.)*. Washington, DC: Author.

American Psychiatric Association (1994). *Diagnostic and statistical manual of mental disorders (4th ed.)*. Washington, DC: Author.

American Psychiatric Association (2000). *Diagnostic and Statistical Manual of Mental Disorders-Text Revision*. Washington, DC: Author

Billu, Y. & Beit-Hallahmi, B. (1989). Dybbuk-Possession as a hysterical symptom: Psychodynamic and socio-cultural factors. *Israel Journal of Psychiatry Related Sciences*. 26(3): 138-49. (abst)

Castillo, R.J. (1994a). Spirit possession in South Asia, dissociation or hysteria? Part 1: Theoretical background. *Culture, Medicine & Psychiatry*. March; 18(1): 1-21.

Castillo, R.J. (1994b). Spirit possession in South Asia, dissociation or hysteria? Part 2: case histories. *Culture, Medicine & Psychiatry*. June; 18(2): 141-62. (abst)

Das, P.S. & Saxena, S. (1991). Classification of dissociative states in DSM-III-R and ICD-10 (1989 draft): A study of Indian out-patients. *British Journal of Psychiatry.* September; 159: 425-7.

Gaw, A.C., Ding, Q., Levine, R.E., & Gaw, H. (1998). The clinical characteristics of Possession Disorder among 20 Chinese patients in the Hebei Province of China. *Psychiatric Services.* Mar; 49(3): 360-5. (abst)

Grisaru, N., Budowski, D., & Witztum, E. (1997). Possession by the Zaramong Ethiopian immigrants to Israel: Psychopathology or Culture Bound Syndrome? *Psychopathology.* 30(4): 223-33.

Kaplan, H.I. & Sadock, B.J. (1998). *Synopsis of Psychiatry (8th Ed.).* Williams & Wilkins; p. 673.

Korolenko, C. & Muhamedzanov, H. (2001). Culture bound mental disorders among the Tatars of the Siberian North. *International Journal of Circumpolar Health.* April; 60(2): 275-9. (abst)

Kua, E.H., Sim, L.P., & Chee, K.T. (1986). A cross-cultural study of the possession-trance in Singapore. *Australia and New Zealand Journal of Psychiatry.* September; 20(3): 361-4.

Nelson, C. (1971). Spirit possession and world view: An illustration from Egypt. *International Journal of Social Psychiatry.* 17:194-209. (abst)

Obeysekere, G. (1970). The idiom of demonic possession: A case study. *Social Sciences and Medicine.* 4:97-111. (abst)

Pereira, S., Bhui, K., & Dein, S. (1995). Making sense of "Possession State": psychopathology and differential diagnosis. [Review]. *British Journal of Hospital Medicine.* June; 53(11): 582-6.

Pinerose, M., Rosselli, D., & Calderson, C. (1998). An epidemic of collective Conversion and Dissociation Disorder in an indigenous group of Colombia: Its relation to cultural change. *Social Sciences and Medicine.* June; 46(11): 1425-8; (abst)

Rhoades, G. F. Jr. (2003, May/June). Culture-bound syndromes. *The International Society for the Study of Dissociation NEWS,* 21, 3.

Sa-edi, G.H. (1975). *Ahle Hava.* Amir Kabir Pub. (Persian book)

Salisbury. R.F. (1968). Possession in the New Guinea Highlands. *International Journal of Social Psychiatry,* 14:85-94. (abst).

Saxena, S. & Prasad, K.V.S.R. (1989). DSM-III subclassification of Dissociative Disorders applied to psychiatric out-patients in India. *American Journal of Psychiatry.* February; 146(2): 261-2.

Shanmugan, T.E. (1981). *Abnormal psychology.* TATA: McGraw-Hill Publishing Co.; p. 171.

Varma, V.K., Bouri, M., & Wig, N.N. (1981). Multiple Personality in India: Comparison with Hysterical Possession State. *American Journal of Psychotherapy.* January; 35(1): 113-20.

World Health Organization (1992). *International Statistical Classification of Diseases and Related Health Problems-Tenth Revision.* Geneva: Author.

Advances in Dissociation Research and Practice in Israel

Eli Somer

SUMMARY. This essay covers the field of dissociation in Israel as reflected in publications by Israeli contributors and their collaborators both in the Hebrew language and in the international literature. With 140 references, this article covers the 24-year history of the field in this Middle Eastern country presenting documentations on dissociation in indigenous Middle Eastern culture, dissociation and the trauma of the Holocaust, a discussion of the "memory wars" in Israel, a portrayal of Israeli training programs in the field, an account of writing and publicity on dissociative disorders, a report on the process of acceptance of the concept in Israel and the development of advocacy in the field, as well as information on controlled Israeli research and clinical publications on dissociation. This literature review seems to indicate that dissociation is a useful paradigm that has aided Israeli scholars in the understanding of disavowed experiences in a variety of contexts. *[Article copies available for a fee from The Haworth Document Delivery Service: 1-800-HAWORTH. E-mail address: <docdelivery@haworthpress.com> Website: <http://www.HaworthPress.com> © 2005 by The Haworth Press, Inc. All rights reserved.]*

Eli Somer, PhD, is affiliated with the University of Haifa, Israel.

Address correspondence to: Eli Somer, PhD, Israel Institute for Treatment and Study of Stress, 5 David Pinski Street, Haifa 34351, Israel.

The author wishes to acknowledge Erez Zwerling for his invaluable assistance with the media and literature search.

[Haworth co-indexing entry note]: "Advances in Dissociation Research and Practice in Israel." Somer, Eli. Co-published simultaneously in *Journal of Trauma Practice* (The Haworth Maltreatment & Trauma Press, an imprint of The Haworth Press, Inc.) Vol. 4, No. 1/2, 2005, pp. 157-178; and: *Trauma and Dissociation in a Cross-Cultural Perspective: Not Just a North American Phenomenon* (ed: George F. Rhoades, Jr., and Vedat Sar) The Haworth Maltreatment & Trauma Press, an imprint of The Haworth Press, Inc., 2005, pp. 157-178. Single or multiple copies of this article are available for a fee from The Haworth Document Delivery Service [1-800-HAWORTH, 9:00 a.m. - 5:00 p.m. (EST). E-mail address: docdelivery@haworthpress.com].

KEYWORDS. Dissociation, Israel, trauma

This essay presents a comprehensive picture of the dissociation field in Israel by describing traditional, popular, clinical and scientific aspects of dissociation in the country. I will present a review of the collective efforts of local academics and clinicians and their international colleagues to study dissociation and its specific manifestations in this heterogeneous culture. Aspects of dissociation that are distinctive of Israeli culture, such as dissociation perspectives of Middle Eastern and Jewish culture, will be described in more detail than more universal topics concerning measurement of dissociation, correlative dissociation research, or clinical case studies.

Dissociation and indigenous Middle Eastern culture. In Jewish families of ancient times and in traditional contemporary Middle Eastern societies, familial needs and social convention have taken precedence over the needs of the individual. Self-esteem, dignity and social identity have been developed by the self-esteem, dignity and social identity of the family. Of the five basic human needs identified by Maslow (1970)– (1) physiological/biological needs; (2) the need for safety; (3) the need to belong and feel loved; (4) the need for personal self-esteem; and (5) the need to self-actualize–the first four have been provided by the traditional Middle Eastern family. However, this support is contingent upon individual compliance with the norms, directives and values of the family. This requires that the right to self-actualization be forfeited and that expression of sexual and aggressive feelings be severely curtailed. For example, Mid-Eastern tradition dictates that the individual expresses only love and positive regard for his or her parents. Expressions of frustration, anger or hatred are forbidden, even if the children are neglected or maltreated (Somer, 1977). These social values place certain individual needs (e.g., sexual needs or the need to vent anger) in conflict with the needs and will of the family. As such, the individual in the traditional Mid-Eastern society is forced to choose between one of two options. Making the conformist choice means that the individual has chosen to comply with the will of the family and to place the needs of the family above those of the individual. The individual can than expect to enjoy familial support and to have his or her needs met by the family. In return, one relinquishes needs pertaining to actualization of the self. Aggressive feelings towards members of the immediate and extended family are functionally repressed. The conformist choice actually

condones intrapsychic dissociation and repression as a means of cir-
cumventing conflict between the person and the society at large.

In contrast, the traditional Mid-Eastern individual who makes the
"self " choice has decided to individuate from the tribe/family by expressing disagreement with family decisions or norms and/or by choos-
ing to determine one's own life style (e.g., move out from the family
compound to live on one's own). These actions will be viewed by the
family as unacceptable, resulting in temporary sanctions and eventually
the withdrawal of familial support. Although this choice typically leads
to decreased intrapsychic repression and dissociation, there is a corresponding increase in conflicts between the person and the society at
large. Because traditional Mid-Eastern societies are so characteristi-
cally familial, self-assertion by oppressed women is typically met by rejection, sanctions, and inevitably by punishment and ostracizing (if not
murder) when sexual issues are involved (Al-Krenawi, 2000; Al-Krenawi,
Maoz, & Shiber, 1995).

These two choices determine whether the individual will face either
internal or external conflict. Opposing the family is very difficult because the individual has internalized traditional values as the result of
lifelong conditioning. The intrapsychic process of repression and dissociation is further facilitated by two socially sanctioned coping strategies, which are particularly evident among the Druze, Christian and
Muslim Arabs of the region and by Jews of Arab descent:

1. Mosaira–the practice of hiding one's true feelings and opinions
   and behaving only in ways that will please others. This strategy
   helps to ensure that socially appropriate behavior will be maintained and that rejection and punishment will be avoided.
2. Istigaba–the custom of criticizing others only in their absence, as
   well as the practice of performing forbidden acts "far from the
   eyes of society." This enables the individual to vent anger and
   gratify forbidden sexual drives and to disavow them when under
   the scrutiny of controlling others (Dwairy, 1993; Dwairy & Van
   Sickle, 1996).

Two main factors may affect the severity of the individual-family
conflict: the level of acculturation and gender. In traditional Mid-Eastern societies, where women face severe oppression and have no control
over significant choices, sanctions against disobedient women often extend to termination of familial support and include home imprisonment,
physical beating, clitoral circumcision, and even threats to their lives if

the "honor of the family" is construed to be threatened. In these societies, complete adherence to existing social expectations is the only choice for females, while Istigaba is not available for venting. The traditional Mid-Eastern woman is forced to regulate the self in order to survive. Under these conditions, the expression of distress is almost always dissociated and somatized (Somer, 1993), particularly if the distress originates in interpersonal conflict. Traditions in these societies allow for dissociated and somatized distress to be expressed in ways that reinforce the supremacy of male-dominated society and validate religion, namely, hysterical conversive, somatoform and possession phenomena (Bilu & Beit Hallahmi, 1989).

Through these phenomena, forbidden behaviors and expressions of affect are then construed as "non-me" experiences that are outside the woman's realm of control. These loci of control are regarded as Dybbuks (Somer, 1997a, 2004), Jinns, spirits or the acts of God (Bilu, 1987, 2000). To deal with these conditions, there is a need to appease God or the possessing agents or to confront them with invocations of God's powers by calling on him and invoking his holy names (Somer & Saadon, 2000). The rituals are normally conducted by representatives of male-dominated religion and society, such as shamans, mystics, rabbis, imams, or Muslim clergy and psychics (Grisaru, Budowski, & Witztum, 1997). Some rituals documented in Israel among Jews from North African descent have been influenced by black African traditions and often involve rhythmic movements and dance accompanied by drum beats (Somer & Saadon, 2000). The desired result is typically a hypnotic trance, which reaches a peak with convulsive movements and loss of memory. Sometimes afflicted women disrobe during the ritual and verbalize profanities that are said to be the demon's words.

Jewish wisdom and dissociation. Jewish thought in the Land of Israel had regarded the self as being made up of subsystems long before Pierre Janet (1859-1947) introduced his dissociation theory and his model of the functional and structural elements of the mind (Janet, 1889). Possession trance in Judaism is probably best understood within the context of Kabbalist polypsychic philosophy. The Kabbalist book *The Zohar* (Book of Radiance, Tishbi, 1982) is a mainstay of Jewish sacred thought and describes the human psyche as being composed of three main souls: *nefesh,* which is a spiritual force that brings the dimension of vitality into being; *ruach,* which is responsible for human emotions and characteristics; and *neshama,* which is a spiritual-intellectual guiding soul whose task is to guide and correct evil traits. Many folkloristic possession tales inspired by Kabbalist tradition contain the term *dybbuk* (in Hebrew the term denotes a clinging, clutching, an adhering agent).

Recently, Somer (2004) analyzed sixteenth-century *dybbuk* accounts from the Near East and demonstrated a striking resemblance between these eyewitness accounts and modern attributes of Dissociative Identity Disorder (DID). Demonic beliefs were strongly held by many Jews who immigrated to modern-day Israel from Arab countries. In Morocco, for example, a former homeland of many Israeli Jews, demons were accorded a central role in structuring and explaining daily events (Crapanzano, 1973). Jews of the Maghreb integrated many demonic traditions of their neighboring Muslims into their spiritual rituals (Ben-Ami, 1969; Bilu, 1980, 1982). In fact, more than half of the 104 ailments identified among patients of Moroccan Jewish traditional healers in Israel turned out to be of demonic causation (Bilu, 1983, 1985). The synthesis of North (Bilu, 1987) and East African influences (Witztum, Grisaru, & Budowski, 1996), Arab influences (Al-Krinawi, 2000; Daie, Witztum, Mark, & Rabinowitz, 1992; Dwairy, 1993), and polypsychic Jewish mystical philosophy (Somer, 2004a; Witztum, Buchbinder, & Van der Hart, 1990) have played an important role in the development of culture-sensitive assessment and treatment techniques not only for (what would be regarded by Western medicine as) hysterical (e.g., Somer, 1993; Van der Hart, Witztum, & Friedman, 1992) and dissociative psychopathology (e.g., Somer, 1997a), but also for psychotic symptomatology (e.g., Greenberg, Witztum, & Buchbinder, 1992) among traditional societies in Israel.

Dissociation and the trauma of the Holocaust. A 1993 examination of approximately 5,000 long-term psychiatric inpatients in Israel identified about 900 Holocaust survivors. Laub (2003) hypothesized that many of these patients could have avoided lengthy, if not lifelong, psychiatric hospitalizations had they been enabled by their therapists (and by society at large) to more openly share their severe persecution history. Instead, their traumatic experiences remained encapsulated, causing the survivors to lead a double life: a robot-like semblance to normality with incessant haunting by nightmares and flashbacks. Dissociation was a central finding in a study on elderly survivors of the Holocaust (Yehuda et al., 1996). The silence of the survivors never meant that the horror of their suffering was absent from behaviors, attachments, and parenting (Durst, 2003; Moskovitz, & Krell, 1990). In fact, their inability to verbalize and openly process their pain and that which they inflicted on the second generation rendered some of their children more fragile and vulnerable. One of the more provocative Israeli studies on survivors of the Holocaust and their offspring by Solomon,

Kotler, and Miculincer (1988) found that children of Holocaust survivors were more likely than other soldiers to develop PTSD following deployment in the Lebanon War. Barocas and Barocas (1983) reported not only on the alarming number of children of survivors seeking and requiring help, but also of the nature of their symptoms. They found that the offspring of Holocaust survivors presented symptomatology and psychiatric features bearing a striking resemblance to the concentration camp survivor syndrome described in the international literature, and that these children showed symptoms that would be expected if they had actually lived through the Holocaust. Yehuda et al. (1998) actually found correlations between the individual PTSD symptoms in the holocaust survivor parents and their children. Positive correlations were present for flashbacks, avoidance of situations that are reminders of the Holocaust, and emotional detachment. Additionally, there was a significant association between dissociative experiences, as reflected by DES scores in parents and children.

Dissociative amnesia among Israeli survivors of the Nazi persecution was also documented in several clinical case studies (e.g., Modai, 1994; Somer, 1994a) and other articles suggesting specific assessment procedures (Van der Hart & Brom, 2000) as well as intervention techniques for the treatment of dissociative survivors of the Nazi genocide (e.g., Somer, 1995). Compelling testimonies from the survivors of the experiments on twins performed in Auschwitz by Dr. Mengele contained descriptions of traumatic dissociation such as:

> A few of the twins insisted that they had no memories of Auschwitz whatsoever. Instead, they dwelt on the sadness of their postwar adult lives–their emotional upheavals, physical breakdowns, and longings for the dead parents they had hardly known. (Lagnado & Dekel, 1991, p. 8)

The coping of Holocaust survivors with traumatic memories is of obvious interest to Israeli clinicians, as reflected in several studies (e.g., Mazor, Ganpel, Enright, & Ornstein, 1990). Attempts have also been made to conceptualize the extraordinary compartmentalization of the horrors endured by persecuted Jewish children in terms of structural dissociation (Tauber, 1966). Among the most interesting inquiries performed in Israel on survivors of the Holocaust are the studies of Kaminer and Lavie on memory of dreams and mental health of survivors (e.g., Kaminer & Lavie, 1991, 1993, 1996; Lavie & Kaminer, 1991). They found that well-adjusted Holocaust survivors managed to banish memories of their wartime tribulations even from their dreams. Sleepers awakened from dreaming sleep in the sleep laboratory normally recall dreams about 80 percent of the time. The well-adjusted survivors, however, did so only about a third of the time. Survivors who had problems with work, family life, or health slept more fitfully and often dreamed that they were in danger or even back in the concentration camp. Dreams of the less-adjusted had significantly higher scores for general anxiety, guilt anxiety, diffused anxiety, general aggression, inwardly directed aggression, and interpersonal conflicts than the controls. The less-adjusted also dreamed significantly more than the other two groups about their childhood.

Despite the evidence that some survivors of the Holocaust repressed their memories of childhood trauma and continuously repressed fresh memories of relevant dream content, the doubts raised in North America about the very existence of repression of trauma and the veracity of repressed memories was faintly echoed in Israel as well.

Echoes of the "memory wars" in Israel. Israel does not tend to be a litigious society, and malpractice compensations awarded by Israeli courts have generally been quite modest. This may explain why, to the best of my knowledge, no damages have ever been awarded to plaintiffs in repressed/recovered memory malpractice suits in Israel. In fact, I am not aware of any such cases ever submitted to local courts. Nevertheless, the recovered memory controversy that has troubled the field in North America (Campbell, 2002) has not completely evaded Israel. In 1997, a conference entitled *Childhood Trauma: Recovered Memory Therapy or False Memory Syndrome?* was organized in Bar Ilan University near Tel Aviv. The keynote speaker was Dr. Elizabeth Loftus. Yielding to the demands of various advocacy groups for equal time in this highly contested issue, the university invited Dr. Richard Kluft to address the audience following Loftus' talk. The organizer of the conference, who also gave the opening address (Nachshon, 1977), presented his viewpoint in one more conference held in Israel during the following year (Nachshon, 1998a). He then proceeded to publish his thoughts locally (Nachshon, 1998b) and internationally (Nachshon, 2000).

It seems that at least one experimental research thesis on false memory utilizing a word recall paradigm was submitted to Bar Ilan University (Goldberg-Busheri, 2002), but this line of inquiry seems to have been largely abandoned. Other than an update on the "false memory syndrome," which was published during the same year by the journal of the Israel Medical Association (Nemetz, 2002), no further Israeli research projects on this issue have been identified. Yet, two influential

Israeli newspapers featured science stories positing that false trauma memories can be installed in the minds of people (Siegel-Itzkovich, 1996; Slonim, 1997). An opposing view explaining the phenomenon of repressed, suppressed, recovered, and delayed reporting of child abuse memories was extensively presented locally and featured in Israel's leading psychotherapy journal (Somer, 1994b; Margalit & Witztum, 1997a, 1997b), as well as published internationally (Somer & Szwarcberg, 2001; Somer & Weiner, 1996), and in a Hebrew article posted on the Internet (Somer, 1997b).

One of the most compelling sources on the validity of repressed memories of trauma has been the field of combat trauma. Israel, a country that has been battling for its existence since its independence in 1948, has borne the consequences of war trauma, making it possible to document combat-induced dissociative amnesia (e.g., Witztum, Margalit, & Van der Hart, 2002), and the reality of forgetting traumatic experiences.

Advances in Israeli training, writing and publicity on dissociative disorders. Although Israeli psychoanalyst Emmanuel Berman wrote some of the first clinical articles on multiple personality disorder (MPD, now termed dissociative identity disorder, DID) ever published in the international clinical literature (Berman, 1973, 1974, 1975, 1981a, 1981b), it was only in 1987 that interest in this phenomenon budded in Israel. Van der Hart gave a two-day workshop on diagnosis and treatment of MPD for members of the Israel Hypnosis Society, and at the Third National Conference of the same society, I presented the first Hebrew language scholarly lecture on the diagnosis and treatment of MPD (Somer, 1987). Two years later, I also published the first Hebrew language peer-reviewed article on MPD (Somer, 1989), which was also commented on by Berman (1989). Since then, numerous in-service workshops and presentations on the topic have been held at the Haifa office of Maytal–Israel Institute for Treatment and Study of Stress.

The 12th International Congress of Hypnosis, held in Jerusalem in July of 1992, gave interested Israeli clinicians an opportunity to attend an MPD clinical workshop given by Dr. Richard P. Kluft (Van der Hart, 1993). Following this workshop, several clinicians expressed an interest in continued education in the field. This curiosity was probably reinforced by the popular non-fiction book on the subconscious mind that was published during the same period by a respected Bar Ilan University psychologist. The book featured a clear account on the differences between repression and dissociation (Orbach, 1992).

On March 22, 1993, I presented the first Hebrew language workshop on the diagnosis and treatment of MPD. I taught the second workshop on this subject in the summer of the same year during the Israel Psychological Society's Annual Workshops. In the late 1990s, learning opportunities in Israel on dissociative disorders expanded to include graduate courses at the University of Haifa and at Bar Ilan University, as well as the official training course for the treatment of dissociative disorders offered in Israel through the International Society for the Study of Dissociation.

Several popular books on MPD sold in Israel during the 1980s and 1990s added to the public's interest in pathological dissociation. Among them were the Hebrew translations of Keyes' *The minds of Billy Milligan* (1995), published in Israel in 1982; Schreiber's *Sybil* (1973), Hebrew version published in 1987; and Fraser's *My father's house: A memoir of incest and healing* (1989), published in Hebrew in 1994. More recently in 2002, Cameron West's *First person plural: My life as a multiple* (1999) was also translated. Another very significant book to survivors, clinicians and scholars of chronic trauma was Herman's classic *Trauma and recovery* (1992), published in Hebrew in 1997.

Since the mid-1990s, when an Israeli organization of incest survivors was formed in Tel Aviv, a newsletter entitled Makhbarote Khesbone (Account Notebooks), containing mostly survivor poetry and art, has been published on a regular basis. Many of the contributions have described the inner world of structural dissociation and various other dissociative experiences. The turn of the millennium was marked by the publication of several compelling and commercial best-selling Hebrew language autobiographical accounts of Israeli survivors in which they described their dissociative experiences and psychopathology (e.g., Read, 2002; Shalev, 2000), recounted their treatment (Bergamn & Sara, 1998) or shared their poetry (Shaz, 1999). Evidence of the growing professional interest and legitimization of post-abusive dissociative pathology is perhaps best demonstrated by the favorable book reviews on Read's (2002) autobiography published in *Sihot–Israel Journal of Psychotherapy* (Yahav, 2003) and in *Psychoactualia*, the newsletter of the Israel Psychological Association (Bar Sadeh, 2004). The latter contained illuminating paragraphs on dissociation. Another influential best-seller in Israel that credibly presented dissociative psychopathology was an "Irving Yalom-style" book that described in two separate chapters interesting vignettes on posttraumatic amnesia and dissociative psychopathology (Yovel, 2001). Finally, in 2004, a comprehensive Hebrew textbook on incest published as a joint venture between a commercial publisher and The Tel Aviv University featured several original chapters on the role of dissociation in the lives of survivors (e.g., Somer, E., 2004b; Somer, L. 2004; Scwarzberg & Somer, 2004).

The Internet, rightfully dubbed "the information super-highway," has also developed into a useful source of Hebrew language information on dissociation. Pamphlets and articles on dissociative psychopathology are available for retrieval from Web sites for survivor support and advocacy (e.g., macom.org.il; voices.co.il; www.sahar.org.il); pharmaceutical companies (e.g., tevalife.co.il); and treatment centers (e.g., maytal.co.il; machoneitan.org.il). This surge in non- and semi-academic writing on severe dissociative disorders has also been accompanied by a plethora of professional writings on the subject published both locally, in Hebrew (e.g., Somer, 1989, 1994b, 1995d), and internationally (e.g., Somer & Nave, 2001; Somer, & Yishai, 1997).

Dissociation: acceptance and advocacy. Further evidence of the budding awareness and interest in dissociative psychopathology in Israel was provided in a survey of the attitudes of 211 practicing clinicians in Israel toward dissociative disorders (DD) and DID (Somer, 2000a). Of the sample, 95.5% percent scored at or above the midpoint on a 5-point Likert scale measuring belief in the validity of DDs; 84.5% declared at least a moderate belief in the validity of DID. The average Israeli clinician surveyed had made 4.8 career-long DD diagnoses and carried an average of 1.05 DD patients in his/her current caseload. The findings of this survey suggested that attitudes of Israeli clinicians were similar to those of North American clinicians, despite the geographical and cultural differences between them.

This growing awareness of the dissociative consequences of severe childhood traumatization was also utilized in a successful lobbying for the extension of the statute of limitations on incest crimes in Israel. In an attempt to interpret to the legislators some of the freeze responses of non-resisting (peri-dissociating) rape victims and in a separate effort to prolong the old 10-year statute of limitations, op-ed articles were published in a leading Israeli newspaper (e.g., Somer, 1993, December 9; Somer, 1994, May 24). Data on peri-traumatic dissociation (Somer, 1994c) and on delayed calls for help from incest survivors to the rape crisis hotlines were presented to members of the parliament's judicial committee (Nimrod & Somer, 1995; Somer, 1994d). Incest victims' apparent aloofness and lack of resistance to alleged defendants' crimes have been difficult for the prosecution to explain to the Israeli courts. A number of workshops conducted by this author for state prosecutors of sex offenders in the mid-1990s aided attorneys to better understand delayed reporting and dissociative behavior that may have wrongly implied compliance. This growing understanding resulted in numerous invited affidavits and expert testimonies that were cited in the verdicts of numerous convicted offenders (e.g., Somer, 1994e).

Advances in Israeli dissociation research. Several instruments measuring dissociation have been translated into Hebrew over the years. Among them are the Dissociative Experiences Scale (H-DES; Somer, 1992); the Adolescent Dissociative Experiences Scale (H-A-DES; Somer, 1996); the Childhood Dissociation Questionnaire (1995b); the Structured Clinical Interview for Dissociative Disoders (H-SCID-D; 1995c); and the Multimodal Inventory of Dissociation (H-MID, 2002a). Research has shown that translated dissociation measures demonstrate strong internal consistencies, statistical reliabilities and construct validities when tested in the culturally diverse Israeli society (Somer & Dell, 2005; Somer, Dolgin, & Saadon, 2001). The most well-known assessment tool in the field, the DES, has been used in several graduate research theses supervised by Bar Ilan University (e.g., Herman, 1994; Krigel-Luski, 2001) and University of Haifa faculty (e.g., Avni, 2000; Bar, 1999; Finkelstein, 2004; Tzarfati, 2001).

The understandable interest of Israeli scholars in the course of PTSD development has steered some local research into the investigation of peri-traumatic antecedents of PTSD. A number of quantitative studies have examined the role of peri-traumatic dissociation in the development of PTSD (e.g., Shalev, Freedman, Peri, Brandes, & Sahar, 1997; Shalev, Peri, & Canetti, 1996) and identified it as significantly predictive of PTSD symptomatology four months following exposure to the traumatic event (Freedman, Brandes, Peri, & Shalev, 1999). Several Israeli qualitative studies have shown that peri-traumatic dissociation plays an important role in the sexual victimization of female clients by their male psychotherapists (e.g., Ben Ari & Somer, 2004; Somer & Nachmani, in press; Somer & Saadon, 1999) and in the coping of emergency room social workers vicariously traumatized during terror attacks (Peled-Avram, Ben-Yizhack, Gagin, Somer, & Buchbinder, 2004; Somer, Buchbinder, Peled-Avram, & Ben-Yizhack, 2004).

The role of dissociation in the etiology of suicide has been the focus of investigation for a Bar Ilan University research group led by Israel Orbach. These academics have shown that the life narrative of a suicidal person can be formulated in terms of a sequence of losses associated with unbearable mental pain, including the belief that a person is unneeded and useless (Orbach, 1994). The loathed self is said to be reified in actual self-hate, and a total mental offence on the self ensues. In a phenomenological investigation into mental pain, Orbach and Mikulincer (2000) concluded that the mental pain syndrome constitutes dissociative aspects that are predictable of suicidality, such as a sense of loss of control, emotional freezing, and estrangement (Orbach, 1994, 1996; Orbach, Kedem, Herman, & Apter, 1995). They have also demonstrated that suicidal individuals experience their body differently from other populations and that these changes are related to suicidal behavior. Their bodily experiences include rejection of the body, detachment, numbness, physical anhedonia, and lack of self-care (e.g., Orbach, Lotem-Peleg, & Kedem, 1995; Orbach, Mikulincer, King, Cohen, & Stein, 1997).

Although this group seemed to be rather unconcerned by the etiology of these dissociative traits, several other Israeli publications attempted to show the link between childhood trauma and dissociative pathology, among them a book review (e.g., Somer, 1997c), literature review articles (e.g., Bar-Guy & Shalev, 2001), and empirical research papers demonstrating significant statistical pathways connecting dissociation with childhood trauma, as well as with distressful introspectiveness and maladaptive daydreaming (Somer, 2002a, 2002b). The interest in the traumatic etiology of dissociative psychopathology was also reflected in several other Israeli research studies showing that posttraumatic dissociation was a predictor of a later proclivity to seek chemical dissociation through opiate use (Avni, 2000, 2002; Somer, 2003, in press; Somer & Avni, 2003) and a probable factor in the tendency of survivors to seek solace in the arms of misguided male therapist offenders (Somer, 1999). The relationship between chronic traumatization and dissociative pathology was extensively described in several Hebrew language literature reviews published in the *Journal of the Israel Medical Association* (Eldar, Stein, Toren, & Witztum, 1997), in the *Israel Journal of Psychotherapy* (Bar-Guy & Shalev, 2001), and in a textbook on the psychological sequels of incest (Somer, 2004b).

Clinical articles. Although several Israeli scholars have contributed significantly to the promotion of the understanding of dissociation among professionals locally and worldwide, an examination of the list of contributors in the reference list of this essay reveals that much of the Israeli writing in the field can be attributed to a small number, most of whom are academics rather than field workers. My examination of the programs offered by local psychiatry, social work and psychology conferences has revealed that the field of dissociation is under-represented in these meetings. The picture is not much different where clinical publications on dissociative psychopathology are concerned. A few Israeli clinicians have contributed to the understanding of such clinical issues as the relationship between hypnosis and structural dissociative phenomena (Arlow, 1992), the relationship between hypnotic trance and dissociation (Somer, 1995d), and the manifestations of dissociation in the artwork of dissociative clients (Somer & Somer, 1997a, 1997b). Clinical articles by Israeli therapists have suggested various treatment strategies, including short-term therapies in posttraumatic conversion reactions (Daie & Witztum, 1991; Grisaru, Gelbar, & Witztum, 1999) and techniques for working with aging survivors (Somer, 2000b), but good case studies and treatment-oriented articles in Hebrew are scarce, possibly reflecting the early evolutionary state of the field in Israel.

CONCLUSION

This essay describes the field of dissociation study in Israel. Well over 100 cited publications addressing a broad array of topics were presented. This literature review seems to indicate that dissociation is a useful paradigm that has aided Israeli scholars in the understanding of disavowed experiences in a variety of contexts. Israeli anthropologists, scholars of religion, personality researchers, clinical social workers, psychoanalysts, clinical psychologists, psychiatrists, substance abuse counselors, sleep disorder specialists, and social activists have shared their observations on the role that dissociation has played in the lives of oppressed and traumatized Israelis. The findings are encouraging. The growing awareness regarding the role of dissociation in the mental health of traumatized Israelis guarantees that earlier attention will be given to unprocessed trauma, thereby offering enhanced chances of recovery. The evidence provided here regarding the usefulness of the dissociative model in an ethnically diverse Middle Eastern country such as Israel also renders further support to the validity of dissociation theory, habitually contested by some North American clinicians and memory scholars. Despite the relative wealth of knowledge on dissociation disseminated by Israeli writers, a good deal has been accomplished by relatively few. Future efforts should be invested in promoting the teaching of dissociative dynamics to Israeli clinicians, with the aim of augmenting diagnostic and treatment skills to offset a pathology mostly associated with oppression and abuse.

REFERENCES

Arlow, J.A. (1992). Altered ego states. *Israel Journal of Psychiatry and Related Sciences, 29*(2), 65-76.

Avni, R. (2000). *The phenomenology of drug abuse among high-dissociating recovering heroin addicts.* Thesis submitted to the University of Haifa.

Avni, R. (2002). Khavayat ha'nitook hamooseget be'emtzoot hasheemoosh be'sumeem [The experience of dissociation achieved through substance use]. *Miksumim–Newsletter of Ministry of Welfare Service for the Treatment Drug Users, 1,* 54-57

Al-Krenawi, A. (2000). *Etno-psykhiatria ba'khevra ha'bedouit-araveet ba'negev* [Ethno-psychiatry among the Bedouin-Arab of the Negev]. Tel-Aviv: Hakibbutz Hameuchad Publishing House.

Al-Krenawi, A., Maoz, B., Shiber, A. (1995). Sheloov ma'arkhote modernioterefooiote im amahmiote-datiote be'tipool nafshee be'bedouiim [The integration of modern-medical systems with folkloristic-religious systems in the psychological treatment of the Bedouin], *Sihot–Israel Journal of Psychotherapy, 10*(1), 42-48.

Bar, E. (1999). *The relationship between self-awareness, dissociation, emotional distress and well-being, and traumatization in women.* Thesis submitted to the University of Haifa.

Bar-Guy, N., & Shalev, A. (2001). Hashpaote shel hit'aleloot beshnote hayaldoot al psikhopathologhia bemvoogarim [The effects of child abuse on adult psychopathology]. *Sihot–Israel Journal of Psychotherapy, 6*(3), 180-194.

Bar Sadeh, N. (2004). *Maya Read–"Shvooya."* Psychoaktualia, (July, 2004 issue), 18-21.

Barocas, H., & Barocas, C. (1983). Wounds of the fathers: The next generation of Holocaust victims. *International Review of Psychoanalysis, 5,* 331-341.

Ben-Ami, I. (1969). Nukhekhoot shedim ba'bah'it ha'yahoodie maroccai [The presence of the demons in the Jewish Moroccan house] *Proceedings of the Fifth World Congress for Judaic Studies.* Jerusalem: The World Organization for Judaic Studies.

Ben Ari, A., & Somer, E. (2004). The aftermath of therapist-client sex: Exploited women struggle with the consequences. *Clinical Psychology and Psychotherapy, 11,* 126-136.

Bergamn, Z., & Sara (1998). *Ahavah zeh loh sukeen* [Love is not a knife]. Tel Aviv: Yediot Aharonot.

Berman, E. (1973). The development and dynamics of multiple personality. Ann Arbor, Michigan: University Microfilms International.

Berman, E. (1974). Multiple personality: Theoretical approaches. *Journal of the Bronx State Hospital, 2,* 99-107.

Berman, E. (1975, August). Tested and documented split personality: Veronica and Nelly. *Psychology Today,* pp. 78-81.

Berman, E. (1981a). Multiple personality: Psychoanalytic perspectives. *International Journal of Psychoanalysis, 62,* 283-300.

Berman, E. (1981b). "Pram lamentis," or she's a young thing and cannot leave her mother. *Family Process*, *20*, 449-451.

Berman, E. (1989). Comments on Eli Somer's article on Multiple Personality. *Sihot– Israel Journal of Psychotherapy*, *3*(3), 225.

Bilu, Y. & Beit Hallahmi, B. (1989). Dybbuk possession as a hysterical symptom. Psychodynamic and socio-cultural factors. *Israel Journal of Psychiatry*, *26*(3), 138-149.

Bilu, Y. (1980). The Moroccan demon in Israel. The case of 'Evil Spirit Disease.' *Ethos*, *8*, 1, 24-38.

Bilu, Y. (1982). Tafkeed hashydeem be'hasbare makhalote bekarave ychooday morocco be'Israel [The role of demons in explicating illnesses among Moroccan Jews in Israel]. *Jerusalem Studies in Jewish Folklore*, *2*, 102-123.

Bilu, Y. (1983). Ha'dybbuk ba'yahadoot. Makhalut nefesh ke'mashuv tarbooti [The Dybbuk in Judaism. Mental disorder as a cultural resource]. *Jerusalem Studies in Jewish Thought*, *2*, 4, 529-563.

Bilu, Y. (1985). The taming of the deviants and beyond. An analysis of Dybbuk Possession and exorcism in Judaism. In: Boyer, L.B., Grolnick, S.A. (Hg.): *The Psychoanalytic Study of Society*, 11. New Jersey (The Analytic Press), 1-32.

Bilu, Y. (1987). Dybbuk possession and mechanisms of internalization and externalization. In: Sandler, J. (Hg.): *Projection, Identification, and Projective Identification*. New York (International Universities Press), 163-178.

Bilu, Y. (2000). Islai, Dybbuk, Zar: Neevdalote tarbootiote ve'hamshikhiyoot historeet be'makhalote ikhooz [Islai, Dybbuk, Zar: Cultural differentiation and historical continuity in possession afflictions in Jewish communities]. *Pe'amim–Studies in Oriental Jewry*, *85*, 131-148.

Campbell, P.C. (2002). Hypnosis, demand characteristics, and "Recovered Memory" Therapy. *Prevention & Treatment*, *5*, Article 40, posted October 18, *http://www.journals. apa.org/prevention/volume5/pre0050040c.html* accessed Oct. 4th, 2004.

Crapanzano, V. (1973). *The Hamadsha: A study in Moroccan ethno-psychiatry*. Berkeley: University of California Press.

Daie, N., & Witztum, E. (1991). Short-term strategic treatment in traumatic conversion reactions. *American Journal of Psychotherapy*, *55*, 335-347.

Daie, N., Witztum, E., Mark, M., & Rabinowitz, S. (1992). The belief in the transmigration of souls: Psychotherapy of a Druze patient with severe anxiety reaction. *British Journal of Medical Psychology*, 65, 119-130.

Durst, N. (2003). Child-Survivors of the Holocaust: Age-specific traumatization and the consequences for therapy. *American Journal of Psychotherapy*, *57*, (4) 499-518.

Dwairy, M., & Van Sickle, T.D. (1996). Western psychotherapy in traditional Arabic societies. *Clinical Psychology Review*, 16 (3), 231-299.

Dwairy, M. (1993). *Mental health among Arabs in Israel* (Hebrew). Paper presented at mental health conference, Nazareth, Israel.

Eldar, Z., Stein, D., Toren, P., & Witztum, E. (1997). Tismonayt hafra'at zehut dissotziyativit be'yeladeem u'mitbagreem [Dissociative Identity Disorder in children and adolescents]. *Harefuah–Journal of the Israel Medical Association*, *133*(1-2), 36-40.

Fraser, S. (1989). *My father's house: A memoir of incest and healing*. London: Virago. The book was published (1994) in Israel in Hebrew by Am Oved.

Finkelstein, M. (2004). *Traumatic stress, coping resources and psychological adjustment among Ethiopian immigrants in Israel*. Doctoral thesis submitted to the University of Haifa.

Freedman, S.A., Brandes, D., Peri, T., & Shalev, A. (1999). Predictors of chronic post-traumatic stress disorder: A prospective study. *British Journal of Psychiatry, 174*, 353-359.

Goldberg-Busheri, M. (2002). *Real and false memories: Discrimination according to accessibility*. Graduate Theses submitted to Bar Ilan University.

Greenberg, D., Witztum, E., & Buchbinder, J., (1992). Mysticism and psychosis: The fate of Ben Zoma. *British Journal of Medical Psychology, 65*, 223-235.

Grisaru N, Budowski D, & Witztum E. (1997). Possession by the 'Zar' among Ethiopian immigrants to Israel: Psychopathology or culture-bound syndrome? *Psychopathology, 30*(4), 223-33.

Grisaru, N., Gelbar, D., & Witztum, E. (1999). Tipool astrateggi meshoolove be'narcoanalysa, be'hafra'a conversiveet posttraumatit [An integrative strategic treatment with narcoanalysis in a posttraumatic conversive disorder]. *Sihot–Israel Journal of Psychotherapy, 13*(2), 135-141.

Herman, L. (1994). *Changes in attitudes toward life and death and in dissociation*. Thesis submitted to Bar Ilan University.

Herman, L. J. (1992). *Trauma and recovery*. NY: Basic Books. The book was published (1997) in Israel in Hebrew by Am Oved.

Janet, P. (1889). *L'Automatisme psychologique*. Paris: Félix Alcan. New edition: Société Pierre Janet, Paris, 1973.

Kaminer, H., & Lavie, P. (1991). Sleep and dreaming in Holocaust survivors. *The Journal of Nervous and Mental Disease, 179* (11), 664-669.

Kaminer, H., & Lavie, P. (1993). Sleep and dreams in well-adjusted and less adjusted Holocaust surviviors. In M. S. Stroebe, W. Stroebe, & R. O. Hansson (Eds.), *Handbook of bereavement: Theory, research, and intervention* (pp. 331-345). Cambridge, MA: Cambridge University Press.

Keyes, D. (1995). *The minds of Billy Milligan*. New York: Bantam, The book was published (1982) in Israel in Hebrew by Cherikover.

Krigel-Luski, Y. (2001). *Reference to the body and investment in it, dissociation and defense mechanisms among adolescent girls diagnosed with Anorexia Nervosa and suicidal girls*. Thesis submitted to Bar Ilan University.

Lagnado, L.M., & Dekel, S.C. (1991). *Children of the flames: Dr. Josef Mengele and the untold story of the twins of Auschwitz*. New York: William and Morrow.

Laub, D. (2003). Video testimony pilot study of psychiatrically hospitalized Holocaust survivors, Holocaust Trauma Project, Yale University Genoside Studies Program, *http://www.yale.edu/gsp/trauma_project/index.html* accessed Oct.1, 2004.

Lavie, P., & Kaminer, H. (1996). Sleep, dreaming, and coping style in Holocaust survivors. In D. Barrett (Ed.), *Trauma and dreams* (pp. 114-124). Cambridge, MA: Harvard University Press.

Lavie, P., & Kaminer, H. (1991). Dreams that poison sleep: Dreaming in Holocaust survivors. *Dreaming: Journal of the Association for the Study of Dreams, 1*(1), 11-21.

Margalit, H., & Witztum, E. (1997a). Trauma, amnesia, ve'dissotziatzia: Heybeteam kliniyim ve'teyoretyim, khaylek beit–Skeerah tayoretit [Trauma, amnesia and dissociation–Clinical and theoretical aspects. Part I: Theoretical revue]. *Sihot–Israel Journal of Psychotherapy, 11* (3), 214-217.

Margalit, C. & Witztum, E. (1997b). Trauma, amnesia, ve'dissotziatzia: Heybeteam kliniyim ve'teyoretyim, khaylek beit–Tey'oor mikray [Trauma, amnesia and dissociation: Clinical and theoretical perspectives. Part two–A case study]. *Sihot–Israel Journal of Psychotherapy, 12*(1), 44-50.

Maslow, A. (1970). *Motivation and personality* (2nd ed.). New York: Harper & Row.

Mazor, A., Ganpel, Y., Enright, R.D., & Ornstein, R. (1990). Holocaust survivors: Coping with posttraumatic memories in childhood and 40 years later. *Journal of Traumatic Stress, 3*, 11-14.

Modai, I. (1994). Forgetting childhood: A defense mechanism against psychosis in a Holocaust survivor. In T. L. Brink, (Ed.), *Holocaust survivors' mental health*. New York: The Haworth Press, Inc.

Moskovitz, S., & Krell, R. (1990). Child survivors of the Holocaust: Psychological adaptations to survival. *Israel Journal of Psychiatry and Related Services, 27*, 81-91.

Nachson, I. (1997). Me'zeekarone mashookhzar le'zeekarone mesooluf ve'khuzarah [From recovered memory to false memory, and back]. Opening address delivered at the meetings of a conference on *Childhood Trauma: Recovered Memory Therapy or False Memory Syndrome?* Ramat-Gan, June, 1997.

Nachson, I. (1998a). Me'zeekarone mashookhzar le'zeekarone mesooluf ve'khuzarah [From recovered memory to false memory and back]. Invited address delivered at a conference on *Therapist-Client Relationships: Ethical and Legal Aspects*. Tel-Aviv, September, 1998.

Nachson, I. (1998b). Me'zeekarone mashookhzar le'zeekarone mesooluf ve'khuzarah [From recovered memory to false memory, and back]. *Psychologia, 7*, 7-23.

Nachson, I. (2000). Truthfulness, deception and self-deception in recovering true and false memories. *International Journal of Victimology, 8*, 1-18.

Nemetz. B. (2002). Tismonayt ha'zikron ha'medoomay–Tmoonut matzav udkanit [The false memory syndrome–A current update]. *Harefuah–Journal of the Israel Medical Association, 141*(8), 726-730.

Nimrod, N., & Somer, E. (1995). Be'Gove Ha'Arayot: Pneeyote telephoniyote le'merkazay ha'seeyooah shel nifgeote gilooy arayote [Incest survivors calls to the rape crisis centers' hotlines in Israel]. Tel Aviv: The Israel Association of Rape Crisis Centers. A statistical report commissioned by the chair of the Knesset's Judiciary Committee and presented to the committee members.

Orbach, I. (1992). *Olamot Nistarim–Hitbonanoot be-T at Hahakara [Hidden worlds–Observations of the sub-conscious]*. Tel Aviv: Schoken.

Orbach, I. (1994). Dissociation, physical pain and suicide: A hypothesis. *Suicide and Life-Threatening Behavior, 24*(1), 68-79.

Orbach, I. (1996) The role of the body experience in self-destruction. *Clin Child Psychol Psychiatry, 1*, 607-619.

Orbach, I., Kedem, P., Herman, L., & Apter, A. (1995). Dissociative tendencies in suicidal, depressed, and normal adolescents. *Journal of Social and Clinical Psychology, 14*(4), 393-408.

Orbach, I., Lotem-Peleg, M., & Kedem, (1995). Attitudes towards the body in suicidal and nonsuicidal adolescents. *Suicide and Life-Threatening Behavior, 25,* 211-221.

Orbach, I., & Mikulincer, M. (2000). Mental pain: Conceptualization and operationalization. Presented at the annual conference of the American Association of Suicidology Los Angeles.

Orbach, I., Mikulincer, M., King, R., Cohen, D., & Stein, D. (1997). Thresholds and tolerance of physical pain in suicidal and nonsuicidal adolescents. *Journal of Consulting and Clinical Psychology, 65,* 646-652.

Peled-Avram, M., Ben-Yizhack, Y., Gagin, R., Somer, E., & Buchbinder, E. (2004). Tgoovote ve'tzrakheem regshee'im shel ovdeem sotzialee'im be'ayrooah rav-nifguyim [Emotional responses and needs of social workers in a mass disaster]. *Hevra U'rvacha (Society and Welfare), 24* (2), 181-200.

Read, M. (2002). Shvooya: Kroneekah shel Gelooy arayot MIktzo'i–Seepoor autobiographi. [Captive: A chronicle of professional incest–An autobiographical account]. Tel Aviv: Tamuz.

Schreiber F.R. (1973). *Sybil: The true story of a woman possesses by sixteen separate personalities.* Chicago: Regnery, The book was published in Israel Hebrew in 1987 by Kineret.

Scwarzberg, S., & Somer, E. (2004). Khaseefut hasode: Gormim meodedim ume'ukvim et gilooy sode hapgiah bekerev korbanote hit'alelute meneet bayaldoot [Breaking the Silence: facilitating and inhibiting factors in the disclosure of incest among survivors of child sexual abuse]. In Z. Seligman and Z. Solomon (Eds.), *Hasode ve'shevroh: Soogiote be'gelooy arayote [Critical and Clinical Perspectives on Incest].* Tel Aviv: Hakibbutz Hameuchad and Tel Aviv University.

Shalev, R. (2000). Behten [Belly]. Tel Aviv: Carmel.

Shalev, A.Y., Freedman, S., Peri, T., Brandes, D., & Sahar, T. (1997). Predicting PTSD in trauma survivors: Evaluation of self-report and clinician-administered instruments. *British Journal of Psychiatry, 170,* 558-564.

Shalev, A.Y., Peri, T., & Canetti, L. (1996). Predictors of PTSD in injured trauma survivors: A prospective study. *American Journal of Psychiatry, 153,* 219-225.

Shaz (1999). *Rikood Ha'mashooga'at [The dance of the madwoman].* Tel Aviv: Hakibutz Ha'meuchad.

Siegel-Itzkovich, J. (1996, May 19). You must remember this. *Jersalem Post,* p. 7.

Slonim, N. (1997, October, 15). Massa Mefookpuck el he'avar [A dubios journey into the past]. *Ha'aretz daily,* p.8.

Solomon, Z., Kotler, M., & Mikulincer, M. (1988). Combat-related posttraumatic stress disorder among second-generation Holocaust survivors: Preliminary findings. *American Journal of Psychiatry, 145,* 865-868.

Somer, E. (1987, November). Ishiyoot meroobut puneem: Akronot Ivkhoon ve'teepool [Multiple personality: Diagnosis and treatment principles]. Paper presented at the *Third National Conference of the Israel Hypnosis Society.* Tel Aviv.

Somer, E. (1989). Ishiyute meroobat puneem: Hearote al Ivkhoon, tipool U'ragushote ha'metapale [Multiple personality: Comments on diagnosis, treatment and therapist's feelings]. *Sihot–Israel Journal of Psychotherapy, 3*(3), 101-106.

Somer, E. (1992). *Soolum Khavayot dissotzyativiot* [Translation into Hebrew and adaptation of the Dissociative Experience Scale (H-DES)] (E.B. Carlson and F.W. Putnam).

Somer, E. (1993). Tismonet Ikhooz be'Ishiyoot histriyonit: Geroosh shedim ve'psikhoterapia [Possession syndrome in a hysterionic personality: Exorcism and psychotherapy]. *Sihot–Israel Journal of Psychotherapy, 8*, 40-47.

Somer, E. (1993, December 9). Ha'makka ha' 81 [The 81st blow, An Op-page article commenting on the Supreme Court's acquittal of a father convicted of incest]. *Ha'aretz Daily Newspaper.*

Somer, E. (1994a). Hypnotherapy and regulated uncovering in the treatment of older survivors of Nazi persecution. In T. L. Brink (Ed.), *Holocaust survivors' mental health* (pp. 47-65). New York: The Haworth Press, Inc.

Somer, E. (1994b). Hizakhroot meookheret behitaleloot bayaldoot: Zikhronot melakhooti'im o ha'etgar haba be'psikhoterapia? [Delayed recall of child abuse: False memories or the next challenge for psychotherapy?]. *Sihot–Israel Journal of Psychotherapy, 9*(1), 46-50.

Somer, E. (1994c). *Tgoovote nufshiyote le'traumat ha'oness* [*Psychological reactions to rape trauma*]. A document presented to members of the Knesset as part of testimony given to the Judicial Committee in session on change of legislation regarding sex offenses.

Somer, E. (1994d). Trauma be'gil ha'yaldoot: Ovdan Zikaron ve'khasita mooshheyt. [Childhood trauma: Delayed recall and reporting]. A position paper commissioned by the National Council for the Protection of the Child for presentation to the Knesset's Judiciary Committee in session on changing the statute of limitations regarding child abuse. Also appears in T. Morag (Ed.), *Repressed testimony or oppressed childhood: On the statute of limitations in cases of sex offences in the family.* Jerusalem: National Council for the Child, Center for Research and Policy.

Somer, E. (1994e). *Yekholet ha'hitnagdoot shel yalda hanimtzeyt be'gilooy arayot* [*The capacity of an incest victim to resist*]. A position paper submitted to the National Council for the Child as part of assistance given to the State Attorney's Office of Criminal Appeal 851/93.

Somer, E. (1994, May 24). Assiyat deen gum begilooy arayote [No statute of limitation for child abuse, An Op-page article advocating a change in the statute of limitation regarding sexual child abuse crimes]. *Ha'aretz Daily Newspaper*, p. 8.

Somer, E. (1995a). Hynotherapy in the treatment of older Holocaust survivors: Overcoming dissociation. In E. Bolcs, M. Guttman, M. Martin, M. Mende, H. Kanitschar, & H. Walter (Eds.), *Hypnosis-connecting discipline: Proceedings of the 6th European Congress of Hypnosis in Psychotherapy and Psychosomatic Medicine* (pp. 213-217). Parkersdorf/Vienna: Medizinisch-Pharmazeutische Verlagsgeselschaft.

Somer, E. (1995b). *Shay'e'lone dissotzyatzya ba'yaldoot* [Translation into Hebrew and adaptation of the Childhood Dissociation Questionnaire] (F. Putnam).

Somer, E. (1995c). *Rayayon klini moovnay le'hafra'ote dissozyativiote* [Translation into Hebrew and adaptation of the Structured Clinical Interview for Dissociative Disoders (SCID-D)] (M. Steinberg).

Somer, E. (1995d). Trauma, trance ve'abreaktzia behafra'at zehoot dissotziativit [Trauma, trance and abreaction in dissociative identity disorder]. *Hypnoza, 1*(1), 8-15.

Somer, E. (1996). *Soolum Khavayot dissotzyativiot-Mitbugreem* [Translation into Hebrew and adaptation of the Adolescent-Dissociative Experience Scale (H-A-DES)] (J. Armstrong, F.W. Putnam and E. B.Carlson).

Somer, E. (1997a). Paranormal and dissociative experiences in middle eastern Jews in Israel: Diagnostic and treatment dilemmas. *Dissociation, 10*(3), 174-181.

Somer, E. (1997b). Zeekarone traumati: Massa Mefookpuck el he'avar oh massa mefah'raykh el avar mefookpuck? *http://www.maytal.co.il/heb_articles/article_8.html* accessed Oct. 6, 2004.

Somer, E. (1997c). Book review on: J. Silberg (Ed.), The Dissociative Child: Diagnosis, treatment and management. *Sihot–Israel Journal of Psychotherapy, 11*(3), 243-245.

Somer, E. (1999). *Yekhaseem Makbeelim: Petooy ve'neetzool meenee be'psikhoterapia ve'yeootz* [Dual Relationships: Seduction and sexual exploitation in counseling and psychotherapy]. Tel Aviv: Papyrus–Tel Aviv University Publishing House.

Somer, E. (2000a). Israeli mental health professionals' attitudes towards dissociative disorders, differential diagnosis considered, and reported incidence. *Journal of Trauma and Dissociation, 1*(1), 21-44.

Somer, E. (2000b). The effects of incest in aging survivors: Psychopathology and treatment issues. *Journal of Clinical Geropsychology, 6*(1), 53-61.

Somer, E. (2002a). *Ha'metzay ha'rov maymady shel dissotzyatzya* [Translation into Hebrew and adaptation of the Multi-modal Inventory of Dissociation (H-MID)] (Paul Dell).

Somer, E. (2002b). Posttraumatic dissociation as a mediator of the effects of trauma on distressful introspectiveness. *Social Behavior and Personality, 30*(7), 671-682.

Somer, E. (2002c). Maladaptive daydreaming: A qualitative inquiry. *Journal of Contemporary Psychotherapy, 32*(2), 195-210.

Somer, E. (2003a). Prediction of abstinence from heroin addiction by childhood trauma, dissociation, and extent of psychosocial treatment. *Addiction Research and Theory, 11*(5), 339-348.

Somer, E. (2004a) Trance possession disorder in Judaism: Sixteenth-century dybbuks in the Near-East. *Journal of Trauma and Dissociation, 5*(2), 131-146.

Somer, E. (2004b). Hitaleloot bayaldoot ve'hafraote disotzyativiot [Childhood trauma and dissociative disorders]. In Zeligman, z., & Solomon, Z. (Eds.) (2004). *Hasode ve'sheevroh: Gilooy arayot [Breaking the secret of incest]*. Tel Aviv: SIfriyat Hapoalim.

Somer, E. (in press). Opiate use disorder and dissociation. In P.F. Dell, & J. O'Neil (Eds.), *Dissociation and the dissociative disorders: DSM-V and beyond.*

Somer, E., & Avni, R. (2003b). Dissociative phenomena among recovering heroin users and their relationship to duration of abstinence. *Journal of Social Work Practice in the Addictions, 3*(1), 25-38.

Somer, E., Buchbinder, E. Peled-Avram, M., & Ben-Yizhack, Y. (2004). The stress and coping of Israeli emergency room social workers following terrorist attacks. *Qualitative Health Research, 14*(10), 1077-1093.

Somer, E., & Dell, P. F. (2005). The development and psychometric characteristics of the Hebrew version of the Multidimensional Inventory of Dissociation (H-MID): A valid and reliable measure of pathological dissociation. *Journal of Trauma and Dissociation*.

Somer, E., Dolgin, M., & Saadon, M. (2001). Validation of the Hebrew version of the Dissociative Experiences Scale (H-DES) in Israel. *Journal of Trauma and Dissociation*, 2(2), 53-66.

Somer, E., & Nave, O. (2001). An ethnographic study of former dissociative disorder patients. *Imagination, Cognition, and Personality*, 20(1), 315-346.

Somer, E., & Nachmani, I. (2005). Constructions of therapist-patient sex: An analysis of retrospective reports by former Israeli patients. *Sexual Abuse: A Journal of Research and Treatment*.

Somer, E., & Saadon, M. (1999). Therapist-client sex: Clients' retrospective reports. *Professional Psychology: Research and Practice*, 30(5), 504-509.

Somer, E., & Saadon, M. (2000). Stambali: Dissociative possession and trance in a Tunisian healing dance. *Transcultural Psychiatry*, 37(4), 579-609.

Somer, L. (2004). Olama hapnimi shel nefga'at gelooy arayote: Iyoorim betzevah uvetzurah metokhe tahalikh shel tipool bemtzaoot yetzirah [The inner world of an incest victim: Illustrations in color and form from an art therapy process. In Z. Scligman and Z. Solomon (Eds.) *Hasode ve'shevroh: Soogiote be'gelooy arayote [Critical and Clinical Perspectives on Incest]*. Tel Aviv: Hakibbutz Hameuchad and Tel Aviv University.

Somer, L., & Somer, E. (1997a). Phenomenological and psychoanalytic perspectives on a spontaneous artistic process during psychotherapy for dissociative identity disorder. *The Arts in Psychotherapy*, 24(5), 419-430.

Somer, L., & Somer, E. (1997b). Heybetim psikhodinami'im shel avodote omanoot be'hafra'at zehoot disotziativit [Pychodynamic perspectives on art work in dissociative identity disorder]. *Sihot–Israel Journal of Psychotherapy*, 11(3), 183-194.

Somer, E., & Szwarcberg, S. (2001). Variables in delayed disclosure of child sexual abuse. *American Journal of Orthopsychiatry*, 71(3), 332-341.

Somer, E., & Yishai, R. (1997). Handwriting examination: Can it help in establishing authenticity in dissociative identity disorder? *Dissociation*, 10(2), 114-119.

Somer, E., & Weiner, A. (1996). Dissociative symptomatology in adolescent diaries of incest victims. *Dissociation*, 9(3), 197-209.

Tauber, Y. (1996). The traumatized child and the adult: Compound personality in child-survivors of the Holocaust. *Israel Journal of Psychiatry and Related Sciences*, 33, 228-238.

Tishbi, Y. (1982). *Torat ha-Zohar [The teachings of the Zohar]*. Jerusalem: Mosad Bialik.

Tzarfati, A. (2001). *Posttraumatic response among soldiers who were injured in military activity: The relation to peritraumatic dissociation and to history of prior trauma*. Thesis submitted to the University of Haifa.

Van der Hart, O. (1993). Multiple Personality in Europe: Impressions. *Dissociation*, 5(2/3), 102-115.

Van der Hart, O., & Brom, D. (2000). When the victim forgets: Trauma-induced amnesia and its assessment in Holocaust survivors. In A. Shalev, R. Yehuda & A.C. McFarlane (Eds.), *International handbook of human response to trauma* (pp. 233-248). New York: Kluwer Academic/Plenum.

Van der Hart, O., Witztum, E., & Friedman, B. (1992). From hysterical psychosis to reactive dissociative psychosis. *Journal of Traumatic Stress, 6*, 43-64.

West, C. (1999). *First Person Plural: My Life as a Multiple*, NY: Hyperion. The book was published (2002) in Israel in Hebrew by Ma'ariv.

Witztum E., Grisaru, N., & Budowski, D. (1996). The 'Zar' possession syndrome among Ethiopian immigrants to Israel: Cultural and clinical aspects. *British Journal of Medical Psychology, (3)*, 207-25.

Witztum, E., Buchbinder, J.T., & Van der Hart, O. (1990). Summoning a punishing angel: Treatment of a depressed patient with dissociative features. *Bulletin of the Menninger Clinic, 54*, 524-537.

Witztum, E., Margalit, C., & Van der Hart, O. (2002). Combat-induced dissociative amnesia: Review and case example of generalized dissociative amnesia. *Journal of Trauma and Dissociation, 3*(2), 35-55.

Yahav, (2003). Book review on "Shvooya" by Maya Read. *Sihot–Israel Journal of Psychotherapy, 17*(3), 111-113.

Yehuda, R., Elkin, et al. (1996). Dissociation in aging Holocaust survivors. *American Journal of Psychiatry, 153*, 935-940.

Yehuda, R., Schmeidler, J., Elkin, A., Houshmand, E., Siever, L., Binder-Brynes, K., Wainberg, M., Aferiot, D., Lehman, A., Guo, L.S., & Yang, R.K., (1998). Phenomenology and psychobiology of the intergenerational response to trauma. In Danieli, Y. (Ed) *Intergenerational Handbook of Multigenerational Legacies of Trauma*. *http://www.trauma-pages.com/yehuda97.htm* retrieved Oct. 1, 2004.

Yovel, Y. (2001). *Se'arat nefesh [Mindstorm]*. Tel Aviv: Keshet.

PART II

PART II

Social Withdrawal in Japanese Youth:
A Case Study
of Thirty-Five Hikikomori Clients

Yuichi Hattori

SUMMARY. With up to 1,400,00 Japanese youth affected, "Hikikomori," or social withdrawal, has become alarmingly common in Japan. Children of traditional middle and upper middle class families, whose parents are civil servants, teachers, farmers, corporate executives, and business owners, are highly likely to develop Hikikomori. Despite near-epidemic proportions and media prominence, few systematic studies have addressed the condition. This case study describes the clinical phenomenology, etiology, and treatment methods of thirty-five clients at a private clinic in Japan. All patients presented with a loss of secure attachment, and two-thirds had dual personality systems. Their primary clinical feature was inability to trust or

Yuichi Hattori, MA, is affiliated with Sayama Psychological Services. 124-191 Aoyagi, Sayama City, Saitama 350-1301, Japan (E-mail: hattoriyuichi@aol.com).

The author offers special thanks to Dr. George F. Rhoades, Jr., Clinical Psychologist, Director of Ola Hou Clinic Psychological Services, and the author's friend in Hawaii. Without his patience and encouragement, this paper would not have been published. The author also extends acknowledgement to Michael Zielenziger, former Tokyo Bureau Chief of Knight Ridder Newspapers, and Melody Girard, a professional proofreader, for their contributions to the refinement of this paper.

This paper is dedicated to the Japanese youths who have been denied their freedom of expression and who long for the liberation of true self in psychological captivity.

[Haworth co-indexing entry note]: "Social Withdrawal in Japanese Youth: A Case Study of Thirty-Five Hikikomori Clients." Hattori, Yuichi. Co-published simultaneously in *Journal of Trauma Practice* (The Haworth Maltreatment & Trauma Press, an imprint of The Haworth Press, Inc.) Vol. 4, No. 3/4, 2005, pp. 181-201; and: *Trauma and Dissociation in a Cross-Cultural Perspective: Not Just a North American Phenomenon* (ed: George F. Rhoades, Jr., and Vedat Sar) The Haworth Maltreatment & Trauma Press, an imprint of The Haworth Press, Inc., 2005, pp. 181-201. Single or multiple copies of this article are available for a fee from The Haworth Document Delivery Service [1-800-HAWORTH, 9:00 a.m. - 5:00 p.m. (EST). E-mail address: docdelivery@haworthpress.com].

relate to others. Families appeared outwardly functional, however, clients reported histories of emotional neglect and abuse. To adapt to emotionally dysfunctional parents, they repressed original identities and authentic feelings and created false front identities. Emotional neglect, absence of parental-child communication, and inhibition of self-expression may underlie Hikikomori. Successful treatment depends on the recovery and healthy attachment of the original identity. Although a progressive condition, treatment prognosis is good with early intervention. *[Article copies available for a fee from The Haworth Document Delivery Service: 1-800-HAWORTH. E-mail address: <docdelivery@haworthpress.com> Website: <http://www.HaworthPress.com> © 2005 by The Haworth Press, Inc. All rights reserved.]*

KEYWORDS. Social withdrawal, Japanese youth, Hikikomori, attachment trauma, distrust of humans, co-dependency, emotional neglect, Ijime, dual personalities, Taijin Kyofusho, phobia of humans, inability to relate to people, distrust of parents, wish to kill parents, domestic violence

Self-imposed confinement, known as "Hikikomori," is surprisingly common in Japan today. Young people with Hikikomori, predominantly males in their teens to thirties, shut themselves off from their siblings, friends, and even their parents, whom they sometimes verbally and physically attack in violent outbursts (Saitama Newspaper, 2001). The estimated incidences of Hikikomori range from 800,000 to 1,400,000, according to the research of Ogi Naoki, an education clinic (Ogi, 2001). The Nationwide Association of Parents of Hikikomori Sufferers, which is known as "Zenkoku Hikikomori Oyano-Kai" or "KHJ Oyano-Kai," claims that 1 million young adults imprison themselves in their rooms for months to years on end (Tabidachi, 2002; Zielenziger, 2002). One government survey found that adults age 21 and above accounted for more than 60% of the persons who suffer this disorder (Asahi Newspaper, 2001; Tokyo Newspaper, 2001). In 2001, as public awareness and media focus intensified, executive members of KHJ Oyano-Kai and concerned politicians started a study group for this apparent national epidemic (Ikegami, 2001).

Masahisa Okuyama, founder of the KHJ Oyano-Kai, warned, "The nation is wasting human resources. It's a disease that can bring the nation to collapse" (Japan Times, 2003). Controversies have arisen, however, over whether the social withdrawal is a manifestation of the "laziness of spoiled youths" or "a new mental disorder" (Katsuyama, 2001; Mainichi Newspaper, 2003; SPA!, 2000; Saitama Newspaper, 2001; Sunday Mainichi, 2001b, May 27; Sunday Mainichi, 2003, March 30; Ueyama, 2001; Yomiuri Newspaper, 2001). Despite numerous medias reports and publications, the author's research of the literature found that few systematic studies have been done so far, and that there is a dearth of scientific information on the clinical phenomenology and etiology of Hikikomori (Aoki, 2002; Ikegami, 2001; Ishikawa, 2002; Ishiya, 2002; Inoue, 2002; Machizawa, 2003; Saitama Newspaper, 2001; Saito, 1998; Saito 2002; Saito, 2003; Sunday Mainichi, 2001a, b, c; Tanaka, 2001; Uchida, K., 2001; Uchida, T., 2001; Ueyama, 2001).

Lagging behind in their awareness of social changes, the majority of Japanese professionals and academics appear to ignore the syndrome. A lack of consensus on the nature of Hikikomori prevails among Japanese professionals (Hattori, Chicago, 2003; Hattori, Melbourne, 2003; Kastuyama, 2001; Sunday Mainichi, 2003, March 30; Ueyama, 2001).

The government maintains that the term "Hikikomori" refers to a state of social withdrawal, not a clinical diagnosis, and that the causes of this disorder are too diverse to identify (Shohatsu, 2001). In 2003, under pressure from concerned parents, the Ministry of Health and Welfare asserted that the following features characterize Hikikomori:

1. The person shuts himself or herself at home for at least six months.
2. The person has no intimate relationships with other than family members.
3. The social withdrawal is not a symptom of other psychotic disorders.
4. The social withdrawal refers to not taking part in any social activities, such as school and work settings (Saito, 2003).

I met my first Hikikomori patient at my private clinic in 2000. The client was a college student who complained of handshaking and emotional exhaustion for unknown reasons. A few weeks later, he withdrew from all interpersonal relationships and stopped attending his college classes. He became suicidal, while also attacking his parents verbally and physically. As his psychotherapy continued, I began to take in more clients with similar symptoms.

The clients came from seemingly well-functioning families. Most of them had no history of physical or sexual abuse. Nevertheless, all of them showed a constellation of trauma-related symptoms. About two-thirds of the study subjects had dual dissociative identities, or dual personalities, as a product of inhibition of self-expression.

Soon, I became the only psychologist in Japan who identified Hikikomori as a trauma-based disorder. This academic isolation motivated me to present my case studies outside Japan, as the mainstreams of the Japanese professional community did not associate Hikikomori with childhood trauma.

This study describes the clinical phenomenology, etiology, and treatment of thirty-five clients at my Tokyo suburban clinic. It is a synthesis of the two noted presentations and several private meetings with English-speaking professionals, mostly members of ISSD. I presented part of this study at two international conferences outside Japan in 2003: International Conference on Trauma, Attachment, and Dissociation in Melbourne, Australia (Hattori, 2003) and the 20th Annual Conference of International Society for the Study of Dissociation (ISSD) in Chicago (Hattori, 2003).

METHOD

Subjects

Thirty-five clients, whose symptoms met the government criteria of Hikikomori, were selected for this study. There were 25 male and 10 female clients, with the mean age at in-take of 21.5 and ranging from age 11 to 35. The subjects for this study were collected between 2000 and 2002.

Procedure

The clients, including dropouts, received at least fifteen 50-minute sessions. Their conversations and clinical records were analyzed to identify any common clinical features, childhood experiences, personal and family history, and treatment methods. I used the Dissociative Experiences Scale (DES), a widely-accepted instrument for detecting dissociative symptoms. The DES, a self-administered dissociative experience screener, consists of 28 items, each with a frequency percentage from 0 to 100%. Good test-retest has been shown for the DES (Bernstein & Putnam, 1986; Strick & Wilcoxon, 1991).

RESULTS

According to the parents, the patients' periods of total social withdrawal ranged from 6 months to 16 years. The average period was hard to determine due to the clients' and their parents' idiosyncratic definitions of social withdrawal. Out of shame feelings, some clients defined their reclusive life as "taking a rest" and refused to see it as Hikikomori, or some parents insisted that their child's years of social isolation was not Hikikomori because he or she had worked intermittently.

Presenting Symptoms

Table 1 reveals presenting symptoms of the subjects. All of the Hikikomori clients find it difficult to trust people (100%), which relates to their interpersonal problems. During treatment, patients frequently showed inhibition of self-expression, loss of secure attachment, estrangement, and a phobia of humans.

Seventy-one percent of the clients presented with a dual system of dissociative identities (dual personalities), possessing both overt and covert symptoms. Overt dissociative identity indicates that the therapist could directly communicate with a dissociative identity. Covert dissociative identity indicates that a client acknowledges the presence of a dissociative identity or "another part of me" and the therapist communicated with the dissociative identity indirectly through the client.

These identity alternations involved not only regression but also switching to another personality state. Typically, parents describing the perceived alternations of their children would say, "My 24-year-old daughter clings to me like an infant. She demands to sleeps with me and my husband," or "When my son gets into violent outburst, he shows a devilish face that I have never seen before. He becomes a totally different person."

According to the parents, their children showed personality changes after social withdrawal had begun. The drastic changes in personality confused the parents, who found it difficult to deal with their unpredictable children. Clinically, these clients were diagnosed with Dissociative Disorder Not Otherwise Specified (DDNOS) involving the dissociative identities (Diagnostic and Statistical Manual of Mental Disorders, DSM-IV, pp. 490-491).

The phobia of humans, known in Japan as "taijin kyofusho," is the second most common feature (71%) among these patients. "Taijin

TABLE 1. Presenting Symptoms

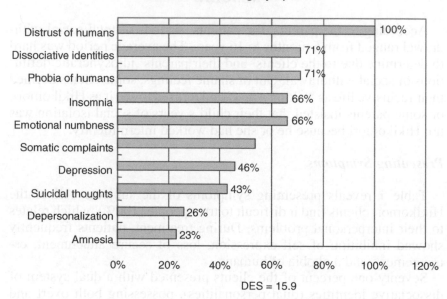

DES = 15.9

Kyofusho" is defined in Diagnostic and Statistical Manual of Mental Disorders 4th Edition (DSM-IV, 1994) as:

> A culturally distinctive phobia in Japan, in some ways resembling Social Phobia as noted in the DSM-IV. This syndrome refers to an individual's intense fear that his or her body, its parts or its functions, displease, embarrass, or are offensive to other people in appearance, odor, facial expressions, or movements. This syndrome is included in the official Japanese diagnostic system for mental disorder. (DSM-IV, p. 849)

Clients displayed a variety of avoidance behaviors, such as taking a walk at midnight to avoid neighbors, not taking phone calls from friends, avoiding crowds, trains or public places. A cognitive schema of distrust and fear of humans usually accompanies their social withdrawals.

Most of the clients did not report the kind of Post-Traumatic Stress Disorder (PTSD) symptoms that are typically related to chronic stressors, or complex trauma. Patients, however, did display a number of post-traumatic symptoms, including insomnia (66%), emotional numbness (66%), somatic complaints (54%), depression (46%), and suicidal thoughts (43%). The clients did not usually associate the PTSD-like symptoms with their past traumas, unless in psychotherapy they were able to explore their past and its possible relationship with the present symptoms.

During treatment, emotional numbness often surfaced as a cover-up symptom. After recovering the repressed emotions, some clients resorted to "self medication" with alcoholic beverages to numb their emotional pain. But none of them became chronic or problem drinkers. This clinical phenomenon suggested that a minimum level of ability to feel emotions is a prerequisite to becoming alcoholic. Upon recovery of the repressed emotions, clients often found themselves facing parricidal wishes, major depression, suicidal tendencies, or somatoform disorders. These responses would explain why the clients resisted recovering their repressed emotions.

The participants' mean DES scores at in-take were 15.9, and ranged from 0 to 41.3. In addition to dissociative identities, some clients reported depersonalization (26%) and amnesia (23%). With the score of 21.8 to 41.3, clients with depersonalization and amnesia tended to score higher on the DES scale than those without these two additional symptoms. Two clients scored 40.3 and 41.3 on the DES scale and were diagnosed with Dissociative Identity Disorder (DID), which involved amnesia after identity alternation. The similar DES scores of these two clients reveal the importance of the overall use of diagnostic criteria in making a diagnosis, rather than relying solely on test cutoff scores.

It is noteworthy that the clients tended to show higher DES scores at the recovery of the original identities. For example, a 31-year-old male client increased his DES score from 9.6 at in-take to 74.6 at the emergence of the original identity. Other clients exhibited score increases. A 21-year-old man's score jumped from 11.4 to 35.4, and a 31-year-old man's scale rose from 10.4 to 48.9 These data suggested that the dissociative clients did not show a full scale of dissociative tendencies at in-take.

Childhood Trauma

Table 2 reviews the types of childhood trauma experienced by the studied clients. Ninety-one percent of the clients reported a history of emotional neglect by parents who were unresponsive or insensitive to their childhood emotional needs.

In the clients studied, emotional neglect may be seen as leading to a sense of emotional abandonment. There was extreme poverty of parent-child interactions in Hikikomori families. Participants stated that

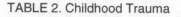

TABLE 2. Childhood Trauma

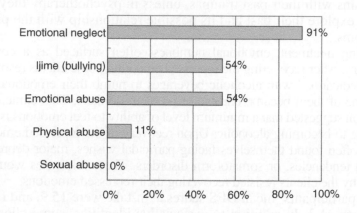

they learned to be quiet and invisible at all times. They reported that their parents:

1. Did not talk to them when they were children.
2. Avoided eye contact with them when they were children and that their mothers were emotionally unavailable for soothing.
3. Ignored them whenever the children displayed emotions or made demands.

Generally, the clients described feeling like emotionally abandoned children. This emotional isolation by the parents fosters the clients' rage, hatred, and even death wishes toward their parents.

In 54% of the cases, the clients reported emotional abuse by their parents, particularly shunning or ignoring the child, which is called "mushi" in Japan. In "mushi," a mother arbitrarily refuses to talk to a child from a few hours to several days–sometimes even for a few weeks. During periods of mushi, the mother refuses to respond to a child's demands or verbal pleadings. She never tells the child the reason for her behavior and never responds if the child asks for an explanation. The clients most commonly report this type of child abuse, a passive-aggressive punishment, which is performed covertly by parents and therefore goes unnoticed by others.

In 54% of the cases, clients were victimized by "ijime" or bullying, in the form of physical and emotional abuse by peers in Japanese elementary, middle, and high schools. Mushi was the most frequently reported form of ijime at school. A victim was ostracized for unknown reasons by a group of peers at school for months, even years. Studied participants said that when a victim subjected himself/herself to ijime, no one helped or attempted to rescue them from this school trauma, not even their friends, teachers, or parents. Parents would typically say, "Stay away from them, and they will not harm you." Some would tell their children, "You must have reasons to be blamed by others." Their distrust of friends, feelings of intense resentment, and loss of emotional bond to their parents appear to be linked to the clients' ijime experiences.

The repeated experiences with mushi reinforced the clients' perception that humans are unpredictable and unreliable. Studied participants tended to assume that people by nature have dual personalities, and that they will suddenly reveal the dark sides of their personalities when offended. Mushi contributed to the clients' fear of humans and exquisite interpersonal sensitivity, which did not accompany a sense of trust, belonging, and intimacy.

In 11% of the cases, the clients said that their parents abused them physically. But none of the abuse instances was ritualistic or sadistic in nature. Most patients stated that their parents "hit" them several times a year. No one, however, reported any injuries from "physical abuse by parents." With this in mind, the so-called "physical abuse" may be more appropriately called "physical discipline."

The clients reported no history of sexual abuse (0%). The studied clients did not report any oral, anal, or vaginal penetrations perpetrated on them during childhood. Sexual abuse does not appear to be an issue in the psychotherapy of Hikikomori.

Parent-Child Relationships

Table 3 illustrated various aspects of parent-child relationships for the studied clients. In 100% of the cases, the clients experienced loss of attachment to their parents, which they expressed as a distrust of their parents. The loss of secure attachment was also related to inhibition of self-expression with parents (89%) and their childhood fear of them (80%). Describing their childhoods as oppressed, study participants stated that they were unable to show their true identity to their parents for fear of rejection. Without healthy attachment, the patients did not seek parental help when they faced distresses, school trauma, or even a life-threatening danger. The inhibition of self-expression may be seen as contributing to the creation of the false front identities (one of the dual personalities).

TABLE 3. Issues of Parent-Child Relationships

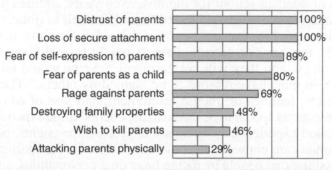

0% 20% 40% 60% 80% 100%120%

In 69% of the cases, the clients expressed intense rage against their parents. This tendency to "vent" their built-up anger and resentments typically occurred upon attaining adolescence and beyond. Forty-six percent of the clients expressed wishes to kill their parents, and 49% of them had a history of destroying house properties, such as furniture, dishes, electric appliances, or damaging house walls in violent outburst.

In 29% of the cases, the Hikikomori patients had a history of attacking their parents physically. The domestic violence reported included hitting a parent's face with a fist, kicking into a parent's body, grabbing the mother's hair, or chasing after a mother. Mothers were the typical targets for this domestic violence. For example, during violent outburst, three male clients, ages 17, 18 and 22 fractured the ribs of one father and two mothers. Some parents confided that they hid kitchen knives and baseball bats in anticipation of their male children attacking them.

Hikikomori patients' parents commonly asked, "Can you tell me when my son is ready for work?" These parents were obsessed with the idea of getting their children back to work or school. They were usually indifferent to their children's feelings, thoughts, and past experiences. Such parents seldom tried to understand the reasons of their child's years of social withdrawal.

The study participants' domestic violence outbursts often appeared to be aimed at opening communication with parents, who would otherwise be unavailable for genuine conversation with their child. Parental lack of empathy and understanding frequently led clients to assert that their parents were incapable of communicating with them. In one instance, a 21-year-old male pinned his unresponsive mother to the wall, squeezed her neck with his hands, and said, "Tell me how you feel about me." The mother said repeatedly, "I'm sorry. I am to blame." Her irrelevant response disappointed him overwhelmingly, and he gave up his desires for communicating with his mother. He called his mother "Puppet" during treatment. Generally, the clients withdrew even more after domestic violence ceased, a response that could be seen as the absence of attachment seeking.

Family History

Table 4 reveals the characteristics of the families of clients. Clients came from middle to upper middle-income families. Ninety-seven percent of the families reported owning their own home. Seventy-seven percent of the fathers had prestigious jobs, such as government employees, teachers, corporate executives, or business owners. The mothers tended to stay at home for housework and child rearing. No families were reported to be on welfare or government assistance.

Despite the relative affluence of their parents, the clients reported having emotionally deprived family environments. In 91% of the cases, the study participants described their fathers as workaholics, uninvolved in child rearing, and the mothers as emotionally unresponsive. Although neglectful of their children's emotional needs, 66% of the parents sought to enroll their children in a prestigious school, and they continued to display an obsession with their children's academic performance.

Most clients studied extra hours at preparatory schools during elementary and middle school. In some cases, parents insisted that their children learn piano, swimming, or English conversation after school, depriving them of any free time. Generally, these achievement oriented parents appeared indifferent to the emotional welfare of their children. Prior to shutting themselves off socially, the children tended to have good grades and academic performance. None of the study participants had any criminal records or confrontations with the legal system, such as police arrest, runaway episodes, or street gang involvement.

In 86% of the cases, the participants gave accounts of marital conflicts between their parents. According to them, their parents did not openly "fight" or argue in home, but the children witnessed "a cold war between parents" that developed over time. These parents can be regarded as traditional Japanese who maintained their marriages without

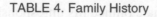

TABLE 4. Family History

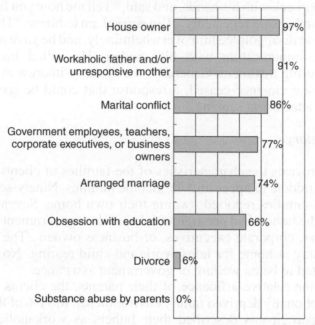

0% 20% 40% 60% 80% 100% 120%

demonstrated affection to each other. Seventy-four percent of their parents' marriages were arranged, and only 6% of the parents were divorced, as opposed to the national average of 25%. All the Hikikomori patients lived with their biological parents, and none resided with a stepparent.

Hikikomori clients did not describe any parental substance abuse. The fathers tended to be workaholics, while the stay-at-home mothers tended to remain emotionally unavailable. Clients growing up in these emotionally deprived environments suffered emotional traumas, related to marital conflicts, obsession with education, mushi–or shunning–and lack of parent-child communication.

In summary, Hikikomori clients in this study do not tend to come from obviously dysfunctional, abusive families. Instead, the clients' middle and upper middle classes families appear to be functional. According to their children, none of the Hikikomori parents had perpetrated any physical or sexual abuse.

Treatment

The treatment utilized was psychotherapy for processing the past traumas, taking both DDNOS and PTSD into consideration. Treatment started with prolonged therapeutic conversations centering on the issue of trust and safety. The clients spent from six months to one year testing the reliability of the therapist, while engaging in pseudo-therapeutic conversations. They often engaged in what the author called "reconnaissance behaviors." Some patients prepared conversation scenarios prior to each session, to observe how the therapist would respond. Others compulsively pleased the therapist until they felt safe with him, rather than reveal their authentic feelings and thoughts.

To avoid offending the therapist, study participants usually smiled when they were angry. Generally, they believed that the therapist had dual personalities. Operating under this assumption, they tended to look for the hidden or the "dark side" of the therapist's personality. This kind of distrustful communication inhibited their anger and unknowingly caused it to build up toward the therapist. During such therapy sessions, the therapist often felt as if he were walking in a minefield, where he had to anticipate the client's unpredictable rejection. This transference, however, indicated that the clients had experienced the same kinds of anxieties with their parents when they were children.

Taking the distrust in humans into consideration, the treatment techniques assume that the client suffers from loss of secure attachment with primary caretakers. Therefore, the recovery of healthy attachment is a major goal in psychotherapy for both the dissociative and nondissociative clients.

The major symptoms of nondissociative clients were PTSD-like symptoms. They were helped to process the abuse memories, particularly traumatic experiences at school. Proceeding under the assumption that clients experienced loss of secure attachment to their parents, the therapist also encouraged them to explore their relationships with parents.

The clients diagnosed with DDNOS presented with a dual system of dissociative identities, which the therapist called "the front personality" and "the original personality." The front personality was seen as a false identity that was artificially created to adapt to the emotionally distant or unresponsive parents. The front personality tended to compulsively conform to what the client believed people expected, and he or she suppressed authentic feelings and thoughts of the original personalities.

The original personality was seen as the authentic identity that had been denied his or her expressions in the real world. The original personality compulsively conforms, via the front personality, to the expectations and demands of the adults around him or her.

The goals of the phase-oriented treatment were: (1) recovery of emotions, (2) recovery of the original identity, (3) forming new attachment with the original identity, and (4) rehabilitation.

Successful treatment depends on the restoration of the original identity and the clinical recovery of the client's emotions. In treatment, a client was helped to attend inward and to seek out and feel repressed emotions. No clients recovered ritual abuse memories of physical and sexual nature, as they had no such histories.

It should be noted that the Hikikomori treatment did not have the risk of the so-called "false memory syndrome," that is, the questionable accuracy of the patient's recovered sexual and physical abuse memories, which have been the subject of debate with cases of DID in North America (Pezdek & Banks, 1998). Sexual abuse has never been an issue in the psychotherapy for Hikikomori clients.

Once a client recovers repressed emotions, he or she is able to restore the original identity that possessed: (1) a desire to live, (2) an ability to relate to people, (3) an ability to make decisions, and (4) an ability to grow. The original identity often emerges as a child personality state, at age 3 or younger. These clients were diagnosed as suffering DDNOS, as they did not experience amnesia after identity alternation. The restoration of the original identity is regarded as vitally important in the client's recovery from withdrawn behaviors, as only the original identity is capable of forming intimate relationships. Without it, the clients will remain withdrawn socially and psychologically. Hence, their total social shutdown was seen as the absence of attachment behavior or intimacy-seeking desire in the client's personality system.

Forming a new attachment requires three major techniques: (1) affectionate eye contact by the therapist with the original personality, (2) communicating verbally with the original personality, and (3) validating the past traumas, most of which were attachment traumas. Affectionate eye contact, wherein the therapist gazes at a client's eyes like the mother of a newborn baby, is clinically important for a new attachment with the original identity, as their parents tended to avoid eye contact. Communicating with the original identity freed the client from the inhibition of self-expression. Validating the past trauma, especially attachment trauma, helped the client feel accepted as a decent human being.

When the original identity formed a new attachment with the therapist, the client was often able to come out of the social withdrawal and became interested in exploring the external world. In the rehabilitation phase, the therapist trained the patient in developing social skills such as making decisions, saying "no," confronting others without explosion of anger, and expressing emotions and thoughts more freely. The therapist may accompany a client in his or her daytime activities, such as visiting a park or public places, or meeting with new people whom the therapist regards as safe for the client.

The same technique applies to the non-dissociative clients, except for the recovery of the original personality.

Hikikomori is treatable. The success of treatment, however, depends on the restoration of the original identity, which a client had not previously expressed to another person. If a client fails to recover the original identity, he or she will remain withdrawn psychologically and socially. A similar principle applies to the non-dissociative clients, that is, if the client fails to recover repressed emotions, he or she will remain withdrawn psychologically and socially. The recovery would take at least two years of weekly sessions. The parents are usually cooperative, since they are afraid of their child's lifetime dependence on them. The rate of dropout is approximately 50%, due to the clients' resistance to recovering repressed emotions and distrust of the therapist.

DISCUSSION

These case studies have found that the major symptom of Hikikomori is distrust of people. The pervasive disturbance in these clients is the inability to trust or relate to people.

With no confidence in other human beings, the patients tend to feel unsafe or unprotected with people. They try hard not to offend others, while they suppress authentic feelings and thoughts in interpersonal relationships. With Hikikomori clients, fear of rejection, criticism, and being disliked usually lay behind their absence of self-expression. The clients withdraw from all relationships when they emotionally burn out from such compulsive compliance to others.

Hikikomori is officially defined as a state of social withdrawal of more than 6 months in duration without psychotic symptoms. People with this condition would seem to have some features in common with other disorders, which may confuse diagnosis. To provide patients with appropriate and effective therapy, professionals must differentiate Hikikomori from other diagnoses.

Initially, the definition of Hikikomori may sound similar to Agoraphobia. In particular, the shut-in behavior of a person with Hikikomori could potentially be confused with symptoms of Agoraphobia, which is clinically the pervasive avoidance of being outside the home or a fear of open places. The diagnosis of Agoraphobia, however, does not include such clinical features as dissociative identities, the phobia of humans, emotional numbness, or other characteristics of Hikikomori.

Unlike an anxiety disorder or phobic avoidance, Hikikomori is a trauma-based disorder, since the clients have histories of complex traumas, mostly from emotional neglect.

In terms of dual personalities, people with Hikikomori are similar to adult children of alcoholics. Charles Whitfield (1989) discusses extensively the dual personality system of the "real self and false self," and the "inner child and co-dependent self," or the "private self and public self " among American patients from dysfunctional families. His psychotherapy focuses on healing the inner child, although he does not address the issue of attachment trauma. This technique is clinically equivalent to the author's recovering and forming a healthy attachment with the client's original identity, which is usually in a child state at emergence. In this study, however, the Hikikomori patients were more severely disturbed than the adult children of alcoholics, who usually do not have the symptom of total social shutdown and are able to form some relationships.

The inhibition of true self and manipulation for parental care is cross-culturally found among children with attachment problems. Beverly James (1994) stated that for an insecurely attached child, "her selfhood is not acceptable to society, her parents, and herself." She pointed out that children assume adaptive roles in dysfunctional families as a survival mechanism. Describing children who ignore their authentic feelings and thoughts in exchange for parental care, James wrote that, "Children's adaptive roles include being overly compliant with abusive parents, being entertainers with distracted parents, being mini-care givers with needy parents" (1994).

The Hikikomori clients' impaired abilities to trust or feel safe with people can be associated with their distrust of parents, their lack of care-free expressions of emotions and thoughts during childhood, and school trauma. Their fear of real or perceived parental abandonment appears connected to attachment problems with their parents. Fear of abandonment and rejection, first by their parents and then by their friends, resulted in the inhibition of their authentic feelings and personal thoughts. The inability to relate to people is believed to originate from attachment trauma (Sable, 2000). Patients couldn't feel safe with the parents, who some clients depicted with dehumanizing statements, such as: "She never appeared real," or "Robots can't raise a human child."

Typically, Hikikomori families are emotionally unsupportive. Most clients described passive-aggressive conflicts between their parents. The husband and father is usually a workaholic, often angry, and frequently away from home. The home mother may desire care from her child, reversing the parent-child role. This reversed role constitutes co-dependency, which Robert Subby defined as "the denial or repression of the real self" (1987).

Co-dependency between the mother and the child was frequently found in the clients' emotionally dysfunctional families. It appears to underlie the intense rage clients feel towards their mothers, which they frequently expressed by this common statement to their mother: "You made me a sick person."

A 28-year-old female client's account of her mother's behavior with her demonstrates the kind of codependent dynamics usually present in Hikikomori families. The mother was frustrated with her own lack of emotional bond with her workaholic husband. After six months of exploring her relationship with her mother, the client identified that her mother was emotionally dependent on the child. During therapy, the client disclosed the following about her mother:

> My mother depended on me for comforting. My mother treated me like her personal teddy bear and used me to satisfy her own emotional needs. She wasn't interested in knowing my feelings and thoughts. I don't think my mother regarded me as a human with free will. She sometimes looked like a zombie to me. I felt emotionally suffocated, as I couldn't communicate with her. I secretly feared my mother, but I tried always to please her. I wanted freedom. I felt emotionally abandoned as a child.

In a Hikikomori family, the parents' pathogenic behaviors leave the client feeling that attachments are not reliable or available for her. She is afraid that telling those from whom she seeks support about her feelings, such as anger or disappointment, will cause them to abandon her.

The patient in such an emotionally unsupportive family has a history of not expressing their original identity to their parents. The inhibition of true self is related to their (1) loss of secure attachment, (2) feelings of being unprotected, (3) creation of a false front identity, (4) relative absence of care-free childhood, (5) distrust of people, and (6) rage and hatred of parents.

Coming from this family environment, the Hikikomori patient enters therapy with belief systems and behaviors that present treatment challenges. The clients' beliefs that human beings are by nature unpredictable and unreliable, combined with their compulsion to please or avoid offending others, makes them poor candidates for certain kinds of therapy.

The client's inability to express authentic emotions and thoughts presented significant challenges in therapy. Group therapy was counterproductive, due to the clients' prevailingly compulsive compliance with others. In a group setting, the clients more strongly suppressed their authentic feelings and thoughts, which reinforced their false front identities. The intense distrust of parents made family therapy impossible, due to the resistance of the clients.

The Japanese public tends to be hostile to Hikikomori and assumes that it is a moral weakness, rather than a legitimate psychological disorder (Hattori, Chicago, 2003; Hattori, Melbourne, 2003; Saito, 1998). Failing to see the real pain these individuals suffer, the man or woman on the street regards people with Hikikomori as spoiled, lazy young people who willfully disregard their parents' wishes and arbitrarily avoid social obligations. In order to avoid criticism and even ostracism, the parents of those with Hikikomori hide their shut-in children from their relatives, neighbors, and their communities (Saitama newspaper, 2001).

Some laypeople organize boot-camp facilities, where parents coerce youth with Hikikomori into military-like training programs. In this setting, the youth are forced to perform manual labor for disciplinary purposes (Osada, 2001). Given the personality traits and belief systems of people with Hikikomori, these "programs" are more likely to harm than heal. Mushi, or shunning, in school is an extension of societal attitudes. This same lack of empathy is also reflected in the passive-aggressive attitude or "Mushi" of the Japanese government that has not allocated a specific budget for the syndrome. Such a social atmosphere would explain why youth with Hikikomori have received so little systematic focus from their countrymen.

CONCLUSIONS

Traditional Japanese families, wherein emotional expressions are inhibited, parent-child interactions are minimized, the welfare of a child has the lowest priority in the family hierarchy, and the role reversal or co-dependency exists between the mother and child are highly likely to produce more youth with Hikikomori. This disorder is more likely to occur among the traditional families of government employees, teachers, farmers, corporate executives, and traditional business owners. In short, Japanese-style oppressive child rearing and education can cause social withdrawal.

The inhibition of self-expression, due to emotional neglect and a lack of communication between parent and a child, apparently can create Hikikomori. Japanese school settings also inhibit self-expression, further reinforcing the child's assumptions about human nature and the social unacceptability of their authentic emotions and thoughts.

The inability to relate to other humans, the primary clinical feature of Hikikomori, disables people in the area of mating and child rearing. Covert Hikikomori may prevail in a larger number than now estimated, and its presence may be linked to the decreases in marriage, birth rates, and population of Japan. With only about 25% of Japanese marriages still arranged, people today marry primarily for love. Without the institution of arranged marriage, young people must form emotional bonds with the opposite sex, which Hikikomori youth are unable to do if left untreated.

Hikikomori is a treatable but progressive disorder. An optimistic prognosis can be expected only with early intervention. People who have had been withdrawn 15 years or more will have a guarded prognosis, as it is more difficult to recover long-repressed feelings and individual thoughts.

With an estimate of 1,400,000 sufferers in mind, this study suggests that Dissociative Disorder Not Otherwise Specified, involving dissociative identities, is mushrooming in the young people of Japan. Regrettably, the mainstream of the Japanese professional community does not share this view. Until the mental health community grasps the true nature and effective treatment of this disorder, hundreds of thousands of Japanese young people will remain locked within the painful isolation of Hikikomori.

REFERENCES

American Psychiatric Association (1994). *Diagnostic and Statistical Manual of Mental Disorders, 4th Edition*. Washington, DC: Author.

Aoki, S. (2002). Futouko, Hikikomori, Kateinai-boryoku No Enjyo (Supports for school truancy, Hikikomori, and domestic violence). *Japanese Journal of Adolescence Psychiatry*, 12(1):76.

Asahi Newspaper (2001). Hikikomori Soudan 6000 Ken (6000 cases of mental health visiting for Hikikomori), May 9.

Bernstein, E., & Putnam, F. W. (1986). Development, reliability and validity of a dissociation scale. *Journal of Nervous and Mental Disease,* 172, 197-202.

Hattori, Y. (2003). Keynote Panel: Social Withdrawal/DDNOS Through Faulty Attachment between Parents and Child in Seemingly Well-Functioning Japanese Families. International Conference on Trauma, Attachment, and Dissociation: Transforming Trauma, Melbourne, Australia. The Delphi Center. September 14, 2003.

Hattori, Y. (2003). Workshop: Treatment of Hikikomori Patients. The 20th International Fall Conference, Chicago. The International Society for the Study of Dissociation (ISSD). November 15, 2003.

Ikegami, M. (2001). Hikikomori Seikanki (Survival Stories of Hikikomori Sufferers). *Shougakukan Bunko.*

Inoue, Y. (2002). Gendai No Seinenki to Hikikomori (The Current Relationship Between Adolescence and Withdrawal in Japan). *Japanese Journal of Adolescence Psychiatry,* 12(1):21-28.

Ishikawa, K. (2002, October). Hikikomori wa Naze Umare Ikanishite Naosunoka (How are Hikikomori sufferers produced and treated?). *Shunjyusha.*

Ishiya, H. (2002). Futouko, Kateinai-boryoku, Hikikomori (School Truancy, Domestic Violence, and Hikikomori). *Japanese Journal of Adolescence Psychiatry,* 2(1):76-77.

James, B. (1994). *Handbook for Treatment of Attachment-Trauma Problems in Children.* The Free Press. New York.

Japan Times (2003). Group seeks care for socially withdrawn. Nao Shimoyachi, staff writer. April 22.

Katsuyama, M. (2001). Hikikomori Calender. Bunshun Nesco.

Machizawa, S. (2003). Hikikomoru Wakamono-tachi (Young People Withdrawing from Society). *Yamato Shobo.*

Mainichi Newspaper (2003). Nihon Byo (Hikikomori as Japanese culture-bound syndrome). Takahiro Takino. February 5.

Ogi, N. (2001). Rinsho Kyoiku Kenkyujo Niji (Clinical Education Research Institute Rainbow). Retrieved April 10th from http//www2.odn.ne.jp

Osada, U. (2001). Oyaga Kawareba Kodomo Mo Kawaru (A change in parents leads to a change in child). Kodansha. Tokyo.

Pezdek, K., & Banks, W. P. (1998). *The Recovered Memory/False Memory Debate.* Academic Press. San Diego, London, Boston, New York, Sydney, Tokyo, & Toronto.

Sable, P. (2000). *Attachment and Adult Psychotherapy.* Northvale: Jason Aronson Inc.

Saitama Newspaper. (2001). Oya Tachi Wa Ugoki Hajimeta: Hikikomori Series (Parents in action: Hikikomori cases), January 19, 20, 21, 23, 24, 25, 26, 27, 28, 29.

Saito, T. (1998). *Shakaiteki Hikikomori* (Social Withdrawal). PHP Institute. Tokyo.

Saito, T. (2002). Shakaiteki Hikikomori No Genjho To Tenbo (Social Withdrawal in Adolescent Japanese). *Japanese Journal of Adolescent Psychiatry.* 12(1): 13-20.

Saito, T. (2003). Hikikomori Bunkaron (Cultural Perspectives of Hikikomori). *Kinokuniya Shoten.*

Shohatsu. (2001). Guideline for social withdrawal of youths in teens and twenties. *Journal of The Ministry of Health and Welfare,* 199, May 8.

SPA! (2000) Hikikomori No Shinjitsu (The reality of Hikikomori). Kazumi Ishimaru, Takako Kurihara, & Naoyuki Shinohara. June 7.

Strick, F. L., & Wilcoxon, A. (1991). A comparison of dissociative experiences in adult female outpatients with and without histories of early incestuous abuse. *Dissociation,* 4(4): 193-199.

Subby, R. (1987). *Lost in the Shuffle.* Health Communications, Inc. Deerfield Beach, Florida.

Sunday Mainichi (weekly magazine; 2001a, May 20). Seikan from Hikikomori (Escape from Hikikomori). Contributed by Masaki Ikegami.

Sunday Mainichi (weekly magazine; 2001b, May 27). Hikikomori To Vietnam Veteran No Kokuji (Similarities between Hikikomori and Vietnam Veterans with PTSD). Contributed by Masaki Ikegami.

Sunday Mainichi (weekly magazine; 2001c, June 5). Free School No Hikikomori Saloon (Casual Meetings for Hikikomori Sufferers at Tokyo Shale). Hikikomori. Contributed by Masaki Ikegami.

Sunday Mainichi (weekly magazine; 2003, March 30), Hikikomori Wa Kyushitsu Subekika Houtte Oku Beki Ka (Should people with Hikikomori be rescued or left alone?).

Tabidachi (2002). Journal of KHJ Oyano Kai (Zenkoku Hikikomori Oyano-Kai). November 14.

Tanaka. C. (2001). Hikikomori No Kazoku Kankei (Family Relationships of Hikikomori Sufferers). Kodansha.

Tokyo Newspaper (2001, May 9). Hikikomori Shakai (Social Withdrawal Society).

Uchida, T. (2001). Hikikomori Karute (Clinical Records of Hikikomori Sufferers). Houken.

Uchida, Y. (2001). Oya Ga Kawareba Ko Mo Kawaru (A child will change if his parents change). Kodansha.

Ueyama, K. (2001). Hikikomori datta boku kara. (I was a Hikikomori sufferer). Kodansha.

Whitfield, L. C. (1989). *Healing the Child Within.* Deerfield Beach: Health Communications, Inc.

Yomiuri Newspaper (2001, April 6). Hikikomori Oya No Sei Sanpi Gekiron (Is Hikikomori caused by parents?)

Zielenziger, M. (2002). Deep pessimism infecting many aspects of Japanese society. *San Jose Mercury News.* December 29, 2002.

Trauma and Dissociation in Aotearoa (New Zealand): The Psyche of a Society

Susan Farrelly
Thomas Rudegeair
Sharon Rickard

SUMMARY. Aotearoa, or the more widely used term, New Zealand (NZ), is a sparsely populated country of four million with a land area roughly the size of California. It is far from the world's centres of power, both geographically and ideologically. Colonisation by the British in the nineteenth century occurred relatively recently and relatively smoothly. The country's indigenous people, the Maori, endured the ordeal of colonisation but today comprise 14.7% of the population (Ministry of Social Development, 2003). Maori, however, are over-represented in prisons and in mental health facilities. Suicide rates, especially among Maori youth, are higher than for non-Maori, as are rates of substance abuse.

Susan Farrelly, MBChB, is Psychiatric Consultant, Cornwall House, Auckland District Health Board, Auckland New Zealand. Thomas Rudegeair, MD, PhD, is Psychiatric Consultant, Te Whetu Tawera, Auckland Hospital, Auckland District Health Board, Auckland, New Zealand. Sharon Rickard, BA, MA(Hons) PGDipClinPsych, is Clinical Psychologist: Head of Te Aho Tapu Trust–Psychological Services, South Auckland.

Address correspondence to: Susan Farrelly, Cornwall House, Aukland District Health Board, Auckland, New Zealand.

[Haworth co-indexing entry note]: "Trauma and Dissociation in Aotearoa (New Zealand): The Psyche of a Society." Farrelly, Susan, Thomas Rudegeair, and Sharon Rickard. Co-published simultaneously in *Journal of Trauma Practice* (The Haworth Maltreatment & Trauma Press, an imprint of The Haworth Press, Inc.) Vol. 4, No. 3/4, 2005, pp. 203-220; and: *Trauma and Dissociation in a Cross-Cultural Perspective: Not Just a North American Phenomenon* (ed: George F. Rhoades, Jr., and Vedat Sar) The Haworth Maltreatment & Trauma Press, an imprint of The Haworth Press, Inc., 2005, pp. 203-220. Single or multiple copies of this article are available for a fee from The Haworth Document Delivery Service [1-800-HAWORTH, 9:00 a.m. - 5:00 p.m. (EST). E-mail address: docdelivery@haworthpress.com].

Health statistics generally are poorer among Maori, including lower life expectancies (Durie, 2001; Ministry of Social Development, 2003; Ministry of Youth Development, 2001). There are, of course, modern-day traumas of all sorts throughout New Zealand society but Maori children are more at risk of illness, intentional injury and sexual abuse (Ministry of Health, 1998). We contend that this social picture is a reflection of the trauma of colonisation transmitted, as trauma often is, through generations. The fundamental trauma to Maori has been cultural and, although remedies have been actively pursued, much remains to be done. Along with the indigenous people, we suggest that the broad NZ society suffers the systemic effects of trauma, many of which are dissociative in nature. Our society's challenge is first to acknowledge the prevalence of trauma-induced dissociation and then to design corrective approaches to reduce the suffering of trauma survivors and to improve the efficiency of our own institutions. *[Article copies available for a fee from The Haworth Document Delivery Service: 1-800-HAWORTH. E-mail address: <docdelivery@haworthpress.com> Website: <http://www.HaworthPress.com> © 2005 by The Haworth Press, Inc. All rights reserved.]*

KEYWORDS. Cultural trauma, New Zealand, dissociation

As we prepared this discussion of the nature of Aotearoa's trauma history and the ways in which dissociation has manifested itself as a consequence, it became clear to us that the understanding of trauma and dissociation within a culture demands an all-encompassing historical exploration. Just as the persistence of dissociation in an individual can only be understood in light of developmental stressors, so too the dissociative aspects of a people are a consequence of the traumas, both acute and chronic, to which whole populations have been exposed. Although this brief exploration is by no means exhaustive, the very act of reviewing Aotearos's cultural evolution has provided new insights for us into the psyche of our rich and extremely multi-cultural society.

AOTEAROA'S TRAUMA HISTORY

Overview

Aotearoa rests safely in the South Pacific some 1500 miles from Australia, the nearest major land mass. As a consequence it has been relatively isolated from the major events that have traumatised Europe, the Middle East, and Asia over the last century. Although Kiwi men, many of whom were Maori, fought and died in wars around the globe (the Maori Battalion suffered especially heavy casualties in World War II), the devastation of modern warfare has never been directly visited upon Aotearoa.

Significant trauma has permeated Aotearoa's history, however, and the prevalence of indices of trauma-related problems indicates that trauma continues to affect many New Zealanders. As in any country with a history of intense colonialism, cultural trauma was visited upon Maori. More recently the country has become a haven for traumatised emigrants from Europe, Asia and North Africa, and the city of Auckland has become the biggest "Pacific Island" city in the world. The resultant economic, cultural and racial diversity has created vitality but has also generated significant social stress. The diversity of traumatised, disenfranchised and impoverished people in Aotearoa poses a serious challenge to the public mental health services.

Brief History of Aotearoa Colonisation and Maori Cultural Trauma

Maori had occupied NZ for at least 800 years when the Dutch explorer, Abel Tasman arrived in 1642 (Walker, 1990). The Maori tribal level of organisation created a mosaic of inter-related and competing groups that extended the full 1600 km length of the North and South Islands. The world of the pre-European Maori was focused around food growing and gathering, with episodic eruptions of inter-group "warfare" over access to resources. As Michael King (2003a) summarises, however,

> So long as the Maori possessed only hand-to-hand weapons and lacked large quantities of portable food, warfare was probably not endemic. It . . . often resulted in the deaths of no more than a handful of combatants. . . . Nor were all Maori forever at war with all other Maori. (p. 83)

Regarding the quality of Maori life, King (2003a) concludes:

> Apart from the times of sporadic inter-tribal conflict, when existence was threatened by violence, enslavement or death, life would have been as culturally rich and as physically pleasant as anywhere else on earth in comparably Neolithic times. (p. 91)

The arrival of the Europeans dramatically altered the Maori way of life: . . . the balances and certitudes developed over at least five centuries of occupation of New Zealand would be . . . seriously challenged in the eighteenth [century]. . . . Europeans would succeed in . . . introducing Maori to . . . all the cultural, technological and pathogenic impedimenta carried by mankind. . . . (p. 91)

But the British version of colonisation implemented in Aotearoa was significantly different from the strategy employed in other countries such as Australia and the United States, where the process was swifter and more physically violent. In Aotearoa a combination of disease, musket warfare, land wars, land legislation and alienation contributed to a decline in the Maori population and ultimately the disappearance of traditional Maori society (Durie, 2001; Walker, 1990). The initial resolution of the Maori-European conflict was relatively benign, however. The 1840 Treaty of Waitangi between the Crown and at least a large subset of North Island Maori chiefs guaranteed Maori Tino Rangatiratanga o õ rãtou wenua o rãtou kãinga me o rãtou taonga katoa," which is interpreted as "the unqualified exercise of chieftainship over their lands, villages and their treasures" (Te Puni Kokiri, 2002). Unfortunately, in the English text "all the rights and powers of sovereignty" were ceded to the Queen of England." (King, 2003b; Orange, 1987; Te Puni Kokiri, 2002). The impact of the Treaty was complex. Wholesale bloodshed was averted but the ambiguous interpretations of its meaning would lead to the undermining of Maori cultural traditions and a resultant cultural trauma that has reverberated down the generations to the 21st century.

Maori were members of local tribal units rather than an overarching national society and thus tended to focus on inter-tribal issues. Even Maori parliamentary representatives were unable to forge a consensus to stand against the initiatives organised to benefit the Europeans and the Maori position quickly eroded.

Central to the emerging cultural trauma was the usurping of Maori lands. Maori were tangata whenua (people of the land) and the concept of legal ownership was alien to them. The English version of the Treaty granted Maori possession but only until they decided to relinquish it. Maori dominion over the land was initially destabilized through the land wars between Maori and British forces. However, far more destructive than guns was the passing of parliamentary acts specifically designed to separate Maori from their land. In particular, the Suppression of Rebellion Act and the New Zealand Settlements Act both passed in 1863 gave the colonial government power to confiscate entire districts from tribes who were 'believed' to be in rebellion (Awatere, 1984; Durie, 2001; Walker, 1990). For example, in the Waikato alone, the government confiscated 887,808 acres. Prior to confiscation the Waikato people had supported themselves comfortably and were able to offer hospitality generously. After confiscation the Waikato people could barely subsist on land of its own and quite apart from loss of income and livelihood, their land loss carried with it an intense sense of deprivation (King, 2003a; Durie, 2001).

Early consequences of Maori disenfranchisement included declining population numbers, due to many causes. As time went on they began to include the loss of language and culture, the overrepresentation of Maori in prisons and mental hospitals, higher levels of suicide, substance abuse, and more medical morbidity. Interestingly, the trend towards increasing rates of psychiatric hospitalisation began around 1970, with lower rates for Maori before that time (Durie, 2001).

The erosion of Maori cultural foundations and the usurping of Maori resources was formally addressed with the passage of the Treaty of Waitangi Act in 1975 which established the Waitangi Tribunal (King, 2003a). In its initial stages the Tribunal could only address claims made from 1975 onwards. In 1985 this was remedied and claims dating back to 1840 were also included. The Tribunal is now a permanent commission of inquiry intended to make recommendations on claims brought by Maori relating to actions or omissions of the Crown that potentially violate the promises made in the Treaty of Waitangi. Significantly, under the auspices of the Tribunal, the rights of Maori moved beyond a narrow interpretation of the Treaty as assuring only Maori rights to physical resources into a broader entitlement to authority over cultural and social "property" as well, including cultural beliefs and practices around mental "illness." Buoyed by the support of the Tribunal, Maori cultural pride and assertiveness has flourished over the last two decades. However, the legacy of colonialism in the form of cultural trauma persists.

THE IMPACT OF CULTURAL TRAUMA

Trauma results in sustained dissociation on many levels. It is interesting, and we think salient, to explore the kinds of societal dissociation which have resulted from the cultural trauma described above. The initial response of Maori to the colonization was, paralleling events in individual trauma situations, a kind of "identification with the aggressor." It was cooperative, opportunistic, and involved a suppression of those characteristics which accentuated difference. Through missionary influence Maori rapidly adopted Western dress, pushed for their children to learn English in school, and began trading, seeing the benefits of selling goods important to the Pakeha (Europeans) and easily obtained by Maori. Initially most Maori lived in rural areas, quite separately from the majority of Pakeha, and interactions with Pakeha were primarily for trading purposes. The Europeans wanted land and food. Maori wanted guns as well as an array of tools unavailable prior to the arrival of European traders. As Maori access to traditional food sources became more difficult, and Pakeha goods more highly prized, young Maori began to shift away from traditional life in communal areas, and into the urban environment. This demanded even more suppression of Maori ways and the success of this strategy was limited. Maori life was very communitarian in philosophy, significantly with regard to land ownership, and measures of achievement. Pakeha society focused on individual ownership and individual measures of achievement. These cultural differences retain huge significance to the present day.

Maori, consequently, who had begun as a very tribal people and had initially resisted integration by remaining on tribal land, gave the superficial appearance of "integration" into the new Pakeha society. This required, however, a powerful suppression of many things Maori. Language was almost entirely lost as parents insisted on their children gaining the benefits of learning the Pakeha language (Benton, 1979; King, 2003a). Assimilation policies and theories of cultural deprivation gave rise to negative stereotyping of Maori. "Not speaking English was seen as a flaw and fluency in Maori was seen to be the cause for deficiency in English. In this way Maori people as well as their language were discriminated against. In becoming more proficient in English they were actually becoming more English and less Maori (Coxon, Jenkins, Marshall & Massey, 1994). By 1995, only 8% of Maori were fluent in their original language (Durie, 2001). Tribal customs and oral histories suffered as the urban shift meant that traditional communal events no longer involved the younger people, who then grew up without the histories and without the language. Maori were good at "being Pakeha," but it gradually became clear to many observers that this was happening at enormous cost.

Maori performance in schools, as a general rule, was often poor for many reasons. Early beliefs regarding Maori school failure were explained as an intellectual deficiency within Maori. By the 1960s Maori educational failure was explained through theories of 'cultural deprivation.' Large families, overcrowding in homes, group-centred ways of living and language problems were all factors indicative of this deprivation. Strategies formulated to address this deprivation amounted to nothing more than an increased imposition of English culture upon Maori pupils (Coxon et al., 1994). There was minimal Maori participation in curriculum design or in the education system in general and Maori children continued to perform poorly. Where parents spoke Maori and children English, their estrangement increased. European emphasis on individual achievement disadvantaged Maori children, and adults, in a competitive Pakeha system. Cultural separateness was enhanced.

In 1874 the New Zealand Herald read " . . . the native race is dying out in New Zealand . . . the fact cannot be disguised that the natives are gradually passing away; and even if no cause should arise to accelerate their decrease, the rate at which they are now disappearing points to their extinction in an exceedingly brief period" (New Zealand Herald, 17 August, 1874). By 1896, the population had decreased to its lowest point, 42,000, and it seemed likely that by the next century Maori would be extinct (Durie, 2001). The passing of the Maori race did not occur, however, and the population decline was halted. By 1936 the Maori population totalled 82,000 and by 1996 an all-time high was recorded with 579,714 claiming Maori ancestry (Durie, 2001). These high numbers mean that the ongoing effects of the trauma are impossible to ignore.

Over time, the suppression of the constituent parts of cultural identity has resulted in a sense of serious disadvantage and deprivation among Maori, with associated rage and resentment and great loss of "mana" (loosely translated as somewhere between power and self esteem). As an added complication for urban Maori, Pakeha governments approved escalating immigration, increasing the country's population and racial complexity. What was initially conceptualised as a "bi-racial" society has become dramatically multi-racial, with increasing inter-racial tensions, and with a shift away from the original emphasis on bi-cultural partnership.

Within this context Maori have developed an increasing awareness of the need for education and the fundamental importance of their own language and cultural connections for the wellbeing of their children. Emphasis on cultural learning has grown among Maori, and led in the early 1970s to the development of kohanga reo (or Maori "language nests") to provide preschool education with a Maori language and cultural context. Over time, with pressure from both Maori and Pakeha educators, Maori language immersion classes have been established within mainstream Pakeha education systems, as well as Kura Kaupapa Maori or Maori language schools with a powerful emphasis on cultural practice. This has raised self esteem and pride among young Maori.

Along with an emphasis on Maori-focused education, attempts at reparation have been made in the realm of mental health, with an overt emphasis on cultural identity and recognition of the need for Maori workers alongside mainstream workers. There has also, more innovatively, been an emphasis on the development of separate Maori mental health streams, so that Maori are given a choice of 'style' of care. This, perhaps ironically, has introduced a dissociative element into the treatment approach to dissociogenic trauma.

Within the approach of psychiatry itself there has developed another type of dissociation. There is now an essential split, in Aotearoa as in many other countries, between practice that recognizes the significance of trauma in the generation of "mental illness" and the prevailing "biopsychosocial" model (a more fundamentally medical way of practice). This translates into a split between those who see addressing trauma as a primary treatment for mental illness, and those who rely heavily, or even exclusively, on pharmacotherapy (Read, Perry, Moskowitz & Connolly, 2001; Read, Mosher & Bentall, 2004).

At the governmental and legal level there are also dissociative elements. There has been major recognition of the cultural trauma in our history and a formal attempt has been made to increase bi-cultural awareness. This effort to enhance recognition between previously isolated societal "alters" strikes us as an important element in a kind of societal dissociative therapy. Classes on the Treaty are now requisite in many institutions such as schools, universities and medical systems. The government has issued a public apology to the Maori people, and the Tribunal constitutes a formal vehicle for hearing and deciding Maori claims under the treaty. Settlements through the Tribunal have served to help reconstitute a sense of pride and Maori cultural identity (King, 2003a). Initially most claims were land related, and settlements were made from "Crown" (i.e., government-owned) lands; more recently cases were of a more subtle nature. The concept of "taonga," broadly translated as treasures, was enshrined in the Treaty and the consequent legal obligations remain a focus for the ongoing attention of the Tribunal. Matters of health, education and conservation have been regarded as relevant in this forum (King, 2003a). Customary rights to fishing grounds, seabed and foreshore ownership, and even Maori television, have been argued in this court.

In line with our understanding of effective treatment for dissociation (either intra-psychic or intra-societal) the next step in the integrative "therapy" of this trauma-induced state must be aimed at increasing mutual empathy and developing an understanding of the mutual history. There must be a focus on shared communication and decision making. Even on this systemic level, recognition of the importance and validity of the essential parts of the whole followed by an emphasis on the facilitation of internal communication and collaboration, toward a mutually beneficial and validating shared end, seems likely to be the effective model for healing a traumatised society.

THE IMPACT OF INDIVIDUAL TRAUMA

Aotearoa, as any country, has a significant degree of the usual trauma seen on an individual level. Although we have a very low murder rate (possibly related to our very stringent gun control laws), there are high rates of physical and sexual assault, child abuse and neglect, and youth suicide (Beautrais, 2000; Fergusson, Horwood & Lynskey, 1996a; Mullen, Martin, Anderson, Romans & Herbison, 1993; Mullen, Martin, Anderson, Romans & Herbison, 1996). As we have already noted, Maori are especially affected as they are over-represented in prison populations and mental health statistics (Durie, 2001; Brinded, Simpson, Laidlaw, Fairly & Malcolm, 2001), show high rates of suicide (New Zealand Health Information Service, 2004), child abuse (Ministry of Health, 1998), and medical morbidity. Maori have higher rates of obesity, smoking, have a shorter lifespan and are significantly more likely to be admitted to hospital compared with non-Maori (Ministry of Social Development, 2003). Maori children are significantly more likely to fail a school entry hearing test than are non-Maori children (Ministry of Health, 1998). Maori are more likely to be disabled and on welfare (Ministry of Social Development, 2003). It is clear that the results of trauma, both cultural and more intimate in origin, are widespread and various and will be demonstrated in our prisons and hospitals. Research done in our own hospitals show clearly that the rate of identified trauma in psychiatric inpatients is very high (Read et al., 2001).

There are also significant elements of systemic dissociation in the addressing of individual trauma. In 1974 the government established a statutory body, known as the Accident Compensation Corporation, whose role is to assess injury and allot appropriate compensation following accidents of all sorts. Initially the concept of injury was purely physical, applied to accidents within and without the workplace. With no allocated budget and a legally defined mandate, funds were raised from employers and employees. The limits of the Corporation's responsibilities are continually tested in court. As a result of this legal process, the brief has been enlarged, first to encompass injury of the emotional and psychological kind, secondary specifically to sexual abuse and later to include Post-Traumatic Stress Disorder (PTSD) secondary to other physical injury. There is still no brief for emotional or psychological harm, secondary to accident, but not related to physical injury, so PTSD alone is not covered.

On the surface, the establishment of the Corporation is a good thing and should ensure that trauma is addressed adequately. However, as a result of the establishment of the ACC, the treatment of the sequelae of childhood abuse most often occurs in the private system, with ACC covering most of the cost of counselling and other costs for abuse-related cases. Partly as a consequence of this, and partly, undoubtedly, as a legacy of the British model of psychiatry practiced here, there is yet another example of a dissociative split at the societal level, this time between trauma work and mainstream psychiatry. Despite an overt policy in mainstream psychiatric practice which mandates the taking of a trauma history on assessment, there is no directive about subsequent recognition or treatment of trauma related issues (Young, Read, Barker-Collo & Harrison, 2001). There is generally little attention paid in mainstream psychiatry to the importance of trauma in presentations to psychiatric services, especially in psychotic disorders. There is often quite overt hostility toward practitioners who choose to work with traumatized patients within the mainstream service, and an underlying ethic of, "it's not really our job." Within the mainstream remarkably few trauma-related diagnoses are formally assigned to patients. Between January 2002 and January 2003 there were only 24 diagnoses of DID made in the entire country within mainstream mental health services (Mental Health Information Collection data from the National Health Information Service, 2004). In a country of four million people, this is a prevalence of .0006%. This clearly indicates a fundamental split in the philosophies of treatment services, and in diagnostic models, between the private ACC funded system, and the public medical-model system.

Despite all of this, the public sector does treat traumatized patients. We have a very functional Dialectical Behavioural Therapy (DBT) treatment stream, and are working on the development of a more integrated, virtual trauma service (in the absence of a separate specifically trauma-focused service), within mainstream psychiatry (Farrelly & Rudegeair, 2004). Dissociation is, in this country, an unpopular concept and meets with both scepticism and hostility. We have made efforts to develop a "dissociation pathway" but thus far even the meetings of the working group have been so fragmented that the same group has never met twice. We have developed a dissociation interest group which meets quasi-regularly to discuss research projects and conceptual matters. It is a very stimulating and productive group, but has little clinical power, in effect, yet another dissociated fragment.

CULTURAL ASPECTS OF DISSOCIATION

As we have discussed, the urbanization of Maori, with the resultant disruption of traditional communal cultural supports, has generated social isolation and impoverishment with the predictable rise in the indices of trauma-related morbidities. One would expect the prevalence of dissociative disorders to be significantly elevated among Maori, but official data in NZ do not support this. We are convinced that this says much more about societal attitudes towards dissociation than it does about Maori intra-psychic structure. As we've pointed out, dissociative disorders are rarely diagnosed in New Zealand and, interestingly, were not even considered as a category in an important survey of mental illness among prison populations in NZ (Brinded et al., 2001). This study of the prevalence of psychiatric illness in NZ prison populations appears to present a golden opportunity to establish prevalence data for dissociative disorders (and trauma) in this most socially important population. Unfortunately, DSM-IV (Diagnostic and Statistical Manual of Mental Disorders, Fourth Edition, American Psychiatric Association [APA], 1994) dissociative disorders were ruled out as possibilities by the diagnostic tool employed by the researchers (the Composite International Diagnostic Interview–CIDI). In addition, the survey did not include questions around the history of physical abuse, sexual abuse, or neglect. Despite the absence of systematic prevalence data our current, admittedly anecdotal, clinical experience suggests significant dissociative symptomatology among Auckland Maori service users.

Although neither DSM-IV (APA, 1994) dissociative disorders nor the importance of individual trauma histories are adequately appreciated among NZ psychiatrists, there are some very encouraging developments. In parallel with, and possibly directly related to, the development of

Maori-focused mental health services there has developed a broader awareness in mainstream psychiatry of the particular ways in which trauma is manifested in Maori. Three such concepts are "mate Maori" in which illness is seen as the result of an infringement of a "tapu" (breach of a rule or restriction), from a "makutu" or curse being invoked by an outsider, "whakamaa" (which has an element of profound shame), and "whakamomori," defined variously as a deep seated underlying sadness, an inbuilt tribal suffering, and grieving without a death (Lawson-Te Aho, 1998a) Although these may present in the form of psychotic illness or be diagnosed as depression, we consider them likely to be dissociative in nature. "Whakamomori" for example may present as suicidal behaviour (and is sometimes used to mean suicide) and the effective treatment is cultural in essence, performed by a 'tohunga' ("expert"). This suicidal grief out of apparent context and responsive to cultural interventions is, we think, best understood as a dissociative illness exacerbated by Maori cultural trauma. Keri Lawson-Te Aho (1998b) agrees, linking Maori suicidal behaviour directly with unresolved collective grief following cultural trauma.

Yearly data for new "sensitive claims" (i.e., abuse-related) to the Accident Compensation Corporation (ACC) reveal a consistent yearly submission rate by Maori that is one and a half times the percentage of Maori in the general population (ACC, 2004). Although claim submission rates are obviously affected by multiple factors, these data reveal that the Maori are seeking assistance for the sequelae of childhood trauma at rates that suggest significant exposure to trauma. Perhaps surprisingly, given this data, diagnosis of Maori with specifically trauma-related diagnoses–Dissociative Identity Disorder (DID), Borderline Personality Disorder, and Post Traumatic Stress Disorder (PTSD)–within mainstream psychiatric services around the country are not disproportionately high (Mental Health Information Collection data from the National Health Information Service, 2004). The potential implications of this should stimulate investigative research.

THE DISSOCIATIVE NATURE OF TRAUMA RESEARCH IN AOTEAROAB

There is a distinctly dissociative phenomenon apparent in the organisation of research in this country. There is a great deal of research looking at trauma from many different and complementary perspectives, funded in many ways, from many sources, and by many routes from a diversity of (often dissociated) departments. For example, here is a lot of research, often statistical in nature, funded and organised directly by a multiplicity of government departments including the Ministries of Health, Social Policy and Development, Youth Development, Justice, Education, Research, Science and Technology, Women's Affairs, Maori Development ("Te Puni Kokiri"), Culture and Heritage. The Ministry of Research, Science and Technology guides the Health Research Council (HRC) which is a purchase agent partly responsible for the Governmental investment in research. The Ministry of Health is responsible for the publication of the Christchurch cohort study, to be described later, which was largely funded by the HRC. It has also published a report called *Our Children's Health* (Ministry of Health, 1998), presenting data in all areas of child health including injury and abuse. Many government departments commission their own research. The Ministry of Social development, for example, publishes a "publication archive" which includes many reports and studies on violence and abuse. The Ministry of Justice also has a research directory listing many studies of violence against women, child sexual abuse, etc. The Mental Health Commission (a governmental body advisory to the Ministry of Health), frequently commissions the writing of position papers on mental health related matters, including a recently published paper on the responsiveness, or the lack thereof, of mental health services to abuse (Wells, 2004).

So, many very different governmental organisations are in some way involved in the engendering and fostering of research on trauma. Much health research is university-based which is paid for by the government. Medical research often occurs in settings quite separate from Universities, e.g., in hospitals and, again, is often funded via the Health Research Council, also a governmental body. There are several major university centres generating trauma research, all with rather different foci. Much of the work has been cited in our discussion above. A brief overview of each follows.

Otago University, in Dunedin, runs a Multidisciplinary Health and Development Research Unit from the Department of Preventive and Social Medicine in the Medical School, under Associate Professor Richie Poulton. This unit has been responsible for a long-running cohort study of approximately 1000 babies who this year will turn 32. They have collected a wide range of psychosocial and biomedical information and published over 850 papers. Of particular interest is a part of the study (Caspi et al., 2002) which looks at violent behaviours in relation to experiences of physical abuse during childhood. Their interesting conclusion is that, although there is clearly a relationship, they have also identified some "protective factor," and have been investigating a gene locus in this respect.

The other major trauma research group in Dunedin was primarily focussed around Professor Paul Mullen (now Professor of Forensic Psychiatry at Monash University, Melbourne, Australia), and Dr. Sarah Romans. They, with various others, have published widely on the longer term effects of childhood sexual abuse in adulthood, usually assessing randomised community samples (e.g., Mullen et al., 1993; Romans, Martin, Anderson, Herbison & Mullen, 1995; Mullen et al., 1996; Kazantzis et al., 2000; Romans, Gendall, Martin & Mullens, 2001).

In Christchurch, where there is a clinical school of the Otago School of Medicine, Professor David Fergusson and John Harwood have repeated the cohort study with more than 1000 children, and have had a slightly different focus. Their cohort is now aged 21. They have explored the prevalence of psychiatric disorders and have looked closely at potential correlates such as ethnicity, trauma in childhood, and socioeconomic disadvantage. They have shown that Maori, and most dramatically Maori men, are consistently at higher risk of mental health problems than non-Maori (e.g., Fergusson, Horwood & Lynskey, 1996a,b).

A second Christchurch-based research group is the Canterbury Suicide Project run by researcher Dr. Annette Beautrais from the Christchurch School of Medicine and Health Sciences. She has published a great deal on suicide and risk factors, and has been the principal investigator on the research project since it began in 1991 (e.g., Beautrais, 2000).

A fourth research group works out of Massey University, in Palmerston North. The Head of Maori Studies is Professor Mason Durie, a psychiatrist and very widely published author on matters Maori. He has multiple areas of research interest, primarily relating to Maori health issues and the ongoing effects of colonisation on health. He, in collaboration with Dr. Chris Cunningham, runs the Research Centre for Public Health Research, along with the Research Centre for Maori Health and Development (e.g., Durie, 1998, 2001).

Massey University's Psychology department also has a focus on trauma in the broader sense and publishes the *Australasian Journal of Disaster and Trauma Studies*. The brief is to cover disasters of the natural, technological and human-generated types, exploring "disaster and trauma mitigation and prevention, response, support, recovery, treatment, policy formulation and planning and their implications at the individual, group, organisational and community level" (*Australasian Journal of Di-*

saster and Trauma Studies website, "About the Journal" Webpage, 1998).

The Psychology Department at the University of Auckland runs a Clinical Psychology doctoral programme. The Head of the programme is Dr. John Read who publishes extensively on the role of trauma, and childhood abuse in particular, in the generation of mental illness. He has done world-leading research, recently confirmed by a British study, showing the prevalence of childhood sexual abuse in both inpatient and outpatient psychiatric populations (see Read & Argyle, 1999; Read, Perry, Moskowitz & Connolly, 2001; Read, Mosher and Bentall, 2004). In the same department is Dr. Andrew Moskowitz (2004), whose primary research interest is in the relationship between dissociation, psychosis and violence.

In Auckland there is also a centre of interest in Kaupapa Maori and Indigenous Peoples' research. Growing out of an awareness of the ongoing need for research, of the traumas of colonisation worldwide, and the limitations of Western-model research methodologies, there is now a move toward "decolonising" research methodologies especially as they pertain to indigenous peoples. Linda Tuhiwai Smith, Associate Professor in Education and Director of the International Research Institute for Maori and Indigenous Education at the University of Auckland is a leader in such thinking in this country. She identifies several health research units around the country as using Kaupapa Maori models. These include Te Pumanawa Hauora, at Massey University, the Eru Pomare Research Centre at the Wellington School of Medicine, (both funded by the Health Research Council), a unit at the Auckland Medical School, and others inside existing centres such as the Alcohol and Public Health Research Centre at the University of Auckland (Smith, 1999).

It is clear from our current exploration that there is an ongoing need for better coordination and "integration" of research into trauma related areas. In a country as small as Aotearoa it does seem at least theoretically possible to produce a coordinated research approach, including Kaupapa Maori research attitudes. It would appear that dissociative elements have frustrated integration at all levels of social organisation.

CONCLUSION

Aotearoa's small population, remote location, and relatively recent and straightforward social history provide an opportunity to examine the impact of cultural trauma on an indigenous people who were dominated but not destroyed, traumatised but not obliterated. We contend that the European usurping of Maori resources, and the evolution of the Maori cultural response to the resultant trauma have shaped the psyche of the society. We have outlined how the indigenous people suffered but survived, attempted assimilation, languished, but ultimately re-asserted their cultural values. We have speculated that the dissociative elements in modern NZ society, detectable as much in our professional and governmental approaches to mental health as they are in the individual psychology of the citizens, are at least in part a consequence of our colonial history and our multi-cultural fabric. It is an exciting time to be confronting the dissociative aspects of NZ society informed by this historical perspective.

REFERENCES

Accident Compensation Commission, *Injury Statistics* (3rd Ed.). 2004. (Section 13.1. Sensitive Claims).

American Psychiatric Association. (1994). *Diagnostic and Statistical Manual, Fourth Edition*, Washington, DC: Author.

Australasian Journal of Disaster and Trauma Studies website, 1998. "About the Journal" webpage, Retrieved. 19 February, 2005, from http://www.massey.ac.nz/~trauma/info/journal.htm

Awatere, D. (1984). *Maori Sovereignty*. Broadsheet. Auckland, NZ.

Beautrais, A.L. (2000). Risk factors for suicide and attempted suicide among young people. *Australian and New Zealand Journal of Psychiatry*, 34, 420-436.

Benton, R. A. (1979) *Maori Language in the Nineteen Seventies*. New Zealand Council for Educational Research. Wellington, NZ.

Brinded, P.M., Simpson, A.I., Laidlaw, T.M., Fairly, N., & Malcolm, F. (2001). Prevalence of psychiatric disorders in New Zealand prisons: A national study. *Australia New Zealand Journal of Psychiatry*, 35, 166-173. Retrieved 19 February, 2005 from http://www.corrections.govt.nz

Caspi, A., McClay, J., Moffitt, T. E., Mill, J.S., Martin, J., Craig, I., Taylor, A., & Poulton, R. (2002). Role of genotype in the cycle of violence in maltreated children. *Science*, 297, 851-854.

Coxon, E., Jenkins, K., Marshall, J., & Massey, L. (1994). *The Politics of Learning and Teaching in Aotearoa–New Zealand*. Dunmore Press Ltd. Palmerston North, NZ.

Durie, M. (1998). *Whaiora: Maori Health Development* (2nd Ed.). Oxford. University Press: Oxford, NY.

Durie, M. (2001). *Mauri Ora: The Dynamics of Maori Health*. Oxford University Press: Oxford.

Farrelly, S., & Rudegeair, T. (2004). A virtual trauma service: Building an island in the mainstream. International Society for the Study of Dissociation conference presentation, New Orleans.

Fergusson, D., Horwood, L.J., & Lynskey, M.T. (1996a). Childhood sexual abuse and psychiatric disorder in young adulthood: Part I: The prevalence of sexual abuse and factors associated with sexual abuse. *Journal of the American Academy of Child and Adolescent Psychiatry*, 35, 1355-1364.

Fergusson, D.M., Horwood, L.J., & Lynskey, M.T. (1996b). Childhood sexual abuse and psychiatric disorder in young adulthood: Part II: Psychiatric outcomes of sexual abuse. *Journal of the American Academy of Child and Adolescent Psychiarty*, 35, 1365-1374.

Kazantzis, N., & Flett, R.A. et al. (2000). Domestic violence, psychological distress and physical illness among New Zealand Women: Results from a community based study. *New Zealand Journal of Psychology*, 29, 67-73.

King, M. (2003a). *The Penguin History of New Zealand*. Penguin Books Ltd., Auckland, NZ.

King, M. (2003b). *Te Puea: A Life*. (4th Ed). Reed Publishing. Auckland, NZ.

Lawson-Te Aho, K. (1998a). A Review of the Evidence: A Background document to Support Kia Tiki Te Ora O Te Taitamariki. Te Puni Kokiri. Wellington, NZ.

Lawson-Te Aho, K. (1998b). Maori Youth Suicide–Colonization, Identity and Maori Development. In Te Pumanawa Hauora (ed.) *Te Oru Rangahau Maori Research and Development Conference 7-9 July 1998 Proceedings* (pp. 218-221). School of Maori Studies, Massey University.

Ministry of Health. (1998). *Our Children's Health*. Retrieved 27 February, 2005 from http://www.moh.govt.nz

Ministry of Social Development. (2003). *The Social Report*. Retrieved 19 February, 2005 from http://www.msd.govt.nz/index2.html

Ministry of Youth Development. (2001). *New Zealand youth suicide prevention strategy*. Retrieved 19 February, 2005 from www.youthaffairs.govt.nz

Moskowitz, A. (2004). Dissociation and violence: A review of the literature. *Trauma, Violence and Abuse*, 5, 21-46.

Mullen, P., Martin, J., Anderson, J., Romans, S., & Herbison, G. (1993). Childhood sexual abuse and mental health in adult life. *British Journal of Psychiatry*, 163, 721-732.

Mullen, P., Martin, J., Anderson, J., Romans, S., & Herbison, G. (1996). The long-term impact of the physical, emotional, and sexual abuse of children: A community study. *Child Abuse & Neglect*, 20, 7-21.

National Health Information Service. (2004). Mental Health Information Collection Data.

New Zealand Herald. (1874). August 17 Edition.

New Zealand Health Information Service. (2004). *MHINC Data*. Retrieved 19 February, 2005 from www.nzhis.govt.nz/stats

Orange, C. (1987). *The Treaty of Waitangi*. Wellington: Allen and Unwin, Port Nicholson Press.

Read, J., & Argyle, N. (1999). Hallucinations, delusions and thought disorders in adult psychiatric inpatients with a history of child abuse. *Psychiatric Services*, 50, 1467-1472.

Read, J., Mosher, L.R., & Bentall, R.P. (Eds.). (2004). *Models of Madness: Psychological, Social and Biological Approaches to Schizophrenia*. New York: Brunner-Routledge.

Read, J., Perry, B., Moskowitz, A., & Connolly, J. (2001). The contribution of early traumatic events to schizophrenia in some patients: A traumagenic neurodevelopmental model. *Psychiatry*, 64.

Romans, S.E., Martin, J.L., Anderson, J.C., Herbison, G.P., & Mullen, P.E. (1995). Sexual abuse in childhood and deliberate self harm. *American Journal of Psychiatry*, 152, 1336-1342.

Romans, S.E., Gendall, K.A., Martin, J.L., & Mullens, P. (2001). Childhood sexual abuse and later disordered eating: A New Zealand epidemiological study. *International Journal of Eating Disorders*, 29, 380-392.

Smith, L. T. (1999). *Decolonising Methodologies*. Dunedin, New Zealand: University of Otago Press.

Te Puni Kokiri. (2002). *He Tirohanga o Kawa ki te Tiriti o Waitangi*. Wellington, NZ.

Walker, R. (1990). *Ka Whawhai Tonu Matou: Struggle Without End*. Penguin Books. Auckland, NZ.

Wells, D. (2004). Disturbing the sound of silence: Mental health services' responsiveness to people with trauma histories. Wellington: Occasional Report, Mental Health Commission.

Young, M., Read, J., Barker-Collo, S., & Harrison, R. (2001). Evaluating and overcoming barriers to taking abuse histories. *Professional Psychology: Research and Practice*, 32, 407-414.

Trauma and Dissociation
in Northern Ireland

Martin J. Dorahy
Michael C. Paterson

SUMMARY. Following a resurgence of militant resistance to British rule among Irish Nationalists in 1916, the landmass of Ireland was divided in 1921. Twenty-six counties gained independence from Britain and become the Republic of Ireland, while 6 counties, in the northeast, remained politically attached to Britain and became known as Northern Ireland. Since the partitioning of Northern Ireland from the Republic, political-motivated violence has been used by those fighting for a united Ireland free of British rule, as well as those defending Northern Ireland's union with Britain. This violence reached a greater intensity and ferocity in the late 1960s with the start of what is referred to as "the

Martin J. Dorahy, PhD, DClinPsych, is affiliated with North & West Belfast Health and Social Services Trust, Belfast, Northern Ireland, and the School of Psychology, The Queen's University of Belfast, Northern Ireland.

Michael C. Paterson, PhD, DClinPsych, is affiliated with TMR Health Professionals, Belfast, Northern Ireland.

Address correspondence to: Martin J. Dorahy, PhD, DClinPsych, 1 Trauma Resource Centre, North & West Belfast Health and Social Services Trust , Belfast, Northern Ireland.

The authors would like to thank Dr. Colin Gorman for his comments on an earlier draft of this piece.

[Haworth co-indexing entry note]: "Trauma and Dissociation in Northern Ireland." Dorahy, Martin J., and Michael C. Paterson. Co-published simultaneously in *Journal of Trauma Practice* (The Haworth Maltreatment & Trauma Press, an imprint of The Haworth Press, Inc.) Vol. 4, No. 3/4, 2005, pp. 221-243; and: *Trauma and Dissociation in a Cross-Cultural Perspective: Not Just a North American Phenomenon* (ed: George F. Rhoades, Jr., and Vedat Sar) The Haworth Maltreatment & Trauma Press, an imprint of The Haworth Press, Inc., 2005, pp. 221-243. Single or multiple copies of this article are available for a fee from The Haworth Document Delivery Service [1-800-HAWORTH, 9:00 a.m. - 5:00 p.m. (EST). E-mail address: docdelivery@haworthpress.com].

Troubles." This piece examines the many manifestations of trauma in Northern Ireland, from the familial and interpersonal to the social and political. Moreover, attention is given to the growing study of dissociation in Northern Ireland. Case examples are used throughout to highlight salient points and demonstrate the human cost of trauma and dissociation. *[Article copies available for a fee from The Haworth Document Delivery Service: 1-800-HAWORTH. E-mail address: <docdelivery@haworthpress. com> Website: <http://www.HaworthPress.com> © 2005 by The Haworth Press, Inc. All rights reserved.]*

KEYWORDS. Dissociation, trauma, Northern Ireland

The Province of Northern Ireland is made up of six counties geographically located in the northeast of the island of Ireland, and separated from mainland Britain by the Irish Sea. The history of Northern Ireland is one of conflict, dislocation and uncertainty (Darby, 1976). Following centuries of turmoil in British-ruled Ireland, Northern Ireland came into existence when in 1921 it was partitioned and politically severed from what is now the Republic of Ireland (Bew, Gibbon, & Patterson, 1996). The creation of a separate state followed several years of political negotiations and bloody battling which commenced with the uprising of Irish nationalists in Dublin in 1916. With political and military momentum building among Irish nationals for another challenge to British rule of Ireland, and the British fully engaged in the war against Germany (World War I), 1916 offered a window of opportunity for those opposed to British sovereignty. The settlement following this conflict was an independent Republic of Ireland minus six of its 32 counties which became the Province of Northern Ireland and remained under the governance of Britain; an arrangement acceptable to Northern Ireland's unionist majority (currently representing 53.13% of the population) but unacceptable to its Irish nationalist (currently 43.76%) minority (Barton, 1999). Until this day, "Nationalist," and the more militant "Republican," political ideologies and strategies favour and fight for a united Ireland free of British rule. "Unionist," and the more militant "Loyalist," ideologies and strategies defend a continuation of British sovereignty, "protecting" the Province against changes in the political status quo. Cairns and Darby (1998) argue that at its most basic level the conflict in Northern Ireland is the struggle between these two viewpoints, which are "underpinned by historical, religious, political, economic and psychological elements" (p. 754). In terms of the religious element, *typically*, Catholics would espouse a Nationalist or Republican viewpoint, whilst Protestants would favour Unionism or Loyalism.

The partitioning of Northern Ireland did little to quell conflict and since the late 1960s the Province has experienced a major re-ignition of politically-motivated violence referred to as the "Troubles." Civil disturbance, sectarian attacks and political unrest initially punctuated the social fabric of Northern Ireland, but are now intricately woven into it and to some extent, in some geographical areas, have been its determinants. In their encyclopaedic volume of deaths *directly* related to the "Troubles" in Northern Ireland from July 1969 until April 2001, McKittrick, Kelters, Feeney and Thornton (2001) tabulate 3,658 (see Fay, Morrissey, & Smyth, 1997, for demographic and geographic details of "Troubles-related" deaths). With a modest population of just over 1.68 million (Northern Ireland Statistics & Research Agency, 2002), "Troubles-related" deaths alone have inflicted a considerable social strain. For comparative purposes, Cairns and Darby (1998) point out that on a pro rata basis, the number of Troubles-related deaths is equivalent to 500,000 in the US and 100,000 in Britain. Victims predominantly are working class males from urban areas (Fay et al., 1997), suggesting that, like the violence more generally, the psychological repercussions of these deaths are not uniformly distributed across geographical location and social classes (Daly, 1999).

Since the mid-1990s progress towards a lasting peace has been assisted by 'ceasefires' from the main Republican paramilitary (i.e., Irish Republican Army, IRA; Irish National Liberation Army, INLA) and Loyalist paramilitary (e.g., Ulster Defence Association, UDA; Ulster Volunteer Force, UVF) organizations. Despite occasional breakdowns in these ceasefires and the on-going activities of smaller 'splinter' groups opposed to the cessation of military operations as a political strategy, bombing raids and attacks on 'legitimate' targets have essentially stopped. The death rates associated with the "Troubles" have simultaneously fallen (Fay, Morrissey, & Smyth, 1999). However, other trappings of paramilitary activity, such as intimidation, punishment attacks, rioting, within-community paramilitary feuds and intelligence gathering, continue.

The "Troubles" have texturized the social and personal lives of Northern Irish people (Cairns & Darby, 1998). For example, one respondent in Fay, Morrissey, Smyth and Wong's (2001) study noted, "The theme of the 'Troubles' is a string of death, injury and tears" (p. 26). For many, the Troubles have been a source of unbearable stress and suffering (Fay et al., 2001). Yet, Troubles-related traumas represent only a proportion of potentially traumatizing events evident in Northern Ireland. The aim of this piece is to outline the nature of the traumatic events most apparent in the Province and examine their link with, and research on, dissociation. This piece is selective rather than comprehensive in assessing trauma types and with the exception of familial/relational traumas (see below) will tend to focus on "Troubles-related" traumas as they are more unique to Northern Ireland.

Consistent with contemporary literature (e.g., APA, 2000; Carlson, 1997) this piece understands trauma as containing two components: (1) a potentially damaging physical event (e.g., a car accident, a bomb exploding, a father incestuously assaulting his daughter) which, (2) by its nature, creates aversive, overwhelming and uncontrollable psychological consequences. Thus, the two components are the physical (objective) event itself (which may also include the *omission* of physical contact in case of neglect, for example) as well as the psychological (subjective) consequences of that event which deem it traumatic. It should be noted from this understanding that an event is classed as psychologically traumatizing based on the severity and type of emotions it elicits, an individual's or society's ability to deal constructively with these emotions and the meaning attributed to the event by one or more individuals. Consequently, an event is defined as traumatizing based on its psychological *outcome* for a person or society. However, for the current purposes, "trauma" will refer to *events* which have considerable potential to evoke ongoing overwhelming, uncontrollable and negative psychological reactions. This will allow the discussion of events such as a bomb blast to be counted as traumatic even though not everybody exposed to it may experience ongoing posttraumatic symptoms or view it as a traumatic event.

TYPES OF TRAUMAS OCCURRING IN NORTHERN IRELAND

Psychological trauma in Northern Ireland can be organized around three superordinate categories: familial/relational, political, and social. These categories provide some necessary structure and clarity but are artificial in nature because in many cases they are overlapping and may be interrelated. For example, familial trauma such as domestic violence may co-vary with the degree of social (e.g., paramilitary feuding) or political (e.g., sectarianism) trauma at a particular moment in time. Nonetheless these categories will help organize and elucidate the type of traumatic events most apparent in Northern Ireland.

Familial/Relational Traumas

Under the heading of familial and relational trauma would fall the childhood abuse and neglect experiences that Briere (2002) has referred to as acts of omission and acts of commission. Acts of omission include childhood neglect by family members or caregivers to children. Acts of commission, according to Briere (2002), refers to abuse perpetrated by adults on a child. This may include sexual and physical assaults, and emotional abuse, such as name calling, belittling and verbal tirades and insults.

In a large scale, Province-wide study cognizant of the well documented difficulties in determining prevalence and incidence of abuse due to factors such as secrecy (e.g., Finkelhor & Hotaling, 1984), Kennedy et al. (1990) set out to determine "the number of children who may have been sexually abused and who were reported prospectively during 1987" (p. 20). In excluding suspected and alleged cases of child sexual abuse, Kennedy et al. found 408 cases where incidence of sexual abuse had been established. Of the 408 established cases, 330 (80.9%) were female. Penetrative sexual contact (e.g., anal intercourse, digital penetration) accounted for most incidences of abuse (265, 65%) and the majority of the 408 cases were abused by a single perpetrator (369, 90.4%) on more than one occasion (284, 69.6%). By and large, perpetrators tended to be male (359, 88%) and non-family members (e.g., neighbour, co-habitee: 220, 53.9%). Due to the stringency of the inclusion criteria and the many social and psychological factors inhibiting reporting of child sexual abuse (see Finkelhor & Hotaling, 1984), these 408 established cases identified in 1987 are a considerable under-representation of incidence (Kennedy et al., 1990). Mackenzie, Blaney, Chivers, and Vincent (1993) have calculated an incidence rate of child sexual abuse based on this sample of 0.9 cases per 1,000. However, using statistical methods to identify cases from those suspected and alleged, the established incidence of child sexual abuse in Northern Ireland was calculated at 1.16 per thousand. For the current purposes these statistics demonstrate that the trauma of childhood sexual abuse is evident in Northern Ireland.

With reference to more contemporary work, in their recent "Full Stop Review," the National Society for the Prevention of Cruelty to Children (NSPCC, 2003) drew on a range of sources for statistics on child abuse and neglect in Northern Ireland. They note that from the 12 months commencing April 1st 2000, 148 children were put on the Child Protection Register for sexual abuse. In addition, 352 children were added to the Register for physical abuse while over 450 were added because of neglect. Eyeballing the most recent police statistics (PSNI, 2003) on "offences against children under the age of 17" shows a reduction in sexual offences (e.g., gross indecency with a child, unlawful carnal knowledge) from 1998/99 (1,037) to 2001/02 (719). However, physical offences (e.g., cruelty to a child, minor assaults) against children under the age of 17 have showed a marked increase from 1998/99 (2,865) to 2001/02 (4,308).

These figures indicated that child abuse and neglect is a reality for many children in Northern Ireland and may represent a considerable etiological or vulnerability factor for the development of mental health difficulties including pathological dissociation. A study of Northern Irish college students utilizing measures of childhood abuse (occurring before 13 years) and dissociation (i.e., Dissociative Experiences Scale; DES) found that childhood emotional abuse, but not childhood sexual or physical abuse, was related to overall dissociation scores (Dorahy, Lewis, Millar, & Gee, 2003).

In the last few years a line of research has been pursued in Northern Ireland on the existence of childhood trauma in people diagnosed with a psychotic illness. This work is concordant with recent studies proffering a connection between childhood abuse and a reasonable percentage of individuals with schizophrenia (e.g., Read, Perry, Moskowitz, & Connolly, 2001) and also overlaps with the literature on the relationship between the positive or first rank (Schneiderian) symptoms of schizophrenia and child abuse (e.g., Read, Agar, Argyle, & Aderhold, 2003; Ross, Anderson, & Clark, 1994). In short, the first study of this type in Northern Ireland (Spence, Shannon, Mulholland, Lynch, & McHugh, 2002) found a history of childhood trauma (e.g., sexual abuse) in 75% of their psychosis sample (n = 40). In addition, the rate of childhood trauma in the psychosis sample was significantly higher than in a psychiatric non-psychotic comparison sample (n = 30). In a second study, individuals with schizophrenia were divided into those with and without a traumatic childhood history (Boyle, Shannon, Mulholland, & Huda, 2003). Those with a traumatic childhood history experienced significantly more dissociative symptoms, as measured by the DES. This difference was not isolated to one particular type of dissociative symptoms. Rather, the schizophrenia sample with a history of childhood trauma displayed significantly higher amnesia, derealization/depersonalisation and imaginative involvement/absorption scores.

Also falling under the heading of familial and relational trauma is domestic violence. Over the years between 1996 and March 2002, annual police statistics (PSNI, 2003) indicate a steady increase in domestic violence call-outs where physical violence was involved (3,681 to 7,749). It remains uncertain whether this trend indicates increased violence within Northern Irish homes or changes in the willingness to report such violence (perhaps due to greater awareness and acceptance of the problem). However, the police have consistently taken a tougher line on domestic violence by removing the perpetrator and prosecuting where evidence exists, which may increase the willingness to report this form of assault. It is accepted that like childhood sexual abuse statistics these figures are unlikely to be an accurate representation of the actual incidence of domestic violence in the Province.

According to female victims of domestic abuse utilizing Women's Aid refuges between April 2001 to March 2002, perpetrators were primarily current boyfriends/partners (51%), with husbands accounting for 32% of those inflicting domestic violence (Northern Ireland Women's Aid Federation, 2002). Some studies have been conducted on the psychological characteristics and mental health problems related to domestic violence in Northern Irish victims (e.g., McClennan, Joseph, & Lewis, 1994). Only one study to date has directly examined dissociative experience among Northern Irish victims of domestic violence (Dorahy, Lewis, & Wolfe, 2002). A comparison of those with a domestic violence history to a general population control group indicated significantly higher trauma and dissociation scores. Most notably, the domestic violence sample reported significantly higher pathological dissociative experience as measured by the Dissociative Experiences Scale-Taxon (DES-T; Waller, Putnam, & Carlson, 1996).

Politically-Motivated Traumas

Politically-motivated traumas relate directly to the use of violence (e.g., bombing campaigns) by paramilitary organizations to bring about or maintain their political goals. In addition, they also relate to sectarian attacks where a civilian is directly targeted by members (often from a paramilitary organization) of the opposing community. These attacks are often retaliatory or designed to intimidate and antagonise, but may also simply be hate-crime, not initiated with a particular overt message in mind (Fay et al., 1999). As with the "Troubles" generally, paramilitary (i.e., terrorist) attacks, sectarian murders and their aftermath have been unevenly distributed across the Province. Some rural areas and urban council wards have escaped much of the conflict. However, Wilson and Cairns (1996) argue that "[T]he variety of types of incident and their seemingly random and unpredictable pattern of occurrence means that everyone living in the Province has been at risk to some extent during their normal day-to-day activities" (p. 19). Fay et al. (1999) point out that 54% of those killed in the "Troubles" have been civilians, and paramilitary organizations have been responsible for just over 80% of all "Troubles-related" deaths. The gruesome nature of countless sectarian murders occupies a psychological space for many people in Northern Ireland. Yet, the incomprehensibility, shame and rage produced by the gravity of numerous incidents inflicting significant casualties, such as "Bloody Sunday," the Remembrance Day bombing in Enniskillen, the Shankill Road bombing, and the Omagh bombing, reverberate both nationally and internationally. In addition, these events also produce considerable psychiatric consequences for many survivors.

Following the Enniskillen Cenotaph bombing during a Remembrance Day memorial service (1987) in which 11 people were killed and scores more seriously injured, Curran and his colleagues were referred 26 adult survivors (Curran et al., 1990). Of these, 13 (50%) were diagnosed with posttraumatic stress disorder (PTSD). In addition, the majority continued to experience the same degree of posttraumatic and general psychiatric symptoms 12 months later. The PTSD rate in this sample was considerably higher than that reported in previous work by this research group (see Loughrey, Curran, & Bell, 1993, below, for summary results of their previous research), a result accounted for by the timing and vicious nature of this attack, according to the authors.

On the 15th of August 1998, and during a ceasefire by mainstream paramilitary groups, a dissident republican organization (the 'Real Irish Republican Army') planted and detonated a bomb in the small market town of Omagh. The bomb killed 29 people plus two unborn babies and injured hundreds of others. The number of casualties has made the Omagh bombing the worst single terrorist incident in Northern Irish history. Those psychologically scarred by the event go well beyond individuals directly exposed to the bomb blast and its immediate aftermath. Studies have found significant psychological distress among health service personnel who, in a professional or civilian capacity, were involved in treating and caring for the bomb victims. Luce, Firth-Cozens, Midgley, and Burges (2002) found health service staff with greater involvement in the care of victims of the Omagh bomb, experienced more severe PTSD symptoms. Not surprisingly, those with a prior exposure to trauma before the Omagh bombing experienced more severe symptoms than those without a trauma history. Staff groups displayed different degrees of PTSD symptom severity, with staff providing less direct and practical help to victims (e.g., domestic staff and home helpers) displaying more severe PTSD symptoms than those in the frontline of treatment, such as doctors. However, doctors were not insusceptible to psychological distress in the aftermath of the Omagh bomb, especially those with less experience (Luce & Firth-Cozens, 2002). Luce et al. (2002) argue that their findings dispel the myth that "professional helpers are somehow immune from suffering the same sort of distress as those they are helping" (p. 29).

The professional mental health response to assist victims in the aftermath of the Omagh Bombing was the development of the multi-disciplinary Community Trauma and Recovery Team. This service was designed to assess the needs of individuals and the community and develop appropriate responses. One of the team's responses was the implementation of cognitive therapy input for individual's suffering PTSD. This work has lead to one of the first effectiveness studies of cognitive therapy for PTSD (Gillespie, Duffy, Hackman, & Clark, 2002). In short, those undergoing cognitive therapy for PTSD displayed a significant reduction in PTSD symptoms, as well as those related to depression and mental health more broadly. Omagh bomb victims with co-morbid psychiatric problems tended to receive more sessions than the average eight given to those with PTSD alone. Yet, the comorbid group were not resistant to improvement with cognitive therapy input. This study demonstrated the effective implementation of psychological techniques for victims of the Omagh bomb.

Community-based surveys of the psychiatric effects of political violence have tended to conclude that the majority of people cope effectively with the added stress of the "Troubles" (Silke, 2003; see Cairns & Wilson, 1993 or Wilson & Cairns, 1996, for review). However, the "Troubles" have been found to make an independent contribution to health problems in areas most affected by "Troubles-related" violence (Smyth, Morrissey, & Hamilton, 2001). Even in areas with intermediate levels of political violence, referrals solely and directly related to the "Troubles" make a significant contribution to psychiatric caseloads (Allen, Cassidy, & Monaghan, 1994). In addition, individuals with a greater exposure to violence display greater psychiatric symptoms.

In a study drawing samples from towns with high and relatively low levels of "Troubles-related" violence, Cairns and Wilson (1984) found greater psychiatric symptoms and more participants above the General Health Questionnaire cut-off for psychiatric morbidity in the high violence area. Moreover, those individuals who lived in the high violence town *and* who perceived their town as experiencing high levels of violence, displayed the most severe psychiatric symptoms. Those denying the true reality of violence in their town experienced less psychological costs. Cairns and Wilson (1984) concluded, "denial of reality is for the people of certain areas of Northern Ireland at least one way to remain stable in a threatening environment" (p. 635). The more stable peace now apparent in Northern Ireland raises questions about the exposure of latent psychological distress given a more predictable and less volatile environment has the capacity to erode denial and make its ongoing use redundant.

Social Traumas

Areas and council wards with high paramilitary membership and sympathies have developed their own kinds of traumatizing social characteristics and realities. The primary function of paramilitary organizations is to fight for, or defend, their ultimate political goal (in the case of republican paramilitaries, a united Ireland, and in the case of loyalist paramilitaries, a Northern Ireland that remains politically attached and loyal to Britain). However, another function of paramilitary groups that developed simultaneously is the defence and protection of their communities from external persecutory sources. External persecutory sources include the apparent "rival" community and also, particularly with republican communities, the security forces such as the police. Perceiving the security forces as threatening has consequences for law enforcement in many rural and urban housing estates and communities. In commenting on the Northern Ireland situation, Fay et al. (1999) noted that a breakdown or erosion in law enforcement is common in contexts marred by civil conflict. In addition, many Northern Irish communities, particularly but not exclusively Catholic, have lost faith in or mistrust the police service. In the absence of trusted state policing, paramilitary organizations have taken to "community policing" (Fay et al., 1999) to curb anti-social behaviour such as drug dealing and so-called "joyriding" (i.e., reckless and often under-age driving in a stolen car). Paramilitary organizations use "punishment attacks" as both a deterrent and penalty for anti-social activities. Punishment attacks may also be used as a means of intimidating those opposed to paramilitary control within their community (Fay et al., 1999). These attacks include grievous assaults to the legs and arms with bats or iron bars and gunshots to the knees, ankles and hands. Between 1993/94 and 2002/03 there have been

247 such attacks on average per year (PSNI, 2003). Bew and Gillespie (1999) have chronicled a number of these attacks and some of the political strategies designed to curb them.

Fay et al. (1999) point out that "[l]ocal communities are divided on the issue of policing of their communities, with some advocating paramilitary policing in the absence of an acceptable state police force, and others, horrified at the brutality of the punishments meted out, and the summary nature of the attribution of guilt" (p. 194). To the authors' knowledge there have been no studies specifically and systemically assessing the psychological effects of punishment attacks (Loughrey et al., 1993 did include victims of punishment attacks in their study but they were incorporated into a larger traumatized sample and not studied selectively or in detail). However, in the clinic, the psychological impact of these attacks is evident. Following a punishment attack one 19-year-old male presented for psychiatric assessment complaining of severe sleep disturbance and agitation. He had been taken from his home, blindfolded, and over a two day period "interrogated" about drug-related activity, and then shot in both ankles and his right hand. He experienced significant emotional numbing and had become socially phobic, fearing another attack. Intrusive and overwhelming re-experiencing of the event had become a feature of his daily life. Despite having some involvement in anti-social behaviour, due to his social network, approximately nine months previously, he had severed connections with this group and had been living a relatively secluded life with his aunt and girlfriend.

Another male referred for psychological assessment experienced dissociative hallucinosis (i.e., hallucinatory-type re-experiencing of dissociated traumatic memories), and intense and disturbing vengeful fantasies. Over a period of nine years he had experienced four separate punishment attacks (e.g., beatings and shootings). He suggested that one of the paramilitary leaders in his community had had a grudge against him since his school years and continued to bully him with these attacks. When in his house, especially when alone and lying on his bed, he could hear footsteps coming up the hall towards him. At these times he believed his attackers were coming back to "finish me off." His waking hours and often his sleep were punctuated with horrific images and fantasies of what he would like to do to these tormenters. Not only did these fantasies distress him, they had an impact on his self-image because he felt ashamed and guilty that he could even have these thoughts and was fearful he might act on them.

Rioting has become commonplace in parts of Northern Ireland. Historically, the onset of the "Troubles" was marked by widespread civil disturbance that stretched police resources. People were forced from their homes if they lived in the other side's area and had to relocate where it was safer. Despite this, communities lived in fear of attack from the other side. This resulted in the construction of peace lines in Belfast to separate loyalist and republican areas. Currently, police carry out 'interface patrols' to ensure this security is not breached; when it is, police officers often come under attack from both sides, resulting in physical and psychological consequences.

By way of example, a 35-year-old police officer was with colleagues in an armoured Land Rover attending to a public order situation in Belfast. The rioting crowd surrounded the vehicle, forced open the officer's door and tried to pull him out. He struggled to remain in the vehicle, wedging his foot and leg in the doorway. Had he been pulled from the vehicle his fate would likely have been death. Fortunately, the driver of the vehicle was able to drive clear, the momentum causing the heavy door to swing shut thus knocking the main assailant off balance and breaking his grip on the officer. Following the incident, the officer had dissociative flashbacks when surrounded by crowds; he avoided shopping with his wife and preferred solitary activities. He also had regular nightmares where he would wake with cramp in his left leg–the one that he had wedged in the doorway during the attack.

THE DISSOCIATIVE RESPONSE TO TRAUMA IN NORTHERN IRELAND

The study of dissociation has received little attention in Northern Ireland (Dorahy & Lewis, 1998) until very recent times. Dorahy and Rhoades (2001) provided a brief overview of the study of dissociation in the Province and this work continues to gradually expand. Empirically, dissociation has been examined at the individual level and those studies not discussed above will be presented now. In addition, a brief theoretical argument will be made for how dissociation may be seen to manifest at the group or communal level.

Personal Level

Posttraumatic stress disorder. If it is accepted that posttraumatic stress disorder (PTSD) is a dissociative disorder (e.g., Nijenhuis, Van der Hart & Steele, 2002), then PTSD is one manifestation of trauma-induced dissociation in Northern Ireland. It had previously been argued that the "Troubles" were not responsible for increased mental health problems and by and large individuals coped effectively with the added stress of the "Troubles," utilizing defences such as denial and distancing to stave off psychiatric illnesses (e.g., Cairns & Wilson, 1989; Curran, 1988; Lyons, 1974). However, in more recent times it has been argued that PTSD is a common psychiatric consequence of the "Troubles" but is underdiagnosed (Daly, 1999), even though general practitioners and occupational health physicians have some knowledge of the core symptom indicators of PTSD (Daly, 1997). Studies examining PTSD in Northern Ireland have routinely found a relationship between trauma exposure and PTSD prevalence. For example, based on medical-legal referrals, Loughrey et al. (1993) assessed for PTSD in "survivors of assassination attempts, paramilitary punishment shootings and beatings, violent assaults, intimidation and exposure to bombings and shootings." They found that 116 (23.2%) of the 499 cases met diagnostic criteria for PTSD and recurrent intrusive recollections and markedly diminished interest were considerably higher in those with PTSD. Paterson, Poole, Trew and Harkin (2001) recorded a higher incidence of PTSD in former police officers who had served longest in what they regarded as "high risk" areas. Fay et al. (2001) found that PTSD symptom indicators (e.g., re-experiencing, arousal) were far more prevalent in individuals from council wards experiencing intense violence compared to those exposed to less violence. Moreover, nearly half of the respondents from high intensity wards experienced PTSD symptoms, whereas only approximately 22% and 12% experienced the same set of symptoms from moderate and low intensity areas, respectively. Other studies have found considerable posttraumatic stress symptoms in individuals bereaved by violence associated with the "Troubles" (e.g., Smyth, Hayes, & Hayes, 1997).

Dissociative disorders. The diagnosis and treatment of dissociative disorders have been relatively uncommon in Northern Ireland (Dorahy & Lewis, 2002), though this may have little bearing on the actual existence of dissociative disorders in the Province (Darves-Bornoz, Degiovanni, & Gaillard, 1995). Northern Irish clinicians tend to believe in the legitimacy of dissociative identity disorder, for example, but believe the condition is relatively rare (Dorahy & Lewis, 2002). Yet, data from a recent study indicates that in Northern Irish psychiatric patients with complex clinical profiles, dissociative disorders, including dissociative identity disorder, are relatively common (Dorahy, Mills, Teggart, O'Kane, &

Mulholland, 2004). Consistent with existing literature, those with dissociative disorders report a history of childhood trauma and many years of misdiagnoses (e.g., Coons, 1994; Putnam, Guroff, Silberman, Barban, & Post, 1986; Swica, Lewis, & Lewis, 1996). Yet, it is unclear what impact, if any, the "Troubles" had on the development of dissociative disorders.

Dissociative coping style. Irwin (1998), among others (e.g., Spiegel, 1986), has advanced the notion of a dissociative coping or dissociative defence style for non-clinical individuals who experience a heightened degree of dissociation. Typically, a dissociative coping style is associated with exposure to traumatic stress. One study in Northern Ireland has examined the relationship between dissociation and exposure to the "Troubles" (Dorahy et al., 2003). Utilising 112 college students who were deemed non-pathological dissociators according to the Bayesian algorithm of their taxon scores (Waller & Ross, 1997), direct exposure to political violence was related to higher DES scores. The calculation of this relationship controlled for the impact of other traumatic experiences (e.g., childhood abuse) on dissociation.

Peritraumatic dissociation. Peritraumatic dissociation, or dissociative experiences at the time of a traumatic event, has received considerable attention over the past 10 years because of its hypothesized ability to predict the development of PTSD. Many studies have supported the contributory influence of peritraumatic dissociation on PTSD development (e.g., Murray, Ehler, & Mayou, 2002; Shalev, Peri, Canetti, & Screiber, 1996). However, some have questioned the direct nature of the association (Marshall & Schell, 2002). Following the Omagh Bomb in 1998, Dorahy, Gilmore, Lewis, and Millar (2000) assessed peritraumatic dissociation as well as posttraumatic and general psychiatric symptoms 8 weeks, 6 months and 12 months after the explosion. Participants directly exposed to the explosion (n = 20) showed significantly higher peritraumatic dissociation scores than those who were residents of Omagh but who were not in the vicinity of the explosion or directly witnessed its immediate aftermath (n = 17). In addition, those directly exposed to the explosion showed significantly more intrusive episodes at six months and avoidance experiences at 12 months. Of the predictor variables assessed at eight weeks (e.g., depression, anxiety, interpersonal sensitivity), peritraumatic dissociation at the time of the explosion was the only predictor of the development of avoidance and intrusion symptoms. Interestingly, general psychiatric symptoms did not differ across samples at any time point. Support from this study for the causal relationship between peritraumatic dissociation and PTSD symptom development is restricted by some of the methodological limitations outlined by Marshall and Schell (2002). For example, there may have been retrospective memory distortions arising from the lag between the event and the initial assessment of peritraumatic dissociation (i.e., eight weeks). Nonetheless, the findings from this Northern Irish study are consistent with previous work showing a relationship between peritraumatic dissociation and PTSD symptom development.

Societal Level: A Theoretical Proposal

If one adopts Nijenhuis, Van der Hart, and Steele's (2002; see also Steele, Van der Hart, & Nijenhuis, 2004) understanding of dissociation as a structured separation of psychobiological (e.g., memories, emotions) subsystems into those aspects which remain attached to the reality and horror of traumatic events and those aspects which defensively distance and actively seek to avoid re-experiencing them, we can begin to understand how dissociation manifests at a social level. The inability to integrate the over-identification with the under-identification of a traumatic event gives rise to and maintains the dissociation. This dissociation is responsible for the characteristic trauma dynamic of oscillating between re-experiencing/reliving, and phobic avoiding and emotional numbing, or as Van der Hart and colleagues describe: between knowing and not knowing. Successful integration of the structured separation entails an autobiographical realization that the traumatic event not only occurred, but was experienced by the individual or community (Steele et al., 2004). For this to happen, defensive avoidance strategies blocking realisation must be overcome, which in the context of continued threat is psychologically unlikely. For this reason a lasting peace in Northern Ireland is integral to psychological healing.

In commenting on the 1994 paramilitary cease-fires and peace negotiations, Fay et al. (1999) point out, "Until then, it was as if we dared not realise the extent of the damage in case we had to live with more of it" (p. 1). Even with the current peace it still seems that some communities cannot afford to *realise* the extent of the damage because due to their geographic location they are still living with the threat of sectarian aggression. This is especially the case in so-called "interface" areas where republican and loyalist communities live side-by-side or in enclaves. Protective behaviours such as intimidation and aggression which are often evoked by living with perceived or actual threat to personal and communal integrity also serve as an avoidance mechanism of personal and communal suffering.

Still now some of the communities which bore the emotional brunt of the "Troubles" appear to try and avoid the traumatic reality of their past by instigating and propagating more predictable, though less frequent, acts of civil and sectarian violence. For example, the Catholic and Protestant street marches during the summer months bring both individuals and communities back in touch with their emotional burden. As a result, the Summer marches trigger the reactivation of defensive actions and projection of hostility and blame at a community and social level (e.g., rioting, street violence), which serves to distance both individuals and communities from their own intense emotional pain brought about by 30 years of fighting and aggression. In the absence of more effective ways of dealing with, or working through, their own trauma, defensive actions such as hostility directed toward the opposing community becomes a bearable and easier alternative. However, the soothing ointment of externalised hostility and defensiveness for emotional suffering demands regular reapplication until the painful and courageous step is taken to discard the ointment and acknowledge, confront, and accept the reality of one's own suffering and pain. This final step of accepting the reality of their own trauma is too overwhelming and agonizing for the moment for some communities and the dissociation that gives rise to the reactivation-inactivation oscillations of re-experiencing and avoidance remains.

The activation of trauma may heighten an individual's awareness of their social identity to the point where there is a clear distinction between "Them" and "Us" categories. The "Them" category relates to the identifiable opposition, the social group which has, or has been perceived to, inflicted the trauma, pain and suffering on the individual's identified community. The "Us" group represents the community the individual identifies with and the group which has been victimized by the "Them" group. In Northern Ireland social identity is typically based on factors pertaining to culture, religion, history and/or political ideology (Cairns & Darby, 1998). Many social indicators have the potential to differentiate people in the two groups including place of education, housing, geographic location of family, sporting activities and a person's name.

There has been considerable work conducted using Social Identity Theory in Northern Ireland because it provides a means of understanding the conflict and the staunch divide between Catholic and Protestant communities (see Trew, 1992, for review; or Bloomer & Weinreich, 2003; Niens, Cairns, & Hewstone, 2003). Social Identity Theory, according to Cairns and Darby (1998), argues that "part of one's self-image is derived from membership in various groups. If one finds oneself as a member of a group from which it is difficult or impossible to leave, the only way to enhance self-esteem is to act to preserve or defend the group's interests" (p. 756). It is proposed here that in Northern Ireland the tendency to strongly identify with one group can be elicited as a defensive reaction to remembering and re-experiencing traumatic pain (i.e., dissociative connectedness; activation of re-experiencing, deactivation of avoidance and numbing). At these times the burden of this pain may be lightened by distinguishing an opposition group, to displace blame and project latent hostility towards, from an identified group where empathic support and social identification can alleviate personal suffering. During times of dissociative disconnectedness where re-experiencing is deactivated and emotional numbing and avoidance are activated a heightened sense of "Us" and "Them" categories is not needed to defend against emotional re-experiencing. In addition, because of their association with "feeling" traumatic pain, these social cognitions may be actively avoided.

In Northern Ireland, the summer is a time of marked increase in tribal displays reasserting group identity, e.g., 12th of July parades throughout Northern Ireland that celebrate the victory in 1690 of the Protestant Prince William of Orange over the Catholic King James. Denial of a perceived right of passage for parades and demonstrations has, in the past, led to civil and street violence, as communities feel they are being re-victimized by the opposing group. The tension at this time is often a cue for the re-experiencing of dissociated traumatic affects and memories. Following from the current argument, it should therefore also be a time where social identity distinctions are at their highest. This hypothesis has not been empirically tested in Northern Ireland (Karen Trew, personal communication, March, 2003). Nonetheless, it is proposed here that structural dissociation on a communal level, the cycling between communal re-experiencing (dissociative connectedness) and communal non-realization and numbing (dissociative disconnectedness) is linked to the social cognitions of social identity disinctions. When communities dissociatively connect with their (unresolved) traumatic pain, social identity distinctions are defensively evoked. When communities are dissociatively disconnected, social identity distinctions are a less evident social cognition.

The benefit of heightened social identification in warding off grief, unresolved trauma, emotional pain and vulnerability are highlighted when an individual feels betrayed by or ostracized from their social group and therefore lacks a social identity or cannot defensively utilize such social cognitions. The main overarching communities in Northern Ireland are: Unionist (pro-Britain), Nationalist (pro-united Ireland), and security forces such as the police. One of the authors (MP) has worked clinically with serving and retired police officers who have been left vulnerable through the withering of their social identity. In the wake of the Belfast Agreement in 1998, a joint political recipe for the road to peace, called the Patten Report, proposed sweeping changes to policing in Northern Ireland that permitted wholesale early retirements and paved the way for a new police service in the Province. This was coupled with prisoner releases where people convicted of terrorist crimes were released under licence (i.e., re-offending would result in a return to prison) and caused numerous officers to question the purpose of their role over the period of the "Troubles." Several of those seen by the author developed posttraumatic symptoms after their early retirement from policing in Northern Ireland; the trigger for each one of them was their perception of betrayal and devaluing of their service. They felt attacked and abased by the very group they defensively relied upon for their social identity. Feeling isolated from, and abandoned by, the group which once provided psychological protection, left these retired officers vulnerable to emotional insult when dissociatively connected with their own trauma.

Police officers and other security force personnel who have developed psychiatric conditions tend to be reticent in who they will accept help from. Background information obtained in a survey of retired Northern Ireland police officers (Paterson et al., 2001) indicated that they would prefer a specialist service for former police officers to help them with their psychological difficulties, not for reasons of security as one may imagine, but rather to access help from people who would understand them (i.e., are part of their "Us" group). Communities in which former political prisoners live tend to provide locally-based psychological support. A former prisoner from the Loyalist community stated, "people here do not trust the NHS (public-funded health service) . . . if they mention something they have been involved in [to helpers from their own community] then it goes no further." In this time of apparent peace, practices for healing the psychologically scarred are causing communities to dissociatively connect with traumatic pain and, thus, defensively evoke social identity distinctions. In those isolated, ostracized, or disenfranchised from their social group such protective responses are not possible.

CONCLUSION

In the novel 'Cal,' a fictionalized tale of a young Northern Irish man reluctantly and somewhat inadvertently caught up in a paramilitary crime and organization, the central female figure, Marcella, writes in her diary, "Violence is a bit like antibodies. Small doses build up until you reject and be immune to the most horrific events" (MacLaverty, 1983, p. 127). The limited research conducted in the Province thus far suggests that dissociation may be one psychological factor that assists in building the antibodies to trauma and violence so their effect is minimized. As well as the interpersonal traumas, such as child abuse and domestic violence, evident in many other communities around the world, Northern Ireland has witnessed sustained political and social violence. In the main, social and psychological factors, such as strong community and family ties, denial, distancing and dissociation have contributed to preserving the mental health of the majority of people in the Province. However, in Northern Irish clinics dissociation may be one pathological consequence of violence and trauma that often goes undetected. Progress towards a lasting peace in Northern Ireland, which still remains on shaky ground, and the development of cross-community trust, openness and empathy are all steps towards a greater awareness of the true extent and nature of psychological damage created by interpersonal, political, and social violence and trauma.

REFERENCES

Allen, J., Cassidy, C., & Monaghan, C. (1994). A community mental health team in Northern Ireland: New referrals as a result of civil disorder. *Irish Journal of Psychological Medicine*, 11, 67-69.

American Psychiatric Association. (2000). *Diagnostic and statistical manual of mental disorders (4th ed.) Text revision*. Washington, DC: Author.

Barton, B. (1999). *A pocket history of Ulster*. Dublin: The O'Brien Press.

Bew, P., Gibbon, P., & Patterson, H. (1996). *Northern Ireland 1921-1996: Political forces and social classes*. London: Serif.

Bew, P., & Gillespie, G. (1999). *Northern Ireland: A chronology of the Troubles 1968-1999*. Dublin: Gill & MacMillan.

Bloomer, F., & Weinreich, P. (2003). Cross-Community Relations Projects and interdependent identities. In O. Hargie & D. Dickson (Eds.), *Researching the Troubles: Social science perspectives on the Northern Ireland conflict* (pp. 141-161). London: Mainstream Publishing.

Boyle, C., Shannon, C., Mulholland, C., & Huda, U. (2003). *Investigation of childhood and adult trauma exposure and symptoms in schizophrenia*. Under review.

Briere, J. (2002). Treating adult survivors of severe childhood abuse and neglect: Further development of an integrated model. In J. E. B. Myers, L. Berliner, J. Briere, C. T. Hendrix, C. Jenny, & T. A. Reid (Eds.), *The APSAC handbook on child maltreatment (2nd Ed)*. London: Sage.

Cairns, E., & Darby, J. (1998). The conflict in Northern Ireland: Causes, consequences, and controls. *American Psychologist*, 53, 754-760.

Cairns, E., & Wilson, R. (1984). The impact of violence on mild psychiatric morbidity in Northern Ireland. *British Journal of Psychiatry*, 145, 631-635.

Cairns, E., & Wilson, R. (1989). Coping with political violence. *Social Science and Medicine*, 28, 621-624.

Cairns, E., & Wilson, R. (1993). Stress, coping and political violence in Northern Ireland. In J. P. Wilson & B. Raphael (Eds.), *International Handbook of Traumatic Stress Syndromes* (pp. 365-376). New York: Plenum Press.

Carlson, E. B. (1997). *Trauma assessment: A clinician's guidei* New York: Guilford Press.

Coons, P. M. (1994). Confirmation of childhood abuse in child and adolescent cases of multiple personality disorder and dissociative disorder not otherwise specified. *Journal of Nervous and Mental Disease*, 182, 461-464.

Curran, P. S. (1988). Psychiatric aspects of terrorist violence: Northern Ireland 1969-1987. *British Journal of Psychiatry*, 153, 470-475.

Curran, P. S., Bell, P., Murray, A., Loughrey, G., Roddy, R., & Rocke, L. G. (1990). Psychological consequences of the Enniskillen bombing. *British Journal of Psychiatry*, 156, 479-482.

Daly, O. E. (1997). Doctors' knowledge of posttraumatic neurosis. *Ulster Medical Journal*, 66, 28-33.

Daly, O. E. (1999). Northern Ireland: The victims. *British Journal of Psychiatry*, 175, 201-204.

Darby, J. (1976). *Conflict in Northern Ireland: The development of a polarised community*. Dublin: Gill & MacMillan.

Darves-Bornoz, J., Degiovanni, A., & Gaillard, P. (1995). Why is dissociative identity disorder infrequent in France [letter]. *American Journal of Psychiatry*, 152, 1530-1531.

Dorahy, M. J., Gilmore, J., Lewis, C. A., & Millar, R. G. (2000). Peritraumatic dissociation and the psychological consequences of personal and social exposure to the Omagh bombing in Northern Ireland. *6th annual conference of the International Society for the Study of Dissociation-UK Branch*. Manchester, UK.

Dorahy, M. J., & Lewis, C. A. (1998). Trauma-induced dissociation and the psychological effects of the "Troubles" in Northern Ireland: An overview and integration. *Irish Journal of Psychology*, 19 (2-3), 332-344.

Dorahy, M. J., & Lewis, C. A. (2002). Dissociative identity disorder in Northern Ireland: A survey of attitudes and experience among clinical psychologists and psychiatrists. *Journal of Nervous and Mental Disease*, 190, 707-710.

Dorahy, M. J., Lewis, C. A., Millar, R. G., & Gee, T. L. (2003). Correlates of non-pathological dissociation in Northern Ireland: The affects of trauma and exposure to political violence. *Journal of Traumatic Stress*, 16, 611-615.

Dorahy, M. J., Lewis, C. A., & Wolfe, F. (In press). Mental health consequences of domestic violence in Nortern Ireland. *Current Psychology.*

Dorahy, M. J., Mills, H., Teggart, C., O'Kane, M., & Mulholland, C. (2004). *Do dissociative disorders exist in Northern Ireland: Blind psychiatric-structured interview assessments of 20 complex psychiatric patients.* Under Review.

Dorahy, M. J., & Rhoades, G. (2001). Trauma treatment and anger management in Northern Ireland. *ISSD News*, 19 (5), 12-13, 15.

Fay, M. T., Morrissey, & Smyth, M. (1997). *The cost of the Troubles. Mapping Troubles-related deaths in Northern Ireland 1969-1994.* Londonderry: INCORE.

Fay, M. T., Morrissey, & Smyth, M. (1999). *Northern Ireland's Troubles: The humancost.* London: Pluto Press.

Fay, M. T., Morrissey, Smyth, M., & Wong, T. (2001). *The cost of the Troubles study.* Report on the Northern Ireland Survey: The experience and impact of the Troubles. Londonderry: INCORE.

Finkelhor, D., & Hotaling, G. T. (1984). Sexual abuse in the National Incidence Study of child abuse and neglect: An appraisal. *Child Abuse and Neglect*, 8, 23-32.

Gillespie, K., Duffy, M., Hackman, A., & Clark, D. M. (2002). Community based cognitive therapy in the treatment of post-traumatic stress disorder following the Omagh bomb. *Behaviour Research and Therapy*, 40, 345-357.

Irwin, H. J. (1998). Affective predictors of dissociation-II: Shame and guilt. *Journal of Clinical Psychology*, 54, 237-245.

Kennedy, M. T., Manwell, M. K. C., MacKenzie, G., Blaney, R., Chivers, A. T., Hay, I., & Vincent, O. E. (1990). *Child sexual abuse in Northern Ireland: A research study of incidence.* Antrim: Greystone Books.

Loughrey, G. C., Curran, P. S., & Bell, P. (1993). Posttraumatic stress disorder and civil violence in Northern Ireland. In J. P. Wilson & B. Raphael (Eds.), *International Handbook of Traumatic Stress Syndromes* (pp. 377-383). New York: Plenum Press.

Luce, A., & Firth-Cozens, J. (2002). Effects of the Omagh bombing on medical staff working in the local NHS trust: A longitudinal survey. *Hospital Medicine Journal*, 63, 44-47.

Luce, A., Firth-Cozens, J., Midgely, S., Burges, C. (2002). After the Omagh bomb: Posttraumatic stress disorder in health service staff. *Journal of Traumatic Stress*, 15, 27-30.

Lyons, H. (1974). Terrorists' bombing and the psychological sequelae. *Journal of the Irish Medical Association*, 67, 15-19.

MacKenzie, G., Blaney, R., Chivers, A., & Vincent, O. E. (1993). The incidence of child sexual abuse in Northern Ireland. *International Journal Epidemiology*, 22, 299-305.

MacLaverty, B. (1983). *Cal.* London; Vintage.

Marshall, G. N., & Schell, T. L. (2002). Reappraising the link between peritraumatic dissociation and PTSD symptom severity: Evidence from a longitudinal study of community violence survivors. *Journal of Abnormal Psychology*, 111, 626-636.

McClennan, H., Joseph, S., & Lewis, C. A. (1994). Causal attributions for marital violence and emotional response by women seeking refuge. *Psychological Reports*, 75, 272-274.

McKittrick, D., Kelters, S., Feeney, B., & Thornton, C. (2001). *Lost lives: The stories of the men, women and children who died as a result of the Northern Ireland troubles*. Edinburgh: Mainstream Publishing Company.

Murray, J., Ehlers, A., & Mayou, R. A. (2002). Dissociation and post-traumatic stress disorder: Two prospective studies of road traffic accident survivors. *British Journal of Psychiatry*, 180, 363-368.

Niens, U., Cairns, E., & Hewstone, M. (2003). Contact and conflict in Northern Ireland. In O. Hargie & D. Dickson (Eds.), *Researching the Troubles: Social science perspectives on the Northern Ireland conflict* (pp. 123-139). London: Mainstream Publishing.

Nijenhuis, E. R. S., Van der Hart, O., & Steele, K. (2002). The emerging psychobiology of trauma-related dissociation and dissociative disorders. In H. D'haenen, J. A. den Boer, & P. Willner (Eds.), *Biological Psychiatry* (pp. 1079-1098). New York: Wiley & Sons, Ltd.

Northern Ireland Statistics & Research Agency (2002). *Northern Ireland Census and Population Report and Mid-Year Estimates*. Belfast: TSO Ireland.

Northern Ireland Women's Aid Federation (2002). *Working to eliminate domestic violence: Annual Report 2001-2002*. Belfast. Author.

NSPCC (2003). *Northern Ireland Full Stop review*. Belfast: NSPCC.

Paterson, M.C., Poole, A.D., Trew, K.J., & Harkin, N. (2001). The psychological and physical health of police officers retired recently from the Royal Ulster Constabulary. *Irish Journal of Psychology*, 22, 1-27

PSNI (2003). *Chief Constable's Annual Report. Police Service of Northern Ireland*.

Putnam, F. W., Guroff, J. J., Silberman, E. K., Barban, L., & Post, R. M. (1986). The clinical phenomenology of multiple personality disorder: Review of 100 recent cases. *Journal of Clinical Psychiatry*, 47, 285-293.

Read, J., Agar, K., Argyle, N., & Aderhold, V. (2003). Sexual and physical abuse during childhood and adulthood as predictors of hallucinations, delusions and thought disorder. *Psychology and Psychotherapy*, 76, 1-22.

Read, J., Perry, B. D., Moskowitz, A., & Connolly, J. (2001). The contribution of early traumatic events to schizophrenia in some patients: A traumagenic neuro-developmental model. *Psychiatry*, 64, 319-345.

Ross, C. A., Anderson, G., & Clark, P. (1994). Childhood abuse and the positive symptoms of schizophrenia. *Hospital and Community Psychiatry*, 45, 489-491.

Shalev, A. Y., Peri, T., Canetti, L., & Screiber, S. (1996). Predictors of PTSD in injured trauma survivors: A prospective study. *American Journal of Psychiatry*, 153, 219-225.

Silke, A. (2003). The psychological cost of terrorism. *Forensic Update*, 72, 23-29.

Smyth, M., Hayes, P., & Hayes, E. (1997). *Posttraumatic stress disorder and the families of the victims of Bloody Sunday: A preliminary study*. Londonderry: Incore.

Smyth, M., Morrissey, M., & Hamilton, J. (2001). *Caring through the Troubles: Health and Social Services in Northern and West Belfast*. Belfast: North & West Belfast Health & Social Services Trust.

Spence, W., Shannon, C., Mulholland, C., Lynch, G., & McHugh, S. (In press). Rates of childhood trauma in a sample of patients with schizophrenia as compared with a sample of patients with non-psychotic psychiatric diagnoses. *Journal of Trauma and Dissociation.*

Spiegel, D. (1986). Dissociating damage. *American Journal of Clinical Hypnosis,* 29, 123-131.

Steele, K., Van der Hart, O., & Nijenhuis, E. R. S. (2004). Phase-oriented treatment of complex dissociative disorders: Overcoming trauma-related phobias. In A. Eckhart-Henn & S. O. Hoffman (Eds.), *Dissoziative Störungen des Bewußtseins* [Dissociative disorders of consciousness] (pp. 357-394). Schattauer-Verlag.

Swica, Y., Lewis, D. O., & Lewis, M. (1996). Child abuse and dissociative identity disorder/multiple personality disorder: The documentation of childhood maltreatment and the corroboration of symptoms. *Child and Adolescent Psychiatric Clinics of North America,* 5, 431-447.

Trew, K. (1992). Social psychological research on the conflict. *The Psychologist,* 5, 342-344.

Waller, N. G., Putnam, F. W., & Carlson, E. B. (1996). Types of dissociation and dissociative types. *Psychological Methods,* 1, 300-321.

Waller, N. G., & Ross, C. A. (1997). The prevalence of pathological dissociation in the general population. *Journal of Abnormal Psychology,* 106, 499-510.

Wilson, R., & Cairns, E. (1996). Coping processes and emotions in relation to political violence in Northern Ireland. In G. Mulhern & S. Joseph (Eds.), *Psychosocial perspectives on stress and trauma: From disaster to political violence* (pp. 19-28). Leicester: British Psychological Press.

Trauma and Dissociation in the Philippines

Heather J. Davediuk Gingrich

SUMMARY. The limited literature on trauma and psychopathology in the Philippines makes virtually no reference to dissociation or dissociative disorders. This article reviews descriptions of religious rituals, reports of spirit possession, case study material, and results from the author's study (Gingrich, 2004). These findings indicate that dissociative phenomena, and dissociative disorders, including dissociative identity disorder, are present in the Philippines. Whether these dissociative experiences manifest themselves in culturally specific or more universal ways is discussed in terms of the Filipino view of self and other aspects of the cultural context. The article places the Philippines in its historical and cultural context, examines the literature on trauma and abuse in the Philippines, discusses local views on dissociation, looks at indicators of a possible link between trauma and dissociation, and makes recommendations for future research. *[Article copies available for a fee from The Haworth Document Delivery Service: 1-800-HAWORTH. E-mail address: <docdelivery@haworthpress.com> Website: <http://www.HaworthPress.com> © 2005 by The Haworth Press, Inc. All rights reserved.]*

Heather J. Davediuk Gingrich, PhD, is affiliated with Denver Seminary, Littleton, CO.

Address correspondence to: Heather J. Davediuk Gingrich, PhD, Denver Seminary, 6399 South Santa Fe Drive, Littleton, CO 30120 (E-mail: heather.gingrich@denverseminary.edu).

The author thanks Edwin T. Decenteceo, PhD, for his comments on an earlier version of this piece, and Andreana Benitez for interviewing M.K. Puente, as well as doing an additional literature search of Filipino authors.

[Haworth co-indexing entry note]: "Trauma and Dissociation in the Philippines." Gingrich, Haether J. Davediuk. Co-published simultaneously in *Journal of Trauma Practice* (The Haworth Maltreatment & Trauma Press, an imprint of The Haworth Press, Inc.) Vol. 4, No. 3/4, 2005, pp. 245-269; and: *Trauma and Dissociation in a Cross-Cultural Perspective: Not Just a North American Phenomenon* (ed: George F. Rhoades, Jr., and Vedat Sar) The Haworth Maltreatment & Trauma Press, an imprint of The Haworth Press, Inc., 2005, pp. 245-269. Single or multiple copies of this article are available for a fee from The Haworth Document Delivery Service [1-800-HAWORTH, 9:00 a.m. - 5:00 p.m. (EST). E-mail address: docdelivery@haworthpress.com].

KEYWORDS. Trauma, dissociation, abuse, Philippines, Asia, spirit possession, altered states of consciousness (ASCs)

From the time she was a teenager, Malou had assumed that the voices she heard in her head belonged to evil spirits. Until recently the voices had always felt manageable; she had simply "rebuked" them in an attempt to make them go away which at least brought temporary relief. Now, however, things had taken a turn for the worse. The voices had become louder, insisting that Malou pay attention to their accusations that she was "bad seed," "worthless," and "ugly." Malou was unable to block out the voices; her former ways of controlling them were no longer working. The feeling that another being wanted to occupy her body was overwhelming and she was more than ever convinced that she was demon possessed. Terrified and desperate, Malou sought help from her church counselor, a Filipino graduate counseling student.

Malou's counselor had taken a course that I taught on psychotherapy with traumatized individuals. The course included a section on the diagnosis and treatment of dissociative disorders. This enabled her to recognize Malou's symptoms as potentially dissociative. She received Malou's permission to talk to the "voices." Within a few minutes a voice, which was of higher pitch than Malou's normal speaking voice, informed the counselor that she was not actually an evil spirit but rather another part of Malou. The voice went on to explain that she merely pretended to be a demon because that is what Malou called her. She was angry that Malou constantly tried to get rid of her rather than give her the attention she desired. Hoping that Malou would no longer be able to ignore her, she decided to try scare tactics. However, she was willing to stop if Malou was willing to communicate with her. As she debriefed with Malou at the end of the session, the counselor gave her opinion that the voice did not seem like an evil spirit to her, and, as a homework assignment, encouraged Malou to attempt to listen to it, in order to better judge for herself what might be happening.

The following week Malou excitedly bounced into the therapy room, smiling and expressing great relief. She explained to the counselor that all week she had repeatedly asked the voice who or what it was. The voice had consistently responded *"Ako rin ikaw!"* translated from Filipinoas, "I am also you!" With laughter Malou said to her counselor "Imagine! All this time I was trying to cast out a demon, when the voice was actually part of me!" Malou went on to describe how the voice seemed to belong to a lost child, a little girl part of her who wanted to be loved, and wanted to play, but instead was rejected and always left alone.

Psychotherapy had just begun for Malou, but the goals would now include finding out more about the function performed by this dissociated part. Malou's psychosocial history revealed sexual abuse in early childhood, family dysfunction, adolescent sexual promiscuity, and adult relationships with men who had been emotionally, physically and sexually abusive. Perhaps then, a link would be discovered between the trauma Malou had experienced and her dissociative symptoms. However, just how this voice related to Malou's life history and current life struggles remained to be seen. It was also not clear whether there was just one voice, or whether other dissociated parts also existed. Nor was it obvious whether this voice actually took executive control of Malou's body and behavior. Initially, therefore, there was insufficient information to determine whether Malou could be diagnosed according to the criteria for dissociative identity disorder (DID) outlined in the *Diagnostic and Statistical Manual of Mental Disorders* (DSM-IV-TR; American Psychiatric Association, 2000), or would be better classified under dissociative disorder not otherwise specified (DDNOS). However, the counselor's ability to recognize and work with pathological dissociation had already been experienced as beneficial by Malou.

I am a Canadian who has taught in a graduate counseling program in the Philippines for eight years. During this time, a number of cases with symptoms suggestive of dissociative disorders, such as DID or DD-NOS, have been brought to supervision sessions by my Filipino students. However, while there have been some research studies done in the areas of trauma and abuse in this country, DID and other dissociative disorders have been basically unacknowledged, and any potential association between trauma and dissociation overlooked.

My growing sense that DID was a valid diagnosis in this country motivated me to do my PhD dissertation research in the area of trauma and dissociation in the Philippines (Gingrich, 2004). Using modified versions of a couple of written instruments as well as a semistructured clinical interview, I was able to identify participants who have DID.[1] The diagnostic interview provided the opportunity for my Filipino assistants and I to witness some identity alteration ("switching") in some of the interviewees. The fact that I chose a non-clinical sample adds further weight to my hypothesis that DID is a valid diagnosis in the Philippines.

In this piece I will attempt to briefly place the Philippines in its historical and cultural context, examine the literature on trauma and abuse in the Philippines, discuss local views on dissociation, and look at indicators of a possible link between trauma and dissociation. Finally, I will offer some considerations for future research.

HISTORICAL/CULTURAL CONTEXT

The Philippines is a country of over 7,000 islands with a population of almost 85 million (Central Intelligence Agency [CIA], 2003). Although Filipinos are mostly of Malay origin, other significant ethnic subgroups (e.g., Negritos from Borneo and Sumatra, Chinese merchants, and Arabs) also immigrated to the Philippine islands, bringing with them religions and cultures that have impacted Filipino culture over the centuries. Magellan arrived on Philippine shores in 1521, beginning 377 years of Spanish colonial rule, which was followed by over 40 years of American occupation that began in 1902, ending with the Japanese occupation during World War II. In the postwar reconstruction era the American influence was strong, remaining even after the establishment of an independent Republic of the Philippines in July 1946. Although the American military bases were closed in 1991, American mass media and culture have a continuing impact.

The cultural diversity of the country is evidenced by the existence of eight major language/ethnic groups, strong regional identities, and 87 languages/dialects in addition to the official languages of English and Filipino (based on Tagalog). As a direct result of Spanish colonial rule, the Philippines has the distinction of being the only Asian country with a Roman Catholic majority (82.9%; National Statistical Coordination Board-Philippines [NSCB], 2004). Another 5.4% (NSCB, 2004) to 9% (CIA, 2003) of the population are Protestant, 5% are Muslim, with the remainder representing a variety of religions, including Buddhism and indigenous religions. Although Filipinos share many cultural commonalities with their Asian neighbors, culturally they are a unique blend of East and West.

The Philippines has experienced much political unrest. President Ferdinand Marcos (1965-1986) declared martial law in 1972, which allowed his government unlimited power to arrest and detain dissenters. Human rights violations, corruption, nepotism, economic decline, and lastly, the assassination of Benigno Aquino, a Marcos opponent, eventually led to a "People's Power" uprising in the mid-1980s. A second "People's Power" uprising ousted Joseph Estrada from the presidency in 2001, halfway through his term. For decades, problems with communist insurgents, Muslim separatists, and military rebels have plagued the country. Recent examples are the Abu Sayaf group, which made international news with its terrorist threats and kidnappings, and an attempted coup by junior military officers in July of 2003. Some of the southern islands of the Philippines have been in a state akin to civil war for decades.

The development of a sense of national identity remains an ongoing task for Filipinos, as they struggle to overcome the effects of colonization, economic and political instability, widespread poverty, and cultural diversity. Specific to the field of psychology, one effect of this struggle for national identity is the existence of a strong movement towards indigenization in psychology. The more radical of these groups, *Sikolohiyang Pilipino* (Filipino Psychology) completely rejects Western psychology as helpful to Filipinos. Proponents argue that Western approaches are problematic in that they perpetuate the colonial status of the Filipino mind, can be used to exploit the masses, and that a psychology developed in and for industrialized countries cannot be imposed on a third world country (Pe-Pua, 1982). Therefore, although many psychologists are trained in North America or Europe, and Western approaches are commonly taught and used within the Philippines, attempts towards indigenization are of considerable influence, particularly in the area of research.

ABUSE AND TRAUMA IN THE PHILIPPINES

My initial exposure to abuse and trauma in the Philippines was through reading about the personal experiences of my students who are primarily pastors, spouses of clergy, or lay leaders in churches or parachurch organizations. In a counseling course I teach, these students are required to write a brief autobiography. In the past I have given a similar assignment to my Canadian students, so I thought I knew what to expect. I have also done clinical work with adult survivors of abuse for over 20 years and believed myself relatively shockproof.

However, as I read the accounts of my Filipino students I was stunned: it seemed as though every one of them had experienced trauma of some variety. Yet this was not a clinical population. Many had suffered the loss of a parent through death during their childhoods, and even greater numbers indicated that one or more of their siblings had died young. Some had parents and grandparents who were imprisoned during the Marcos regime, while others wrote of stepping over dead bodies in the streets as they ran from communist rebels. Others had barely escaped with their lives, leaving houses, land and everything they owned to flee by night with their families in order to avoid assassination by rivals for local government positions.

As a North American, I also struggled to come to grips with some local practices of which I had become aware. For example, I discovered that a not uncommon means of discipline, particularly outside of urban centers, is to place a child inside an empty rice sack, close the top, hang it on a tree, then beat the sack with a stick, eventually freeing the child after several hours. A less dramatic, yet still painful punishment is forcing a child to kneel upright on hard, uncooked mongo beans or salt for hours on end.

I have no trouble defining the above disciplinary practices as abusive. What has been less clear to me, as a foreigner in this country, is whether one can consistently label as abuse other culturally prevalent practices, such as the genital fondling of children for the purpose of soothing, or pulling down underpants as a way of teasing. Some of the students confirmed that they have experienced these kinds of incidents as abusive, while others have accepted them as normative, claiming to not have been affected by them. There is no ambiguity, however, in the numerous descriptions of incest, sexual assault and family violence contained within the students' autobiographies.

Categories of Abuse and Trauma

Child abuse and domestic violence. There is general agreement in the literature that child abuse and domestic violence are major social problems in the Philippines. These include sexual abuse (e.g., rape, incest, attempted rape), physical abuse and maltreatment, sexual exploitation (e.g., prostitution, pedophilia, pornography), neglect, child labor exploitation, illegal recruitment, trafficking, emotional abuse, children in situations of armed conflict, street children, and spouse abuse (e.g., Bautista, Roldan, & Garces-Bacsal, 2001; Carandang, 2002; Child Protection Unit, Philippine General Hospital, 2003; de la Cruz, Protacio, Balanon, Yacat, & Francisco, 2001; Guerrero & Sobritchea, 1997; Protacio-Marcelino, de la Cruz, Balanon, Camacho, & Yacat, 2000; Umali-Suico, 2002). These categories often are determined by the international advocacy groups (e.g., UNICEF) which provide funding for much of the research that is done.

Natural disasters. Due to the geographical and geological character-istics of the Philippines, the country is subject to natural disasters including typhoons, flooding, landslides, earthquakes and volcanic erup-tions. Sometimes a region has not had a chance to recover from one such catastrophe before another follows on its heels. Given the economic de-privation and harsh social conditions already existing in the Philippines, communities hit by such catastrophes are often unable to cope (Ignacio & Perlas, 1994).

Abuses of human rights. As mentioned earlier, there were numerous abuses of human rights reported under the dictatorship of President Marcos (1972-1986). Some studies have been done on the rehabilitation of ex-political detainees from this era, who were often noted as victims of torture (e.g., Decenteceo, 1997; Decenteceo, Cristobal, & Lao-Manalo, 1989). Another example of a frequent human rights violation during the Marcos regime was the phenomenon of "involuntary disappearance," that is, "a sudden and forcible disappearance of a real or alleged political person, but detention is not acknowledged" (Bacalso, 1993, p. 31). Some studies reported on the treatment of families and children who were made to disappear in this way (e.g., Bacalso, 1993; Decenteceo, 1993).

Civil war. There have been two ongoing situations of internal armed conflict that have existed for more than the past three decades, particu-larly in the southern part of the Philippine islands. One of these has been between government armed forces and the revolutionary army of the Communist Party of the Philippines, and the other between government forces and groups of Muslim extremists. These conflicts have resulted in the displacement of millions of people from their homes, but even those not displaced have been affected in numerous ways, including suffering the effects of psychological trauma (Dulce, 1993). For exam-ple, there is documentation that the military have used torture of both adults and children as a way to terrorize the rural people and attempt to discourage them from joining the rebel groups (Protacio-Marcelino, de la Cruz, Camacho, & Balanon, 2003). The use of child soldiers in some of these rebel groups is another way in which these armed conflicts have affected children (Protacio-De Castro, 2001).

Problems in the Literature on Child Abuse

The literature on trauma and abuse within the Philippines is limited. For example, research on family violence has just begun (Guerrero & Sobritchea, 1997). It is also hard to get an accurate sense of the inci-dence, causes, or nature of the phenomena because the literature is fraught with so many difficulties. A number of these have been identi-fied by Protacio-Marcelino and colleagues (2000) in their literature review of 189 published and unpublished studies on child abuse in the Philippines.

One of the problematic issues is that different upper age limits have been used in the definition of a child. No standard age existed prior to September 2, 1990 when the UN Convention on the Rights of the Child defined a child as anyone under the age of 18. Consequently, the use of varying age groupings between studies make comparisons between them difficult, dramatically affecting figures on incidence (Protacio-Marcelino et al., 2000).

Protacio-Marcelino et al. (2000) also observe that a variety of terms have been used in the child abuse literature, and that the use of particular terms change over time. This creates confusion in how problems are defined. As a consequence, estimates of incidence are hard to compare. The term *street children*, for example, has referred to different categories of children over the years. An additional complicating factor is that the term *street children* overlaps with the categories of *working children*, *prostituted children* and *youth offenders*. Similar difficulties surround the use of the terms *child labor* versus *child work*, and *child prostitution*, *sexually exploited children* and *sexually abused children* (Protacio-Marcelino et al., 2000).

The data may also lack representativeness. Most studies on child abuse have been conducted in large urban centers such as metro Manila. It is only recently that provincial and regional studies have been done. However, the metro Manila data are often taken to represent the national situation (Protacio-Marcelino et al., 2000).

Specific categories of abuse tend to have been researched to the exclusion of others, in part because child abuse research has been so dependent on what foreign organizations are willing to fund. The tendency in the Philippines has been for many nongovernment organizations (NGOs) to understand child abuse as synonymous with *children in especially difficult circumstances*, that is, to see it as a feature of some other phenomenon such as child labor or child prostitution, rather than as a distinct social phenomenon. However, formerly unacknowledged abuse, including children in bonded labor and in domestic work, abuse in the family, abuse in schools, and abuse by members of the clergy, has begun to be reported at alarming rates (Protacio-Marcelino et al., 2000).

DISSOCIATION IN THE PHILIPPINES

As I pointed out in the introduction to this piece, dissociation does not appear to be a term that is used by clinicians or researchers in the

Philippines. Most professional publications in the country have been written in English. However, there has been some literature written in Filipino. I obtained the help of a native-born Filipino research assistant to do an additional search of this literature, but she too was unable to find any direct references to dissociation in local published or unpublished works.

References have been made, however, to phenomena that could be considered dissociative, although the authors themselves do not use the term dissociation to describe them. An expression that has appeared in the literature is *altered states of consciousness* (ASCs), particularly when used in the context of religious rituals and experiences of spirit possession. I will discuss each of these areas in light of their relevance to the topic of dissociation in the Philippines.

Religious Rituals

There appears to be a high degree of religious ritual in the Philippines. Examples of this are a dance as part of rites for the dead (Ramos, n.d.), experiences of faith healing and ecstatic preaching (Marasigan, 1978), and the shamanic rituals practiced among the Kalinga and Mandaya tribes (Gelido, 1978). Pertierra (1988), in an anthropological study of Zamora, Ilocos Sur, described many local rituals, from a simple name-changing rite for children, to more complex rituals.

Levin (n.d. b), in an unpublished paper entitled "Oraciones as a psychological phenomenon," discussed how the reading of *oraciones* (prayers) induced an ASC. She proposed that the rapid reading of long tracts of prayer produced hyperventilation, which, in conjunction with the rhythms of the *oraciones* as they were repeated aloud, produced an ASC. Levin hypothesized that specific secret key words within the *oraciones*, which are passed down from teacher to student, also contributed to the development of the ASC. As support for this idea, she described how certain words (e.g., *obra, poder, aleluha, misericordia)* triggered an ASC in some Filipino villagers.

In another paper, Levin (n.d. a) described her eyewitness account of a trance-like condition induced by the rhythm of a group of people praying the rosary in cadence. Levin believed that this experience of group hypnosis was an example of ancient shamanic practices that have been de-mythologized to fit into the existing framework of the Roman Catholic Church.

In a study by Marasigan (1986), a type of group hypnotic induction was described as a "meditative state of consciousness" (p. 21). While in this state, a community group was told that they would see a symbol of some kind in their dreams as a way of determining God's will for their community.

Jaime C. Bulatao, a Jesuit priest as well as a clinical psychologist (trained in the United States), is considered the expert on ASCs as they are experienced in the Philippines. An elderly man now, Father Bulatao is one of the founders of psychology in the Philippines, and has written in the areas of mysticism, religion, theology, and spirituality, as they relate to the Filipino psyche. Bulatao (1992) gave several examples of self-induced ASCs for religious purposes: mediums in *Espiritistas* (a religious sect); a woman who would go into a trance at church every Good Friday; and devotees who have sometimes seen the face of Christ come alive when they have looked at an image of Christ after three days of spiritual exercises and lack of sleep. He also considered aspects of charismatic religious experience to be ASCs.

Bulatao (1992) made the observation that Filipinos easily enter into ASCs. He also believes that this is a desirable aspect of Filipino culture. He wrote that:

> Filipinos are rich in possessing a tremendous mental power, which is the ability to shift easily their state of consciousness. Unfortunately they are not always aware of this power and as a result have created theologies involving spirits, devils, *kulam*, visions, etc., mostly under the guise of some form of religion. It is time that the Filipino come to realize his own ability, that what he has is not a mysterious paranormal, supernatural, unmanageable something but a real power–controllable, researchable, normal. (p. 90)

I believe that the above descriptions of ASCs in Filipino religious rituals could be interpreted as examples of dissociative experiences. Viewed in this light, Bulatao has not merely attempted to explain dissociative experiences in Filipinos, but has also declared that Filipinos should take pride in their ability to dissociate.

Spirit Possession

Bulatao has viewed the Christian Filipino as being ultimately animistic as a result of the legacy of pre-Spanish ancestors (1992). From what Bulatao has reported, the typical Filipino mixes orthodox Roman Catholicism with other beliefs about the spirit world, including: belief in a world of spirits that coexist with the world of matter; a belief in God as chief among spirits, with Christ being a spirit with a definite form, such as the *Santo NiZo* (Infant Jesus) or *Nazareno* (The Nazarene); a belief in saints that take forms like those of their statues; a belief in elemental spirits (e.g., *taong lupa, nuno sa punso, duende*), who live in rivers, fields, balete trees and anthills, and require humans to "ask permission" for them to pass by or pour water; and a belief in spirits as the souls of dead humans. Many unexplained phenomena are seen as works of spirits, so that rituals are required to determine the reason the spirits are upset and to find the means for their placation.

Enriquez, Balde, and Bernando (1989) described other commonly held Filipino beliefs connected with the supernatural or spirit world, including: voodoo (*kulam*), *usog* (transfer of heat from one person with usog to another with negative consequences for the latter), use of a talisman (e.g., *anting-anting*), charms (e.g., *gayuma*), psychic surgery, and a type of premonition or intuition of danger known as *kutob* which involves dissociation of affect.

In the Philippines, it is commonly believed that psychological problems diagnosed in the West as schizophrenia, depression, and so on, are caused by spirits (Bulatao, 1992). Bulatao made the observation that spirit possession in the Philippines is so widespread that it can be regarded as culturally normal. Depending upon the identity of the possessing spirit, it could be welcomed, disliked or feared, so it is necessary to know who was doing the possessing. The most common spirits that "possess" Filipinos are saints, as well as lower spirits (e.g., *engkanto, ada, lamang lupa*). Certain people (e.g., the Catholic priest, *arbularyo* or native healers, and faith healers) are purported to have certain powers over spirits, and may voluntarily seek spirit possession (e.g., medium in *Espiritistas*) in order to help heal others. As these spirits are believed to provide the power for the cure, they are considered desirable. Bulatao wrote that such benevolent possessions have become institutionalized in Filipino culture, as a way of devotees getting advice or healing. For these reasons he has regarded this type of spirit possession as culturally adaptive. Those spirits seen as undesirable have been cured through local techniques and rituals aimed at some form of exorcism (Bautista, 1998; Bulatao, 1992).

Although the common people interpret possession literally, Bulatao pointed out that spirit possession could be understood psychodynamically. He suggested, "any experience that has become a part of oneself can become a possessing object" (Bulatao, 1987, p. 7). For example, spirit possession which is interpreted as possession by the *Santo NiZo* (Infant Jesus), could actually be possession by one's child self. Possession by the *Santo NiZo* could be seen, therefore, as a form of regression back to childhood. Consequently, psychological techniques for recovering repressed material could be used to deal with this type of possession (Bulatao, 1987).

However, since he has seen spirit possession as fundamentally a psychological phenomenon as opposed to a religious one, Bulatao (1992) has advocated treatment through "psychological exorcism" (p. 58). That is, even under circumstances in which the exorcism has been regarded as a religious rite, Bulatao has been aware that he has actually been making a psychological intervention. In other words, the one afflicted may have believed that actual spirits had been exorcised, when in actuality the ritual could have been explained psychologically. Bulatao thus has advocated intervening in ways that would fit the conceptual understandings of the culture, rather than challenging the whole cultural background by offering an entirely new perspective.

The concept of spirit possession has been reported to exist not only within Roman Catholicism and indigenous religions, but also as part of the belief system of Filipino protestant evangelicals. Bautista (1998) in a study on spirit possession within evangelical churches in the Philippines, suggested that some cases would fit into the DSM classification system. Other cases could be considered culture-bound syndromes characterized as "a non-psychiatric though abnormal state, of relatively short duration (as compared to psychiatric cases requiring protracted therapy)" that "may be interpreted within the culture within which it operates" (p. 184). Bautista thus used somewhat different terminology than Bulatao, but seemed to agree with his basic premises.

Spirit Possession or DID?

In an interview conducted with Bulatao (personal communication, March 13, 2001), he acknowledged that spirit possession could be considered the form that DID takes in the Philippines. However, he did not see a diagnosis of DID as necessary or even helpful in this country, primarily because he had found that psychological exorcism worked well. He told me that he had initially corrected people who called him an exorcist, making sure they knew that he was working as a clinical psychologist rather than as a priest when he dealt with cases of spirit possession. However, as time went by he had stopped fighting the label, recognizing that his reputation as an exorcist could actually be a positive contributing factor to the healing process.

The literature in the Philippines has not addressed the issue of the differential diagnosis of spirit possession and dissociative identity disorder (DID); in fact, DID is not mentioned in any context. However, in the international literature the differential diagnosis of spirit possession and DID is viewed as particularly difficult because of the many similarities between the symptoms of each. Some authors identify identity alteration as perhaps the most striking similarity, that is, a spirit possessed individual would often behave as though they were a different person (e.g., Akhtar, 1988; Bulatao, 1992; Cramer, 1980; Marasigan, 1978; Pama, 1999; Somer, 1997; Suwanlert, 1976), which included talking and behaving like a child (Bulatao, 1987; Kahana, 1985). These descriptions are reminiscent of what has been written about the dissociated identities of DID patients (e.g., Friesen, 1991; Putnam, 1997; Ross, 1989).

There are other similarities between those who believe themselves to be possessed by spirits and those diagnosed with DID. Somer (1997) discussed an Italian study by Ferracti, Saceo, and Lazzari. The researchers looked at the psychological test results of ten persons undergoing exorcisms for demonic trance possession states, finding that they had many traits in common with DID patients. It has been suggested that the only difference between DID and possession is in cases of voluntary possession (Downs, Dahmer, & Battle, 1990). Das and Saxena (1991) equated possession syndrome with multiple personality disorder in India. But whereas DID would be considered psychopathological, possession cannot always be viewed as problematic (Hale & Pinninti, 1994).

As mentioned earlier, Bulatao has made the assertion that DID in the Philippines is subsumed under the label of spirit possession, with psychological exorcism being the treatment of choice. In fact, in a personal communication, he did not acknowledge the possibility of DID presenting in a fashion other than as spirit possession (March 13, 2001). I wonder, however, if Bulatao's conclusions are in part the result of the circumstances under which he has come into contact with these phenomena. He encountered cases of possession primarily in his work as a priest (personal communication, March 3, 2001 and August 8, 2002). Thus, these were usually single, brief sessions without the opportunity for follow-up. From the descriptions Bulatao provided, I doubt that these cases would meet the *DSM-IV* criteria for DID (although they could be considered as examples of dissociative experiences or even dissociative disorders). Therefore, it would be uncertain whether the technique of psychological exorcism would be as successful with cases of spirit possession that more closely resemble DID.

Having been somewhat influenced, although not totally convinced, by Bulatao's conceptualizations of DID as spirit possession, I went into my own doctoral dissertation research study (Gingrich, 2004) expecting to find at least some examples of spirit possession which met *DSM-IV* criteria for DID. To my surprise, although a number of participants met *DSM-IV* criteria for DID, none presented as spirit possessed. This finding, in conjunction with the observations made from cases presented to me in supervision sessions by student interns, suggests that DID is a relevant diagnosis in the Philippines, and that its manifestation is broader than the phenomenon of spirit possession alone.

TRAUMA AND DISSOCIATION: EVIDENCE FOR A LINK

As mentioned earlier, with the exception of my own dissertation research (Gingrich, 2004), there have been no research studies that have explicitly focused on dissociation or the possible association between trauma and dissociation in the Philippines. Dissociation has also not been mentioned as a symptom in the local literature on trauma and abuse, including publications on the effects of natural disasters such as earthquakes (e.g., Carandang, 1996; Ignacio & Perlas, 1994), the psychological aspects of rehabilitation of ex-political detainees (e.g., Decenteceo et al., 1989), the impact on victims of the manifold varieties of child abuse found in the Philippines (e.g., Protacio-Marcelino et al., 2000), and the effects on both child and adult victims of family violence (e.g., Guerrero & Sobritchea, 1997).

There are, however, indications that dissociative symptoms are present in trauma survivors, even if not interpreted as such by authors. Bautista et al. (2001) gave an example in the case description of a young boy who had been regularly beaten and almost killed by his drug addicted father before seeking refuge in the street. In the following observations made by the researchers, there are indications of possible intra-interview amnesia, dissociation of affect, entering into spontaneous trance states, and even a hint of potential identity alteration. Bautista et al. (2001) wrote:

> Joselito relates his story sans [sic] emotions. He appeared "spaced-out." He looked at his interviewer blankly, as if he were peering into empty space. He did not pay much attention to what was being asked him. He would say something but would say something utterly different when asked about it again. From time to time

he would be occupied playing with his chain. Sometimes, his attention would drift somewhere else. His statements have very little connection with each other. His speech is garbled and incoherent. He would also get a trifle impatient when asked for clarifications . . . He recalls that the saddest experience he had was when he missed his mother terribly but could not go home because his father might kill him when he sees him. He was teary-eyed when he recalled this but he immediately diverted his attention somewhere else as if avoiding the issue. This was the first time he showed some form of emotion but he doused it off right away. (pp. 86-87)

Another investigator (Gonzalez-Fernando, 2000), in a phenomenological study on the inner world of girl child prostitutes, even more clearly describe dissociative symptoms. She actually utilized the term dissociation at one point, although she stopped short of determining a diagnosis of DID or another dissociative disorder. Initially all her subjects denied having been prostitutes despite corroborating evidence to the contrary. Whether this was evidence of dissociation or conscious disavowal of the experience is unknown. However a common tendency to "block out whole episodes in their lives" was observed (p. 77). This resulted in an "*almost absent sense of chronology. . . .*" She added that, "the girls could not give us a coherent, intact, integrated view of their own lives" (p. 78). Amnesia thus seemed to have been a frequently observed symptom.

One girl was described as going "bland" when asked about prostitution experiences. "Whenever the subject came up, she would suddenly stare into the distance, as if going into reverie; her mouth would move, as if speaking to herself absentmindedly, but without any sound; this would go on until the interviewer would call her attention–then she would 'snap back,' as if coming alive again" (p. 77). This type of trance state is very similar to what I have observed in my dissociative clients.

Dissociation of affect was described by Gonzalez-Fernando (2000) as a "highly noticeable lack or 'flatness' of affect" (p. 78) when the girls studied spoke of intense feelings or were describing traumatic situations. Gonzalez-Fernando concluded that the girls' most basic dynamic was that:

In their inner life, these girls are split in two. It is as if they have two separate existences, two personas, two lives–the one they really had and would rather forget, and the one they wish they could have but deep-down are afraid they never could. This 'split' (dissociation) is so pervasive that each of the girls would say something (completely positive or completely negative) about sexuality at one point of the interview, only to express something totally its opposite at another point. (p. 84)

Gonzalez-Fernando (2000) did not diagnose these girls as having DID. However, it seems probable that they would fit into the *DSM-IV* category of DID or DDNOS.

In an interview, M. L. Arellano-Carandang (personal communication, August 7, 2003) elaborated on the research done by Gonzalez- Fernando (2000). Dr. Carandang is a clinical psychologist who supervised Gonzalez-Fernando's research. She described how in addition to the dissociative symptoms referred to by Gonzalez-Fernando, many of the prostituted children would blink their eyes, pause, then their facial expression would change. I noted to Carandang that this sounded very much like the "switches" I have observed in my own DID clients.

When asked why the research team did not see this as a potential instance of DID or another dissociative disorder, Carandang's response was that to talk of dissociative disorders seemed almost "taboo" among mental health professionals in the Philippines; that to label what they were seeing in this manner seemed too extreme. Carandang commented that the way most Filipino psychologists and psychiatrists learn about dissociation is through textbooks, books, and films such as *The Three Faces of Eve* (Thigpen & Cleckley, 1957) and *Sybil* (Schreiber, 1973), which tend to sensationalize dissociation. She went on to say that this perhaps explains why her research team talked all around the issue without explicitly identifying it. They used phrases descriptive of dissociation (e.g., using the word "split," and saying "there are two sides to them"). But when they were tempted to label it as dissociation they reacted: "That's too much! It can't be!" Carandang laughingly admitted that the way they as researchers finally dealt with this dilemma was to describe what they were seeing as "very similar" to dissociation. For example, Gonzalez-Fernando (2000) noted: "However, their emotions did not match their words–there was anger and pain, but it was not there *now*; they seemed to be *reporting* it, talking *about* it, but *not feeling* it then and there, very similar to the process of dissociation" (p. 78).

Researcher-clinician M. K. Puente (personal communication, June 13, 2003), had no reservation in using the term dissociation to describe some of her observations of her Filipino child clients. Puente is a former student of Carandang's as well as a contributor to a book edited by

Carandang which reports on some studies conducted on abused children in difficult circumstances in the Philippines (Carandang, 2002), Puente spent some time studying in the United States, where she received specialized training and gained further clinical experience at a trauma center. While there, the researcher-clinician gained exposure to clients with dissociative symptoms, both as they manifested in diagnosed dissociative disorders, and as symptoms of post-traumatic stress disorder (PTSD). Perhaps her training in identifying dissociation in the United States has allowed Puente to be less hesitant than her Filipino colleagues to utilize the term *dissociation* as a diagnostic label.

Puente made the point that sometimes children are branded as liars when it may be that they are actually dissociating, especially if they had been traumatized earlier. Her impression was that this tendency for dissociative children to be called liars may be even more common in the Philippines than in the United States. Puento also commented that Filipino children with a trauma history often tend to deny that they have been abused, that is, they are amnestic for their trauma, despite confirmed reports by parents of specific incidents.

This tendency for many Filipino children to not acknowledge their abuse, despite corroborating evidence to the contrary, was also noted by M. C. De Ungria (personal communication, July 16, 2003). De Ungria is a researcher who is currently attempting to make sense of data indicating that many traumatized children in the Philippines make such denials. When I mentioned my dissertation research to her, she wondered whether dissociation could possibly explain this phenomenon.

In conjunction with my own study, I think the descriptions offered by these authors and clinicians add weight to my conclusion that dissociative disorders, including cases of classical DID presentation, are valid diagnoses in the Philippines. They also support the theory that dissociation is associated with some forms of childhood trauma. What needs further clarification is the nature of the association: What types of trauma are potentially linked to dissociation?[2] What symptoms of dissociation are the most salient in those who have been traumatized?

OBSERVATIONS AND RECOMMENDATIONS

It is clear that trauma and child abuse are issues of social concern in the Philippines. It is also apparent that Filipinos experience dissociation, although the local literature refers to altered states of consciousness rather than labeling these phenomena as dissociative. Dissociative states have been particularly noted in reference to religious rituals and spirit possession. However, nothing has been published specifically regarding DID, dissociative disorders, or a trauma-dissociation link in the Philippines.

Nonetheless, I believe that there are strong indications that DID and other dissociative disorders are valid diagnoses in the Philippines. These manifest at times through symptoms very similar to those found in the West. On other occasions, they manifest in more culturally specific forms such as spirit possession. There also appears to be some anecdotal evidence, in addition to the findings from my own study, which point to an association between trauma and dissociation. However, the frequency with which dissociative disorders occur in the Philippines is unknown, and the exact nature of the association between dissociation and trauma requires further investigation.

I am aware that I am approaching these issues as an outsider in that I myself am not Filipino. However, since the dearth of relevant research makes coming to definitive conclusions impossible, perhaps I can offer some suggestions regarding specific areas that I feel merit further examination. I would also like to offer some reflections as to what further research could reveal with regards to both dissociation and a trauma-dissociation link.

I believe that it would be useful to determine which forms of dissociation should be considered normal versus which constitute psychopathology within Philippine culture. This is especially important if Bulatao (1992) is correct in his assertion that Filipinos dissociate more easily than do those from other cultural backgrounds. While Bulatao has done some work in this area, there is still much potential for Filipino researchers to explore it in more depth.

It could also be helpful to explore how dissociation and a trauma-dissociation link could be impacted by the Filipino view of self. The self-construals of Filipinos can be seen as more interdependent and less independent than those of Westerners (Sta. Maria, 1999). Filipinos, however, are Asians who have been tremendously influenced by Spanish and American cultures (dominant Western cultures in their respective eras). Therefore, Filipinos could be considered more individualistic than would be typical of other Asians.

There are some indications in the international literature that different cultural self-construals influence the nature of the trauma-dissociation link, as well as the form that pathological dissociation takes. I will briefly refer to some of this literature in order to make some projections as to what might be found in the Philippine context with respect to these areas.

Lewis-Fernandez (1994) wrote that the Western view of self could be important in the potential development of DID. He suggested that because of the Western view of a bounded, individualistic self, "greater psychological violence would be required in order to overcome the cultural barrier against dissociation of the self and produce identity alteration. Consequently, the resulting effect (a *shattered* self) would be more pathological and pervasive" (p. 160). He went on to say that this may explain the association between extreme trauma and DID in the West.

If the Lewis-Fernadez view is correct, a Filipino could potentially develop DID without the same degree of trauma that would be necessary for its development in the West. A corollary might be that DID in the Philippines may not indicate the same level of pathology as DID in the West, therefore, it may also be less difficult to treat.

How individuals in a given culture construe the self can also influence the way in which pathological dissociation manifests. There has been some evidence in the literature to indicate that in cultures where self-construals are more interdependent, cases of DID exist but to a lesser degree than in similar populations in the West. For example, a study by Umesue, Matsuo, Iwata, and Tashiro (1996) showed that while DID has been identified in Japan, diagnoses of dissociative disorder not otherwise specified (DDNOS), which do not quite fit the *DSM-IV* criteria for DID, were proportionately more common in Japan than in the West.

If it is true that self-construals are determining factors in whether DID or DDNOS are more frequently found in a particular culture, perhaps the prevalence of DID in the Philippines will be found to be less than in the West because Filipinos are more interdependent than are Westerners. However, as mentioned earlier, Filipinos in some ways are a mixture of East and West, and therefore are more independent than other Asians such as the Japanese. For this reason DID could potentially be more prevalent in the Philippines than in other Asian countries.

Lewis-Fernandez (1994) addressed how distinctive cultural factors can influence the frequency with which pathological dissociation manifests as spirit possession in a given culture. He wrote that identity alteration in the form of spirit possession would more likely be experienced in a culture where there is greater permeability of the self, as well as more pervasive spiritual notions of causality. Identity alteration in the form of spirit possession may then be culturally accepted as an expression of suffering, but would not require the extreme trauma prerequisite to DID found in the West. Lewis-Fernandez also suggested that spirit possession tends to be more transient, and less severe pathologically. Bulatao (personal communication, August 8, 2002) has made similar observations regarding the transience and severity of pathology of spirit possession in the Philippines. Lewis-Fernandez' view is also congruent with that of Adityanjee, Raju, and Khandelwal (1989), who wrote that possession syndrome in India and DID in the West "represent parallel dissociative disorders with similar etiologies despite some major differences in clinical profiles" (p. 1610).

The high capacity to dissociate among Filipinos, together with a strong, if not always explicit, belief in the spirit world, leads to a hypothesis that spirit possession will continue to be one way in which dissociative symptoms manifest themselves in the Philippines. As A. C. Gaw, Ding, Levine, and H. Gaw (1998) put it: "If a general belief in possession is combined with a propensity to dissociate, the likelihood of developing any dissociative disorder attributed to possession is increased" (p. 364). However, as mentioned earlier, one has to be cautious in assuming that all forms of spirit possession in the Philippines are necessarily pathological.

As Western influence increases in the Philippines, as is the trend in other developing countries, it may be hypothesized further that the incidence of spirit possession will decrease. At the same time, there will likely be an increase in diagnosed cases of DID. This prediction is consistent with the observation that, historically, possessions have decreased in industrialized societies with more Western-oriented values (Begelman, 1993; Somer, 1997). In developing nations where belief in possession is more likely to exist, cases of spirit possession have been found to be more common (Alexander & Das, 1997). Adityanjee et al. (1989) predicted that this will be the trend for their country, India.

There also has been research in some countries (e.g., Akhtar, 1988) to support an association between a higher incidence of spirit possession among the less formally educated, lower socioeconomic classes and a greater frequency of DID among those in the middle and upper classes. It is thus possible that a similar pattern might be found in the Philippines. Results from my own research with freshmen from a premiere university seem to bear this out. No student presented as spirit possessed, while there were some who fit the criteria for a diagnosis of DID.

As a Canadian who has worked and studied in the Philippines for the past 8 years, I would encourage Filipino researchers to take on the challenge of attempting to find their own answers to some of the many questions concerning trauma and dissociation in the Philippines. I recognize that national researchers may need to be convinced that these questions are worth answering. I also understand that the indigenization movement in psychology, by viewing DID and other dissociative disorders as Western, may prematurely reject useful aspects of the full range of dissociative phenomena. Perhaps the reason that Bulatao's conceptualizations of ASCs and spirit possession have gained broad acceptance among Filipino professionals is that his views are consistent with the aims of indigenization.

If future research confirms that there is indeed an association between trauma and dissociation in the Philippines, there are implications for diagnosis and treatment. Dissociative symptoms, for example, could potentially alert mental health professionals to the possibility that an individual has experienced trauma. In addition, accurate diagnosis of dissociative disorders is also an important step towards providing the best help possible to trauma survivors.

Potentially the international community could also make a contribution towards research in this area. Perhaps international agencies and NGOs, some of whom already fund much of the research on child abuse in the Philippines, could specifically support local research on trauma and dissociation. If these organizations become convinced of the benefit of doing this research, they could possibly fund training in the identification and treatment of dissociative disorders in addition to funding the research itself.

Dissociative disorders, including DID are treatable, but in order to intervene effectively, Filipino mental health professionals may need to broaden their awareness of dissociative disorders in the Philippines. The task will then be to interact with Filipino researchers and clinicians regarding how to identify and treat DID and other dissociative disorders and encourage them to find meaningful ways to apply this knowledge to their culture and fellow Filipinos.

NOTES

1. From a total sample of 459 first year Filipino university students, 30 high dissociators and 30 low-moderate dissociators were selected for interviews using the *Structured Clinical Interview for DSM-IV Dissociative Disorders* (SCID-D-R; Steinberg, 1993) based on their scores on the *Dissociative Experiences Scale* (DES; Putnam, 1989), *Somatoform Dissociation Questionnaire-5* (SDQ-5; Nijenhuis, 1999) and *Multidimensional Inventory of Dissociation* (MID; Dell, 2003). Out of the 60 par-

ticipants interviewed, 19 were identified as having dissociative disorders (7 DID, 10 DDNOS, 2 dissociative amnesia).

2. The results of my study (Gingrich, 2004) showed a clear trauma-dissociation link. The historical presence of various types of trauma, over-all child abuse, emotional trauma, sexual trauma, and bodily threat from a person/intense pain were significant associations. However, as this study was exploratory in nature, much more work needs to be done in this area.

REFERENCES

Adityanjee, R., Raju, G. S. P., & Khandelwal, S. K. (1989). Current status of multiple personality disorder in India. *American Journal of Psychiatry, 146,* 1607-1610.

Akhtar, S. (1988). Four culture-bound psychiatric syndromes in India. *Journal of Social Psychiatry, 34,* 70-74.

Alexander, P. J., & Das, J. A. (1997). Limited utility of ICD-10 and DSM-IV classification of dissociative and conversion disorders in India. *Acta Psychiatrica Scandinavica, 95,* 177-182.

American Psychiatric Association. (2000). *The diagnostic and statistical manual of mental disorders* (4th ed., text revision). Washington, DC: Author.

Bacalso, A. (1993). The political phenomenon of making people disappear. *Human Rights Forum, 3,* 31-37.

Bautista, V. V. (1998). View of *sapi* by evangelical churchworkers: Some implications for psychopathology and counseling. In A. B. I. Bernardo, N. A. Daya, & A. A. Tan (Eds.), *Understanding behavior bridging cultures: Readings on an emerging global psychology* (pp. 175-184).

Bautista, V., Roldan, A., & Garces-Bacsal, M. (2001). *Working with abused children from the lenses of resilience and contextualization.* Quezon City, Philippines: University of the Philippines Center for Integrative and Development Studies Psychosocial Trauma and Human Rights Program, and Save the Children Sweden.

Begelman, D. A. (1993). Possession: Interdisciplinary roots. *Dissociation, 6*(4), 201-221.

Bulatao, J. C. (1987). Modes of mind: Experience and theory of consciousness and its alternative states. *Philippine Journal of Psychology, 20,* 3-30.

Bulatao, J. C. (1992). *Phenomena and their interpretation: Landmark essays 1957-1989.* Manila, Philippines: Ateneo de Manila University Press.

Carandang, M. L. A. (1996). *Pakikipagkapwa-Damdamin (Accompanying survivors of disasters).* Makati City, Philippines: Bookmark, Inc.

Carandang, M. L. A. (Ed.). (2002). *Children in pain: Studies on children who are abused, and are living in poverty, prison and prostitution.* Quezon City, Philippines: Psychological Association of the Philippines.

Central Intelligence Agency. (n.d.). *The world factbook.* Retrieved August 14, 2003, from http://www.cia.gov/cia/publications/factbook/geos/rp.html

Child Protection Unit, Philippine General Hospital. (2003). *Annual report.* Manila, Philippines: Author.

Cramer, M. (1980). Psychopathology and shamanism in rural Mexico: A case study of spirit possession. *British Journal of Medical Psychology, 53*, 67-73.

Das, P. S., & Saxena, S. (1991). Classification of dissociative states in DSM-III-R and ICD-10 (1989 Draft): A study of Indian out-patients. *British Journal of Psychiatry, 149*(10), 425-427).

Decenteceo, E. T. (1993). Counseling victims: The children of disappeared persons. *Human Rights Forum, 3*, 39-46.

Decenteceo, E. T. (1997). *Rehab: Psychosocial rehabilitation for social transformation.* Quezon City, Philippines: BUKAL.

Decenteceo, E. T., Cristobal, M., & Lao-Manalo, R. (1989). *Ex-political detainees: Psychological aspects of rehabilitation.* Quezon City, Philippines: BALAY.

de la Cruz, M. T., Protacio, E. P., Balanon, F. A. G., Yacat, J. A., & Francisco, C. T. (2001). *Trust and power: Child abuse in the eyes of the child and the parent.* Quezon City, Philippines: Save the Children UK and United Nations Children's Fund.

Dell, P. F. *Multidimensional Inventory of Dissociation (MID): A comprehensive self-report instrument for pathological dissociation. Journal of Trauma & Dissociation.*

Downs, J., Dahmer, S. K., Battle, A. O. (1990, September). Multiple personality disorder in India [Letter to the Editor]. *American Journal of Psychiatry, 1260.*

Dulce, C. B. (1993). Internal refugees in the Philippines: No escape from war. *Human Rights Forum, 3*, 5-16.

Enriquez, V., Balde, P. J., & Bernardo, M. A. (1989). *Ang kababalaghan at and parasikolohiya.* Philippines: New Horizons Press.

Friesen, J. (1991). *Uncovering the mystery of MPD.* Nashville, TN: Thomas Nelson.

Gaw, A. C., Ding, Q., Levine, R. E., & Gaw, H. (1998). The clinical characteristics of possession disorder among 20 Chinese patients in the Hebei province of China. *Psychiatric Services, 49*(3), 360-365.

Gelido, M. (1978). Two popular religious practices: Faith healing and ecstatic preaching. *Philippine Priests Forum, 10*, 14-22.

Gingrich, H. J. (2004). *Dissociation in a student sample in the Philippines.* Unpublished doctoral dissertation, University of the Philippines, Quezon City, Philippines.

Gonzalez-Fernando, P. (2000). *Pagkatao, pagkababae, at seksuwalidad* (Self-concept, womanhood, and sexuality): A phenomenological study of the inner world of the girl child prostitute. *Philippine Journal of Psychology, 33*(1), 67-91.

Guerrero, S., & Sobritchea (Ed.). (1997). *Breaking the silence: The realities of family violence in the Philippines and recommendations for change.* Manila, Philippines: United Nations Children's Fund.

Hale, A. S., & Pinninti, N. R. (1994). Exorcism-resistant ghost possession treated with clopenthixol. *British Journal of Psychiatry, 165*(3), 386-8.

Ingacio, L. L., & Perlas, A. P. (1994). *From victims to survivors.* Manila, Philippines: University of the Philippines Manila Information, Publication and Public Affairs Office.

Kahana, Y. (1985). The Zar spirits, a category of magic in the system of mental health care in Ethiopia. *International Journal of Social Psychiatry, 31,* 125-143.

Levin, M. A. (n.d. a). Mahika. In *Tinipon ni Dr. Violeta V. Bautista Sikolohiya ng Relihiyon I* (unpublished collection of student papers), 26-40.

Levin, M. A. (n.d. b). Oraciones as a psychological phenomenon. In *Tinipon ni Dr. Violeta V. Bautista Sikolohiya ng Relihiyon I* (unpublished collection of student papers), 41-93.

Lewis-Fernandez, R. (1994). Culture and dissociation: A comparison of *ataque de nervios* among Puerto Ricans and possession syndrome in India. In D. Spiegel (Ed.), *Dissociation: Culture, mind, and body* (pp. 123-167). Washington, DC: American Psychiatric Press.

Marasigan, V. (1978). Tagalog ecstatics. *Philippine Priests Forum, 10,* 23-32.

Marasigan, V. (1986). Local forms of prayer: Dreams. *Ministry Today, 2*(1), 21-23.

National Statistical Coordination Board–Philippines. (2004, January). Retrieved Oct. 28, 2004, from http://www.nscb.gov.ph/view/people.asp

Nijenhuis, E. R. S. (1999). *Somatoform dissociation: Phenomena, measurement, and theoretical issues.* Assen, Netherlands: Van Gorcum.

Pama, H. (1999). Diskurso tungkol sa damdamin, salita at gawa ng kapatirang sa Bundok. Unpublished thesis. University of the Philippines, Quezon City, Philippines.

Pe-Pua, R. (Ed.). (1982). *Filipino psychology: Theory, method and application.* Quezon City, Philippines: University of the Philippines Press.

Pertierra, R. (1988). *Religion, politics, and rationality in a Philippine community.* Quezon City: Ateneo de Manila University Press.

Protacio-De Castro, E. (2001). Children in armed conflict situations: Focus on child soldiers in the Philippines. Retrieved August 14, 2003, from http://www.childprotection.org/ph

Protacio-Marcelino, E., de la Cruz, M. T., Balanon, F. A.., Camacho, A. Z., & Yacat, J. A. (2000). *Child abuse in the Philippines: An integrated literature review and annotated bibliography.* Quezon City, Philippines: University of the Philippines Center for Integrative and Development Studies.

Protacio-Marcelino, E., de la Cruz, M. T., Camacho, A. Z.,& Balanon, F. A. Torture of children in situations of armed conflict. Retrieved August 14, 2003, from http://www.childprotection.org/ph/monthlyfeatures/tortureofchildren.doc

Putnam, F. W. (1989). *Diagnosis and treatment of multiple personality disorder.* New York: Guilford Press.

Putnam, F. W. (1997). *Dissociation in children and adolescents.* New York: Guilford.

Ramos, M. B. (n.d.). Belief in ghouls in contemporary Philippine society. *Western Folklore, 27*(3), 184-190.

Ross, C. A. (1989). *Multiple personality disorder: Diagnosis, clinical features, and treatment.* New York: John Wiley & Sons.

Schrieber, F. R. (1973). *Sybil.* New York: Warner Books.

Somer, E. (1997). Paranormal and dissociative experiences in middle-eastern Jews in Israel: Diagnostic and treatment dilemmas. *Dissociation, 10*(3), 174-181.

Sta, Maria, M. (1999). Filipinos' representations for the self. *Philippine Journal of Psychology, 32*(2), 53-88.

Steinberg, M. (1993). *Structured clinical interview for DSM-IV dissociative disorders (SCID-D)*. Washington, DC: American Psychiatric Press.

Suwanlert, S. (1976). Neurotic and psychotic states attributed to Thai "Phii Pob" spirit possession. *Australian and New Zealand Journal of Psychiatry, 10,* 119-123.

Thigpen, C. H., & Cleckley, H. (1957). *The three faces of Eve*. New York: McGraw-Hill.

Umali-Suico, (2002). A case study of sexual exploitation of children in the Philippines: The role of evangelical churches. *Journal of Asian Mission, 4,* 217-242.

Umesue, M., Matsuo, T., Iwata, N., & Tashiro, N. (1996). Dissociative disorders in Japan: A pilot study with the Dissociative Experiences Scale and a semi-structured interview. *Dissociation, 9*(3), 182-189.

From Obscurity to Daylight:
The Study of Dissociation in Puerto Rico

Alfonso Martínez-Taboas

SUMMARY. The study of dissociation and dissociative disorders in Puerto Rico began in the 1980s. Initially the literature was limited to case-studies and anecdotal reports. In the 1990s a plethora of more sophisticated studies began to be published, including the reliability and validity of some well-known dissociative instruments and scales, including the Dissociative Experiences Scale. Also, some doctoral students in clinical psychology decided to conduct their research dissertations on dissociative disorders. Beginning with the new century, more sophisticated research methodologies are being applied to the study of dissociation in Puerto Rico, including some recent epidemiological findings with youths. Although still limited, the data-base on dissociation in Puerto Rico has been increasing rapidly. The article concludes with some reflections on how to be successful in obtaining support for future studies. *[Article copies available for a fee from The Haworth Document Delivery Service: 1-800-HAWORTH. E-mail address: <docdelivery@haworthpress. com> Website: <http://www.HaworthPress.com> © 2005 by The Haworth Press, Inc. All rights reserved.]*

Alfonso Martínez-Taboas, PhD, is affilaited with Carlos Albizu University.

Address correspondence to: Alfonso Martínez-Taboas, PhD, Parque del Río, Vía del Parque Street, #151, Trujillo Alto, Puerto Rico 00976.

[Haworth co-indexing entry note]: "From Obscurity to Daylight: The Study of Dissociation in Puerto Rico." Martínez-Taboas, Alfonso. Co-published simultaneously in *Journal of Trauma Practice* (The Haworth Maltreatment & Trauma Press, an imprint of The Haworth Press, Inc.) Vol. 4, No. 3/4, 2005, pp. 271-285; and: *Trauma and Dissociation in a Cross-Cultural Perspective: Not Just a North American Phenomenon* (ed: George F. Rhoades, Jr., and Vedat Sar) The Haworth Maltreatment & Trauma Press, an imprint of The Haworth Press, Inc., 2005, pp. 271-285. Single or multiple copies of this article are available for a fee from The Haworth Document Delivery Service [1-800-HAWORTH, 9:00 a.m. - 5:00 p.m. (EST). E-mail address: docdelivery@haworthpress.com].

KEYWORDS. Dissociative disorders, childhood trauma, Dissociative Experiences Scale

In this piece my intention is to present the progression and brief overview of the clinical and research efforts that have been conducted regarding dissociation and dissociative disorders (DD) in Puerto Rico. Puerto Rico is a Caribbean island with a population of 3,878,532 persons (2003 estimate). The primary ethnicity is Hispanic and, although Spanish and English are the official languages, Spanish is the dominant one. English is spoken by 25% of the population. Similar to other Latin American countries, Catholicism is the main religion on the island.

THE CLINICAL YEARS: 1986-1994

Probably the first Spanish article on dissociation was published in 1986 in a major psychological/psychiatric journal in Latin America (Martínez-Taboas). The paper reviewed the main characteristics of dissociative patients. The discussion of psychological trauma and its aftermath were completely absent from Latin American professional literature until the early 1990s (Martínez-Taboas, 1991b; Farrington, 1991). Apparently, there was scant interest and resources directed to understand and solve an endemic situation that was obviously noticeable in many Latin American countries.

In 1988, I encountered my first Dissociative Identity Disorder (DID) patient. As recounted in my book (Martínez-Taboas, 1990), the case surged in an unexpected manner in the clinical evaluation of a 25-year-old woman that was taking part of a vocational assessment. As part of her history, she recounted that she was physically and sexually abused as a child, but insisted that she didn't wanted to talk about her horrible past. I respected her decision. Minutes later, when I was administering the Thematic Apperception Test (a projective test), she told me that she didn't want to see the pictures of the TAT as they were evoking in her some unpleasant childhood memories. I encouraged her to continue her response to the cards, when suddenly she hung her head for a moment, staring at the ground. When she lifted her head, she said: "Why are you annoying her?" At first I didn't understand what was happening. I thought I hadn't heard her correctly, so I encouraged her to continue with the next TAT card. But the response came immediately: "You do not see that all this is making her suffer. I will not permit you to continue to make her suffer." When I heard this, I not only noticed that Migdalia was now speaking in the third person ("she"), but her tone of voice had become more gruff and less melodious. Her facial expression also changed. It had become alarmingly angry. For that reason I asked Migdalia: "What do you mean that the test makes you suffer?" The answer came without delay: "I am not Migdalia . . . I am Pedro" (Martinez-Taboas, 1990, 1995a).

Migdalia was my first DID patient. In the following two years, there came to my attention two additional DID patients. In 1990, I wrote a book (Martínez-Taboas, 1990) that reviewed the international literature on DID and my work with these three patients. Dr. Richard Kluft read an English synopsis of the book and agreed to write the prologue for the book. My book was very well received in Puerto Rico, where more than 2,000 copies were sold, many of them to psychologists and to graduate students. The book became required reading in some graduate courses in Puerto Rico.

Following the publication of the book I began to offer different workshops and conferences on Dissociative Disorders. The response was amazing, with conferences being usually extremely well attended and the interest in dissociation began to expand.

It became apparent that Latin American clinicians and researchers would benefit from material from American (USA) authorities. I obtained permission from Dr. Richard Kluft to make a translation from an unpublished paper on family violence and dissociation. I translated the article to Spanish and it was duly published in a special issue on trauma in a prestigious Mexican journal (Kluft, 1991).

In 1989 I published my first article in the journal *Dissociation* (Martínez-Taboas) detailing the preliminary observations of my first three cases of DID. Two years later, I published a paper that followed the first series of cases of DID in Puerto Rico (Martínez-Taboas, 1991a). In this paper, I systematically analyzed 15 DID cases that were referred to me and that I studied in detail. The results revealed (Table 1) that DID cases in Puerto Rico were nearly identical to DID cases in USA or Canada. The main difference found in our case load was that the mean number of alters was only four, in contrast to the mean number of 13-15 alters reported by clinicians in the USA and Canada (Putnam, Guroff, Silberman, Barban & Post, 1986; Ross, Norton & Wozney, 1989).

Two years later, Martínez-Taboas and Cruz-Igartúa (1993) published, in a major Puerto Rican medical journal, their experience with dissociative patients in one of the principal private psychiatric hospitals in Puerto Rico. Their experience indicated that DID patients were often

TABLE 1. Some Major Clinical Findings with 15 Cases of DID in Puerto Rico.

Variable or Symptom	%
Women	93%
Sexual Abuse	73%
Physical Abuse	60%
Recurrent Headaches	100%
Amnesias	93%
Depression	93%
Suicidal Attempts	80%
Somatization	73%
Seizures	67%
Voices	60%
Depersonalization	53%
Sexual Dysfunction	50%
Mutilations	47%

ostracized by the medical staff; provoked strong counter-transferences in some mental-health providers; and were often excessively over medicated to control unusual dissociative symptoms.

THE RESEARCH YEARS: 1995-2005

From 1995 to the present time a group of psychologists and psychiatrists began to conduct more systematic research on dissociation and its disorders. In 1995, the first report on the use of the Dissociative Experiences Scale (DES) in Puerto Rico (Martínez-Taboas, 1995b) along with the Spanish DES (Martínez-Taboas, 1990) was published The investigation involved a control group of 46 undergraduate students, a comparison group of 15 panic disorder patients, and 16 DID patients. The results indicated the following mean DES scores: (1) students: 17.4; (2) panic disorder: 22.6; (3) DID patients: 60.3. The results were very similar to those reported in various countries (Boon & Draijer, 1993; Ensink & Otterloo, 1989; Ross, Ryan, Anderson, Ross & Hardy, 1989) and highlighted the notion that dissociative patients usually have high scores on the DES. In fact, 100% of the DID group produced scores above a cut-off DES score of 35. None of the control group produced such scores, and only 13% of the panic disorders patients scored a DES score above 35.

That same year, six prominent psychologists and psychiatrists in Puerto Rico wrote a paper titled: *What a group of clinicians have learned about multiple personality disorder in Puerto Rico* (Martínez-Taboas et al., 1995). The paper presented the following ten conclusions:

1. DID appears to be an uncommon disorder in Puerto Rico, but is not as extremely rare as some assume.
2. Childhood trauma and/or abuse is highly prevalent in patients diagnosed with DID.
3. Verification of the abusive experiences was found in the majority of cases treated.
4. None of the DID patients treated had alleged that they were abused in a satanic ritual.
5. The mean number of alter personalities per patient was lower than the number reported in North America and Europe.
6. The use of the DES appears to be a promising instrument in the detection of DID with Hispanics.
7. Most of the DD patients had been in the mental health system for more than five years without remission of symptoms and with diverse diagnosis such as epilepsy, depression with psychotic traits, and schizophrenia.
8. Hypnosis was rarely used in the clinical detection of DID.
9. The limited experience with children and adolescents diagnosed with DID suggested that that their clinical course is more benign than that of adults DID patients.
10. Most of us had encountered colleagues with marked hostility and irrational resistance to the DID diagnosis of our patients.

In 1996 the *American Journal of Psychotherapy* published a paper (Martínez-Taboas, 1996) about two clinical cases in Puerto Rico that produced convincing evidence that the scenes produced during the abreaction of repressed memories corresponded to independently corroborated historical facts. In one of these cases, Madeline (the patient) presented an alter personality of a little girl that adamantly insisted that she was repeatedly raped by a cousin. The alter made many curious drawings wherein the cousin used some elaborate ropes to immobilize her to the bed, but Madeline had no memory for such abusive experiences. After consulting with the therapist and her mother, she traveled to the USA with the intention to talk personally with the alleged abuser who was then living in New York City. During the conversation with him, he at first reluctantly admitted and then further elaborated the abusive acts. The cousin then reportedly assumed that the patient had come to New York to provoke him to continue the sexual relationship. When Madeline understood the latter assumption, she fled from his house in terror.

In 1997 a more rigorous examination of the use of the DES was conducted in Puerto Rico (Martínez-Taboas & Bernal, 2000). This research involved 198 undergraduate students mainly from the University of Puerto Rico. The research was designed to test the hypothesis that higher DES scores were related to psychopathology and to sexual and other types of abuse. The results supported this hypothesis in four ways. First, the overall mean DES score for the whole sample was 14.8, which was consistent the international literature. Second, it was found that DES scores were significantly higher in those participants that endorsed some type of abuse ($p < .01$). Third, we also found that as the frequency of the abuse increased, the DES scores also significantly increased. For example, the group with no abuse obtained a score of 11.87; slight abuse 16.34; frequent abuse 22.36. There was a significant difference between the first group and the last group ($p < .002$). Lastly, the DES was found to be associated with reports of childhood sexual abuse (r = .35, $p < .01$). The use of the Beck Depression Inventory obtained a low and non-significant correlation with sexual abuse (r = .11). This investigation produced a more solid ground for the use of the DES in Puerto Rico.

Recently, Francia-Martinez, Roca de Torres, Alvarado, Martínez-Taboas and Sayers (2003) reported the frequency of self-reported childhood abuse experience of psychiatric inpatients, and the presence of dissociative symptoms. The subjects studied included 100 Puerto Rican inpatients, who were mostly hospitalized for a mood disorder. The dependent variables were the DES, the DES-Taxon and the Questionnaire of Experiences of Dissociation (QED; Riley, 1988). Seventy-eight of the participants reported some type of abusive experience, 38% reported extreme and frequent abuse, and 40% reported being sexually abused during childhood. The findings showed a correlation between greater frequency of the abusive experiences and higher levels of dissociative symptoms. The mean DES scores for the three levels of abuse experiences were: No Abuse 26.83; Slight Abuse 29.44; Severe Abuse 37.84. With the QED a similar finding occurred: No Abuse 11.35; Slight Abuse 14.24; Severe Abuse 15.06. When we compared the mean score of the DES for those participants that specifically reported some type of abusive sexual experience in childhood we obtained a significant difference in the DES ($p < .001$) between those that reported (M = 38.06) and those that do not reported (M = 28.37) such abuse. Of interest is that we obtained a significant correlation between the DES and the QED of r = .69 (*p* < .01).

Our research with the DES became well known in Puerto Rico as we reported the results in major conferences in Puerto Rico and because various graduate students at the University of Puerto Rico and the Carlos Albizu University decided to use and incorporate the DES on their doctoral dissertations. Table 2 presents the results of the DES with a wide variety of clinical populations in Puerto Rico.

Reyes-Pérez, Martínez-Taboas and Ledesma-Amador (2005) conducted a rigorous study with the Child Dissociative Checklist (CDC). For this study we selected three groups of children: a control group of 33 children; an Attention Deficit-Hyperactive Disorder (ADHD) group of 30 children; and a group of 31 children with documented abuse histories (mainly sexual abuse). The results showed that the mean CDC was as follow: control group: 2.88; ADHD group 7.43; abuse group 12.03. The group with documented abuse obtained a significant difference from children in the other two groups (p < .05). Fifty-five percent of the children in the abuse group obtained a score at or above the suggested cut-off score of 12 for pathological dissociation, but no child obtained such a score in the control group and only 17% in the ADHD group. Furthermore, 23% of the abused group obtained a score above 18, which have been found exclusively in cases of children with dissociative disorders (Putnam, 1997). No child in the other two groups obtained such scores. Our results with the CDC are very similar to research conducted by Zoroglu, Tuzun, Ozturk and Sar (2002) in Turkey.

An important area of research in Puerto Rico has recently been conducted on a short form of the Adolescent Dissociative Experiences Scale (ADES). In the first of two studies (Martínez-Taboas et al., 2004) eight items were selected to assess pathological forms of dissociative symptoms, similar to the eight items that comprise the DES-Taxon (Waller, Putnam & Carlson, 1996). The scale was administered to a representative sample of 459 medically indigent adolescents, ages 11 to 17, who received mental health services in Puerto Rico. Results indicated that the ADES-8 demonstrated satisfactory internal consistency (Cronbach's alpha .77) and test-retest reliability (.78). As expected, most adolescents evidenced very low scores, with nearly half (46%) scoring zero on the eight items. The scale showed expected patterns of convergent validity with variables that are hypothesized to be intimately related to dissociative disorders, such as psychiatric impairment, comorbidity, and abusive experiences. Logistic regression analyses

TABLE 2. The Use of the Dissociative Experience Scale in Puerto Rico with Specific Populations.

Participants	N	Mean
Non-clinical groups		
Martínez-Taboas (1995b)	46	17
Martínez-Taboas & Bernal (2000)	198	14
Menéndez-Brunet et al. (2003)	30	9
Sexually Abused Persons		
Menéndez-Brunet et al. (2002)	33	21
Ledesma-Amador (1996)	27	37
Colberg-Toro (2000)	6	20
Dissociative Identity Disoder		
Martínez-Taboas (1991)	16	60
Psychiatric Inpatients		
Francia-Martínez et al. (2003)	100	33
Psychiatric Outpatients		
Menéndez-Brunet et al. (2002)	30	18

suggested that a cutoff score of 3 on the ADES-8 was the best screening rule for identifying persons with higher values on the convergent validity variables. The findings of this epidemiological investigation provide support for the clinical and research use of the ADES-8 as a screening instrument for dissociative disorders in referred youths.

In a second study (Martínez-Taboas et al., 2004), the ADES-8 was administered to a representative island-wide household probability sample of youths aged 11 to 17 years of the Puerto Rican population. We investigated the relationship between scores on the ADES-8 and different types of victimization experiences. This time, a majority of the youths (53%) scored zero on the eight items. Only 44 youths (4.93%) scored above the suggested cutoff of 3. The results highlighted that 43 (98%) of the 44 youths with a score of 3 or more on the ADES-8 reported some type of victimization, versus 54% of those with a lower score ($p < .000$). In a bivariate logistic regression analysis of mean ADES-8 scores with external validators, all five abuse variables (emotional abuse, physical abuse, neglect, sexual abuse, exposure to violence) were significantly associated with the dissociation factor. Also, we documented that as the frequency of abuse became more frequent and severe, there was a greater likelihood that the respondents reported dissociative symptoms. The multivariate logistic regression analysis indicated that two variables, physical abuse and exposure to violence remained significant. Once again, it was observed that, in both variables, as the frequency/severity level of abuse increased, the greater the chances of experiencing dissociative symptoms. Results from this investigation are consistent with other international epidemiological research in highlighting the fact that pathological forms of dissociation are found in about 1-4% of representative community populations and that dissociation scores are significantly related to a wide-variety of victimization experiences (Akyuz, Dogan, Sar, Yargic & Tutkun, 1999; Vanderlinden, Van Dyck, Vandereycken & Vertommen, 1993; Mulder, Beautrais, Joyce & Fregusson, 1998, Maaranen, et al., 2004).

MISCELLANEOUS RESEARCH TOPICS

Méndez, Martínez-Taboas and Pedrosa (2000) conducted a mail survey study among Puerto Rican licensed psychologists to ascertain their attitudes, beliefs and experiences with DID. The following results were found:

1. Almost all (95.5%) of the participants reported that DID as a clinical entity definitely or probably existed. In contrast, 4.5% indicated that they did not accept the diagnosis.
2. A majority of psychologists (66%) admitted that their knowledge base on dissociation was poor.
3. Seventy-three percent indicated that they did not receive any training on DD in their graduate training. Only 3.8% informed that they learned much about DD in their graduate studies.
4. Utilizing clinical vignettes, it was discovered that those clinicians who indicated no clinical training in DD during graduate school, showed more doubts or reservations about the DID diagnosis ($p < .02$).

Ochoa, Martínez-Taboas and Pedrosa (2002) studied the repressed or delayed memories of sexual abuse of 35 women with documented sexual abuse. In this study, 45.7% of the participants indicated partial memory difficulties in recovering the memories of abuse. There was also statistical evidence that multiple episodes of abuse, sexual abuse during childhood and sexual abuse perpetrated by family members were related to the phenomena of partial memory difficulties ($p < .05$). Thirty-eight percent of the participants reported that they had obtained definitive evidence that the abuse had occurred. Finally, the participants with repressed memories indicated that their memories were typically recovered after another traumatic or stressful event, which were typically accompanied by severe somatic and emotional symptoms.

Martínez-Taboas (2002) investigated the clinical utility of using a hypnotic protocol with patients with psychogenic seizures (PS or pseudo-epileptic seizures). Eight patients with a clinical profile suggesting the presence of PS were given a hypnotic suggestion in which they were to go back in time to the exact moment of their last seizure. They were asked to concentrate their attention on any unusual feelings or bodily sensation. All eight patients presented a PS during the age regression protocol. In six cases, independent testimony from family members corroborated the morphological similarity of the induced attack and the one presented in their natural environment. Also, the seizures ended abruptly after a command was given to stop them. It was argued that a simple hypnotic procedure can be useful as a diagnostic tool in the differentiation of epileptic from PS attacks.

Menéndez-Brunet and Martínez-Taboas (2003) conducted a study to explore the clinical utility of the Spanish version of the Trauma Symptom Inventory (Briere, 1995) and the DES with 25 women survivors of sexual abuse. Two comparison groups were used: a group of 30 women who were receiving psychotherapy but with no history of sexual abuse and a control group of 30 women with no history of sexual abuse or psychopathology. The results indicated that the TSI discriminated the group of women with sexual abuse from the control group in all clinical variables. The TSI also discriminated the abuse group from the psychotherapy group on some clinical variables. The DES score was significantly higher in the sexual abused group as compared with the control group ($p < .006$). A statistical significant correlation ($r = .65; p < .01$) was also found between the DES and the Dissociation Scale of the TSI.

FINAL REFLECTIONS

In this piece I have presented the research and publications on dissociation conducted in Puerto Rico. Based on the research presented, the following conclusions are respectfully offered:

1. The DES is a useful clinical screening instrument to detect persons with dissociative and traumatic profiles with a Hispanic population.

2. The Spanish DES scores are very similar to those published in other countries.
3. The Spanish DES is significantly correlated with other dissociative instruments. In the case of the Dissociation Scale of the Trauma Symptom Inventory, a correlation of .65 was found with the DES. In the case of the Spanish DES and the Questionnaire of Experiences of Dissociation a correlation of .69 was obtained. Both were significant at $p < .01$.
4. A preliminary study indicates that the CDC is also useful as a screening instrument to detect dissociation in Hispanic children.
5. Dissociative Identity Disorder patients in Puerto Rico present a nearly identical psychological profile with patients in other countries. The main difference being the mean number of alter identities ($M = 3$).
6. Epidemiological studies conducted in Puerto Rico utilizing the ADES-8 studied a large island-wide probabilistic household sample, permitting generalizations to Hispanic youths age 11 to 17. Also, participants were assessed with culturally sensitive clinical instruments that were translated and adapted for Hispanic children, permitting the valid assessment of the psychological functioning of the participants (Canino et al., 2004).
7. The results with the ADES-8 clearly point to the fact that nearly 100% of adolescents with high scores on the ADES-8 report a history of victimization and trauma. Moreover, as the severity and frequency of abuse increased, the ADES-8 total scores increased.
8. Contrary to the experience of many other psychologists that intensively work with dissociation, in the past 14 years I have very few unpleasant experiences with skeptical colleagues. I can only recall one very unpleasant experience in my years of presenting at conferences, workshops and teaching at universities in Puerto Rico. When I was teaching at the University of Puerto Rico, another professor asserted that my first book was an invention and a fraud. I confronted the professor and offered to have a public debate on dissociation and that if he continued to use innuendo and defamation I would sue him. The professor ceased from commenting on my book.
9. One of the most important and rewarding personal experiences is that there are now a considerable number of colleagues (psychologists and psychiatrists) who recognize and incorporate the concept and diagnosis of dissociation in their clinical or research work.

The dissociation work and research in Puerto Rico could be a model for colleagues who work in other Latin American countries. With very few economic resources, a growing number of colleagues and I have established a foundation for knowledge of dissociation in Puerto Rico. The success of the Puerto Rican work is based on five points:

1. Publish your results in a systematic and productive manner. Submit your research data and/or clinical experience to the prominent psychiatric and psychological journals in your country and when possible to international journals.
2. In my experience, the publication of books has been pivotal in generating interest in Puerto Rican colleagues to dissociation. So, if possible, try to publish a book length monograph about your research and/or clinical experience.
3. Present your findings at prominent national conferences and more importantly one-day or two-day seminars.
4. Teach undergraduate or graduate courses on psychology at your local university. You then have the opportunity to insert training on trauma and dissociation to students that may be more open to new possibilities and concepts.
5. Conduct systematic research with DD. This may be encouraged by enlisting graduate students to conduct their research dissertation on dissociation and establish contact with respected and experienced researchers in your area and propose ideas about how to conduct research with dissociative scales or instruments. My own experience working with the staff at the Behavioral Sciences Research Institute, Medical Sciences Campus, University of Puerto Rico was very productive.

The study of dissociation in Puerto Rico has just begun. An area for future research is the impact of psychotherapy or pharmacotherapy with DD patients. My hope is that the next decade will allow the opportunity to expand and refine what we have accomplished to date.

REFERENCES

Akyuz, G., Dogan, O., Sar, V., Yargic, L. I., & Tutkun, H. (1999). Frequency of dissociative identity disorder in the general population of Turkey. *Comprehensive Psychiatry, 40*, 151-159.

Boon, S., & Draijer, N. (1993). Multiple personality disorder in the Netherlands: A clinical investigation of 71 patients. *American Journal of Psychiatry, 150*, 489-494.

Briere, J. (1995). *Trauma Symptom Inventory (TSI): Professional Manual*. Odessa, FL: Psychological Assessment Resources.

Canino, G., Shrout, P., Rubio-Stipec, M., Bird, H. R., Bravo, M., Ramírez, R., Chavez, L., Alegría, M., Bauermeister, J. J., Hohmann, A., Ribera, J., García, P., & Martínez-Taboas, A. (2004). DSM-IV rates of child and adolescent disorders in Puerto Rico: Prevalence, correlates, service use and the effects of impairment. *Archives of General Psychiatry, 61*, 85-93.

Colberg-Toro, E. (2000). Efectos de una terapia de grupo para sobrevivientes de abuso sexual considerando variables del contexto sociocultural. [Effects of group therapy in sexual abuse survivors, incorporating the socio-cultural context]. Unpublished doctoral dissertation, Centro Caribeño de Estudios Postgraduados, San Juan, Puerto Rico.

Ensink, B. J., & Otterloo, D. (1989). A validation of the Dissociative Experiences Scale in the Netherlands. *Dissociation, 2*, 221-223.

Farrington, K. (1991). La relación entre el estrés y la violencia doméstica: Conceptualizaciones y hallazgos actuales. [The relationship between stress and domestic violence: Current concepts and research]. *Revista Intercontinental de Psicología y Educación, 4*, 87-103.

Francia-Martínez, M., Roca de Torres, I., Alvarado, C. S., Martínez-Taboas, A., & Sayers, S. (2003). Dissociation, depression and trauma in psychiatric inpatients in Puerto Rico. *Journal of Trauma and Dissociation, 4*, 47-61.

Kluft, R. P. (1991). La violencia familiar y el desorden de personalidad múltiple. [Family violence and multiple personality disorder]. *Revista Intercontinental de Psicología y Educación, 4*, 29-55.

Ledesma-Amador, D. (1996). *Niveles de disociación en mujeres víctimas de violencia doméstica y en mujeres sobrevivientes de abuso sexual.* [Levels of dissociation in female victims of domestic violence and survivors of sexual abuse]. Unpublished doctoral dissertation, Centro Caribeño de Estudios Postgraduados, San Juan, Puerto Rico.

Maaranen, P., Tanskanen, A., Haatainen, K., Koivumaa-Honkanen, H., Hintikka, K., & Viinamaki, H. (2004). Somatoform dissociation and adverse childhood experiences in the general population. *Journal of Nervous and Mental Disease, 192*, 337-342.

Martínez-Taboas, A. (1986). Personalidad múltiple. [Multiple personality]. *Avances en Psicología Clínica Latinoamericana, 4*, 19-41.

Martínez-Taboas, A. (1989). Preliminarly observations on multiple personality disorder in Puerto Rico. *Dissociation, 2*, 128-131.

Martínez-Taboas, A. (1990). *Personalidad múltiple: Una exploración psicológica.* [Multiple personality: A psychological exploration]. San Juan, P.R.: Publicaciones Puertorriqueñas.

Martínez-Taboas, A. (1991a). Multiple personality in Puerto Rico: Analysis of fifteen cases. *Dissociation, 4*, 189-192.

Martínez-Taboas, A. (1991b). Introducción a la temática de violencia familiar. [Introduction to the issue of family violence]. *Revista Intercontinental de Psicología y Educación, 4*, 7-12.

Martínez-Taboas, A. (1995a). *Multiple personality: An Hispanic perspective.* San Juan, P.R.: Puente Publications.

Martínez-Taboas, A. (1995b). The use of the Dissociative Experiences Scale in Puerto Rico. *Dissociation, 8*, 13-17.

Martínez-Taboas, A. (1996). Repressed memories: Some clinical data contributing toward its elucidation. *American Journal of Psychotherapy, 50*, 217-230.

Martínez-Taboas, A. (2002). The role of hypnosis in the diagnosis and treatment of psychogenic seizures. *American Journal of Clinical Hypnosis, 45*, 11-20.

Martínez-Taboas, A., & Bernal, G. (2000). Dissociation, psychopathology and abusive experiences in a non-clinical university student group. *Cultural Diversity and Mental Health, 6*, 32-41.

Martínez-Taboas, A., Camino, R., Cruz-Igartúa, A., Francia, M., Gelpi, E., & Rodríguez-Cay, J. (1995). What a group of clinicians have learned about multiple personality disorder in Puerto Rico. *Revista Puertorriqueña de Psicología, 10*, 197-213.

Martínez-Taboas, A., Shrout, P. E., Canino, G., Chavez, L., Ramirez, R., Bravo, M., Bauermeister, J. J., & Ribera, J. C. (2004). The psychometric properties of a shortened version of the Spanish Adolescent Dissociative Experiences Scale. *Journal of Trauma & Dissociation, 5*, 33-54.

Martínez-Taboas, A., & Cruz-Igartúa, A. (1993). Algunas consideraciones sobre el manejo hospitalario de pacientes con el trastorno de personalidad múltiple. [Some observations concerning the inpatient management of patients with multiple personality]. *Revista de la Asociación Médica de Puerto Rico, 85*, 142-146.

Martínez-Taboas, A., Shrout, P. E., Canino, G., Chavez, L. M., Ramírez, R., Bravo, M., Bauermeister, J. J., & Ribera, J. C. (2004). The psychometric properties of a shortened version of the Spanish Adolescent Dissociative Experiences Scale. *Journal of Trauma & Dissociation, 5*, 33-54.

Méndez, N., Martínez-Taboas, A., & Pedrosa, O. (2000). Experiencias, creencias y actitudes de los psicólogos en Puerto Rico con el trastorno de identidad disociativa. [Experiences, beliefs and attitudes of Puerto Rican psychologists with dissociative identity disorder]. *Ciencias de la Conducta, 15*, 69-84.

Menéndez-Brunet, E., & Martínez-Taboas, A. (2003). La utilización del Inventario de Síntomas de Trauma y la Escala de Experiencias Disociativas en una muestra de adultas sobrevivientes de abuso sexual. [The utilization of the Traumatic Symptom Inventory and the Dissociative Experiences Scale with survivors of sexual abuse]. *Revista Puertorriqueña de Psicología, 14*, 85-106.

Mulder, R. T., Beautrais, A. L., Joyce, P. R., & Fergusson, D. M. (1998). Relationship between dissociation, childhood sexual abuse, childhood physical abuse, and mental illness in a general population sample. *American Journal of Psychiatry, 155*, 806-811.

Ochoa, T., Martínez-Taboas, A., & Pedrosa, O. (2002). Memorias de experiencias traumáticas en una muestra de mujeres puertorriqueñas abusadas sexualmente. [Memories of traumatic experiences in Puerto Rican female patients with a history of sexual abuse]. *Ciencias de la Conducta, 17*, 1-11.

Putnam, F. W., Guroff, J. J., Silberman, E. K., Barbau, L., & Posr, R. M. (1986). The clinical phenomenology of multiple personality disorder: Review of 100 recent cases. *Journal of Clinical Psychiatry, 47*, 285-293.

Putnam, F. W. (1997). *Dissociation in children and adolescents.* New York: Guilford.

Reyes-Pérez, C., Martínez-Taboas, A., & Ledesma-Amador, D. (2005). Dissociative experiences in children with abuse histories: A replication in Puerto Rico. *Journal of Trauma & Dissociation, 6,* 99-112.

Riley, K. C. (1988). Measurement of dissociation. *Journal of Nervous and Mental Disease, 176,* 449-450.

Ross, C. A., Norton, G. R., & Wozney, K. (1989). Multiple personality disorder: An analysis of 236 cases. *Canadian Journal of Psychiatry, 34,* 413-418.

Ross, C. A., Ryan, L., Anderson, G., Ross, D., & Hardy, L. (1989). Dissociative experiences in adolescents and college students. *Dissociation, 2,* 240-242.

Vanderlinden, J., Van Dyck, R., Vandereycken, W., & Vertommen, H. (1993). Trauma and psychological dysfunctioning in the general population of the Netherlands. *Hospital and Community Psychiatry, 44,* 786-788.

Waller, N. G., Putnam, F. W., & Carlson, E. B. (1996). Types of dissociation and dissociative types: A taxometric analysis of dissociative experiences. *Psychological Methods, 1,* 300-321.

Zoroglu, S. S., Tuzun, U., Ozturk, M., & Sar, V. (2002). Reliability and validity of the Turkish version of the Child Dissociative Checklist. *Journal of Trauma and Dissociation, 3,* 37-49.

The "Apparently Normal" Family:
A Contemporary Agent
of Transgenerational Trauma
and Dissociation

Erdinc Ozturk
Vedat Sar

SUMMARY. Fifty first-degree relatives of 24 Turkish dissociative patients and 50 Turkish non-clinical controls were screened for childhood traumas, dissociative experiences/disorders, and borderline personality disorder/criteria. The Dissociative Experiences Scale, the borderline personality disorder section of the Structured Clinical Interview for DSM-IV Personality Disorders, the Childhood Trauma Questionnaire, and a structured history form were admistered to all participants. Family members

Erdinc Ozturk, PhD, is Psychologist, and Vedat Sar, MD, is Professor of Psychiatry and Director, Clinical Psychotherapy Unit and Dissociative Disorders Program, Department of Psychiatry, Istanbul University Istanbul Medical Faculty Hospital, Istanbul, Turkey.

Address correspondence to: Erdinc Ozturk, PhD, Istanbul Tip Fakultesi Psikiyatri Klinigi 34390, Capa Istanbul, Turkey (E-mail: erdincozturk@klinikpsikoterapi.com).

An earlier version of this paper, *Frequency of childhood trauma and dissociative disorders among first-degree relatives of dissociative patients*, was presented December 3, 2001 at the 18th Annual Conference of the International Society for the Study of Dissociation, New Orleans, LA.

[Haworth co-indexing entry note]: "The 'Apparently Normal' Family: A Contemporary Agent of Transgenerational Trauma and Dissociation." Ozturk, Erdinc, and Vedat Sar. Co-published simultaneously in *Journal of Trauma Practice* (The Haworth Maltreatment & Trauma Press, an imprint of The Haworth Press, Inc.) Vol. 4, No. 3/4, 2005, pp. 287-303; and: *Trauma and Dissociation in a Cross-Cultural Perspective: Not Just a North American Phenomenon* (ed: George F. Rhoades, Jr., and Vedat Sar) The Haworth Maltreatment & Trauma Press, an imprint of The Haworth Press, Inc., 2005, pp. 287-303. Single or multiple copies of this article are available for a fee from The Haworth Document Delivery Service [1-800-HAWORTH, 9:00 a.m. - 5:00 p.m. (EST). E-mail address: docdelivery@haworthpress.com].

had dissociative experiences, borderline personality disorder criteria (subtreshold scores included), and childhood traumas more frequently than the normal control group. Family members with a Dissociative Experiences Scale score 25 and above (N = 3) were evaluated using the Structured Clinical Interview for DSM-IV Dissociative Disorders. None of the family members were diagnosed as having a dissociative disorder and/or borderline personality disorder on a clinical level. Our findings suggest that these apparently normal families of dissociative patients need to be evaluated for trauma-related family dynamics overall and for hidden subclinical psychopathology. *[Article copies available for a fee from The Haworth Document Delivery Service: 1-800-HAWORTH. E-mail address: <docdelivery@haworthpress.com> Website: <http://www.HaworthPress.com>*

KEYWORDS. Family, dissociation, trauma, borderline personality disorder, transgenerational

Neurosis is intimately bound up with the problem of our time and really represents an unsuccessful attempt on the part of the individual to solve the general problem in his own person. Neurosis is self-division.

Carl Gustav Jung
"On the Psychology of the Unconscious" (1912)

Psychiatric disorders run in families; both bio-genetical and psychological factors being responsible for this well-known phenomenon. The demonstration of familial transmission contributes to the validity of a diagnostic category in psychiatry. Unfortunately, large scale data concerning family history of dissociative disorders are rather scarce. In a preliminary study, Braun (1985) observed that there is evidence of significant dissociation and/or multiple personality disorder in the families of at least 12 of his 18 multiple personality disorder patients. Kluft (1984) found multiple personality disorder in one or both parents of 40% of his childhood multiple personality disorder cases.

High rates of childhood abuse and/or neglect have been reported as central to dissociative disorders (Chu & Dill, & 1990; Chu, Frey, Ganzel, & Matthews, 1999; Ogawa, Sroufe, Weinfield, Carlson, & Egeland, 1997). Research on childhood traumas among psychiatric patients has typically considered certain types of childhood abuse (sexual, emotional, or physical) and neglect (physical or emotional). Most empirical studies were restricted to these well defined types of childhood traumas. This focused approach has been clearly helpful in demonstration of the importance of childhood trauma in clinical psychiatry. However, studies on family dynamics as the context where childhood traumas happen (Gold, 2000) and on possible relationship traumas in dysfunctional families have lagged behind the research on childhood abuse and neglect.

This study concerns the prevalence of dissociative experiences, dissociative disorders, and childhood traumas among first-degree relatives of dissociative patients. We consider this approach as a first step in exploration of family characteristics of dissociative patients. In consideration of the wide phenomenological overlap and the common history of frequent childhood traumas between dissociative disorders and borderline personality disorder (Sar et al., 2003), we also screened Borderline Personality Disorder criteria among family members. They were then compared with a non-clinical control group matched for age and gender.

METHOD

Participants

First-degree relatives of all the dissociative patients being treated at the Dissociative Disorders Program of the Istanbul University Medical Faculty Hospital during the two-month study period, were considered for participation in the study (May 2001). There were 29 dissociative patients at the outpatient treatment program at that time of the study. Five patients were excluded from the study, as they did not have any contact with their family members. The remaining 24 dissociative patients were considered for the study. Eighteen of the patients had the diagnosis of Dissociative Identity Disorder (DID) and six were diagnosed as Dissociative Disorder, Not Otherwise Specified (DDNOS). Nineteen of the patients (79.2%) were female, the mean age of the patients was 24.2 (SD = 6.0) and mean education was 10.7 years (SD = 2.5).

The original study group was comprised of 109 first-degree relatives of 24 dissociative patients. Three fathers were deceased and 10 siblings were excluded as they were under 18 years of age. The target group finally consisted of 96 family members.

Forty-six members of the target group could not be contacted due to following reasons: direct refusal by the patient (N = 6), direct refusal by the family member (N = 6), poor physical condition (N = 4), inability to get permission to leave the workplace (N = 8), no contact between patient and relative (N = 2), living a far distance (N = 16), unknown reasons (N = 4). Statistically, there was no significant difference between excluded family members and the study group on the variables of age, gender, income, and education level.

In conclusion, 50 (52.1%) family members participated in the final study, including 20 mothers, 10 fathers, and 20 siblings. Twenty-seven of the subjects (54.0 %) were female, mean age was 41.1 (SD = 13.8) and the mean education level was 8.3 years (SD = 3.9).

Assessment Instruments

1. The Dissociative Experiences Scale (DES-II) is a self-report instrument that evaluates the severity of dissociative psychopathology (Bernstein & Putnam, 1986; Carlson & Putnam, 1993). The Turkish version has a test-retest reliability of 0.77 (Sar et al., 1997). It distinguishes patients with dissociative identity disorder from those with other psychiatric disorders with a sensitivity of 0.85 and specificity of 0.77 (Sar et al., 1997; Yargic, Tutkun, & Sar, 1995).

2. The Structured Clinical Interview for DSM-IV Dissociative Disorders (SCID-D) is a semi-structured interview developed by Steinberg (1994). It is used to make DSM-IV diagnoses of all dissociative disorders. The Turkish version of the SCID-D (Sar, Tutkun, Yargic, Kundakci, & Kiziltan,1996) was validated on 40 patients with a dissociative disorder and 40 controls yielding an 100% agreement in the presence and absence of a dissociative disorder (Kundakci, Sar, Kiziltan, Yargic, & Tutkun, 1998). Inter-rater reliability of the Turkish SCID-D was evaluated by 4 psychiatrists using 10 videotaped interviews with patients with either dissociative disorder or other psychiatric disorders. The sole discrepancy between raters was observed on the type of the dissociative disorder in one patient who was assessed as having either DID or DDNOS.

3. The Structured Clinical Interview for DSM-III-IV Personality Disorders (SCID-II) is a semi-structured interview (Spitzer, Williams, & Gibbon, 1987). It serves as a diagnostic instrument for personality disorders on axis II of the DSM-IV. The section for

Borderline Personality Disorder was administered in this study. The Turkish version (Coskunol, Bagdiken, Sorias, & Saygili, 1994) of this section has a reliability of 0.95 (kappa).

4. The Childhood Trauma Questionnaire (CTQ) is a 53-item self-report instrument developed by Bernstein and colleagues (Bernstein et al., 1994) which evaluates childhood emotional, physical, sexual abuse and childhood physical and emotional neglect. Possible scores for each type of childhood trauma range from 1 to 5. The sum of the scores derived from each trauma type provides the total score ranging from 5 to 25. The Cronbach's alpha for the factors related to each trauma type ranges from 0.79 to 0.94, indicating high internal consistency (Bernstein et al., 1994). The scale also demonstrated good test-retest reliability over a 2- to 6-month interval (intraclass correlation = 0.88). A separate history-form gathering information about the details of the traumatic experiences, self-mutilative behavior and suicide attempts was also administered to all patients. The definitions by Walker et al. (Walker, Bonner, & Kaufmann, 1988) and by Brown and Anderson (1991) for childhood abuse and neglect were used in this history-form.

Procedure

The 50 family members were evaluated using the DES, SCID-II, CTQ, and the structured history form. Three family members who had a DES score 25 or above were evaluated using the SCID-D.

RESULTS

All the dissociative patients studied reported at least one type of childhood abuse and/or neglect. Eighty-seven percent of the patients reported at least one type of childhood abuse and/or neglect that originated within their family of origin. Sixty-four percent of the family members in this study reported at least one type of childhood abuse and/or neglect, whereas this rate was 36.0% (a significant difference) for the control group. All but one type of childhood traumas (sexual abuse; Table 1) were found more frequently in the family member group than control group. None of the family members reported incest in his/her childhood, whereas 52.2% of the dissociative patients reported incest.

TABLE 1. Frequency of childhood trauma and self-destructive behavior among family members of dissociative patients

Childhood trauma, suicide, and self-mutilation	Dissociative patients N = 24 (*) %	Family members N = 50 %	Normal controls for family members N = 50 %	Family members vs controls X^2 (df = 48) p
Emotional neglect	16 - 69.6	21 - 42.0	4 - 8.0	15.41 - 0.001
Emotional abuse	16 - 69.6	14 - 28.0	2 - 4.0	10.71 - 0.001
Physical abuse	16 - 69.6	19 - 38.0	6 - 12.0	9.01 - 0.003
Any type of abuse or neglect	23 - 100.0	32 - 64.0	18 - 36.0	7.84 - 0.005
Physical neglect	8 - 34.8	19 - 38.0	9 - 18.0	4.96 - 0.026
Sexual abuse (incl. incest)	20 - 87.0	4 - 8.0	2 - 4.0	Fisher's exact test n.s.
Incest	12 - 52.2	0 - 0.0	1 - 2.0	Fisher's exact test n.s.
Suicide attempt	21 - 91.3	7 - 14.0	2 - 4.0	Fisher's exact test n.s.
Self-mutilation	20 - 87.0	6 - 12.0	1 - 2.0	Fisher's exact test n.s.

(*) One patient refused to report

Table 2 demonstrates a significant difference on childhood trauma scores between family members and controls as measured by the CTQ. In addition, family members were found to have had significantly more dissociative experiences than the normal control group. On the CTQ, only physical neglect was found to be significantly correlated with the DES total score (r = 0.50, n = 50, p < 0.001). Family members also demonstrated DSM-IV Borderline Personality Disorder criteria (subtreshold scores are included) more frequently than controls.

Despite these significant differences between study group and controls, none of the first degree relatives of dissociative patients had sufficient symptoms to meet the DSM-IV criteria of a dissociative disorder and/or Borderline Personality Disorder.

Three family members had a DES score above 25.0. which has been considered a useful cut-off level for dissociative disorders in previous studies. The first person was the highly functioning sister of a female DID patient. Although she had dissociative experiences (DES = 25.7, SCID-D = 9, CTQ = 9.9), they were not sufficient to get a dissociative disorder diagnosis. The second subject was a brother of a female DID patient. He was the perpetrator of sexual abuse on the DID patient, in a family seen as highly incestuous. He had high absorption tendency

TABLE 2. Severity of childhood trauma (CTQ scores) and dissociative experiences (DES) among family members of dissociative patients and controls

CTQ Scores	Relatives (N = 50) mean	SD	Controls (N = 50) mean	SD	t (df = 98)	p
Emotional abuse	1.8	- 0.7	1.1	- 0.2	6.02	- 0.001
Physical abuse	1.6	- 0.8	1.1	- 0.2	4.17	- 0.001
Physical neglect	1.4	- 0.4	1.1	- 0.1	3.99	- 0.001
Total CTQ score	8.7	- 2.3	6.9	- 1.0	5.21	- 0.001
Emotional neglect	2.9	- 0.8	2.5	- 0.8	2.93	- 0.004
Sexual abuse	1.1	- 0.3	1.1	- 0.2	0.35	- n.s.
Minimization/denial of childhood trauma	0.1	- 0.3	0.2	- 0.5	0.98	- n.s.
DES score	8.3	- 7.1	4.8	- 2.6	3.31	- 0.001
Borderline criteria endorsed (including subtreshold scores)	0.6	- 1.0	0.2	- 0.7	2.75	- 0.007

(DES = 31.1, SCID-D = 6, CTQ = 9.3). The third family member was the mother of a male DDNOS patient. This subject had derealization without depersonalization, mild amnesia, identity confusion, and alteration due to chronic major depression reportedly due to long-term marital problems (DES = 26.8, SCID-D = 10, CTQ = 6.7).

The family members group overall reported frequent mood fluctuations, intense anger and inability to control anger, transient dissociative experiences or paranoid ideas, and identity confusion more frequently than controls (Table 3). Some of these features were correlated with certain types of childhood trauma, e.g., frequent mood fluctuations with all types of childhood trauma except sexual abuse, and identity confusion with emotional abuse. In contrast, anger and transient dissociative/paranoid symptoms among family member were not correlated with any type of childhood trauma (Table 4).

DISCUSSION

One limitation of this study was the high rate (47.9%) of family members who could not be contacted. Although none of the contacted family members were diagnosed as having a dissociative disorder and/or borderline personality disorder, there may have been subjects

TABLE 3. DSM-IV borderline personality disorder criteria among family members of dissociative patients and controls (subtreshold scores included)

Borderline criteria	Family members (N = 50)		Controls (N = 50)			
	Ort.	SS	Ort.	SS	t(sd = 98)	p
Frequent mood swings	1.88	0.66	1.30	0.54	4.80	0.001
Intense anger or lack of control of anger	1.52	0.65	1.06	0.31	4.53	0.001
Transient dissociative or paranoid symptoms	1.40	0.61	1.04	0.20	3.99	0.001
Identity confusion	1.22	0.51	1.02	0.14	2.69	0.008
Impulsive or unpredicted behavior	1.22	0.58	1.08	0.27	1.76	n.s.
Intense but unstable relationships	1.28	0.50	1.14	0.40	1.55	n.s.
Physically self-damaging acts	1.16	0.42	1.06	0.24	1.46	n.s.
Efforts to avoid abandonment	1.18	0.39	1.08	0.34	1.37	n.s.
Chronic feelings of emptiness and boredom	1.76	0.74	1.60	0.61	1.18	n.s.
Total number of borderline personality disorder criteria	0.62	0.99	0.16	0.65	2.75	0.007

among excluded family members who would have been diagnosed as such. On the other hand, some family members who participated in the study may have dissimulated their dissociative experiences.

In spite of these limitations, these 'apparently normal' families significantly differed from controls on several variables. The family members reported signficantly more dissociative experiences, subthreshold borderline criteria, and childhood traumata than the control subjects. Thus, we conclude that the dissociative patients had a distinct fate concerning development of a clinical psychiatric disorder despite some commonalities that they share with their first-degree relatives. In consideration of this reality, we believe that the family as a whole was a pathological agent and the index patient fulfilled a social role in this system. In addition this asymmetry in dissociative psychopathology among family members may be seen as a system which itself is dissociated.

Dissociative Family Chaos and Apparently Normal Family

Family members reported frequent mood swings, intense anger and inability to control anger, transient dissociative experiences or paranoid

TABLE 4. Correlations (Pearson's r) between childhood trauma (CTQ scores) and DSM-IV borderline personality disorder criteria (subthreshold scores included) among family members (N = 50)

DSM-IV BPD criteria	CTQ Total	CTQ Sexual abuse	CTQ Physical abuse	CTQ Emotional abuse	CTQ Emotional neglect	CTQ Physical neglect	CTQ Minimization/ Denial of Childhood Trauma
Frequent mood swings	0.39 **	−0.16	0.32 *	0.31*	0.32 *	0.48**	0.17
Intense anger or lack of control of anger	0.13	0.04	0.10	0.25	−0.01	0.13	0.11
Transient dissociative or paranoid symptoms	0.05	−0.11	0.05	0.02	0.03	0.18	0.05
Identity confusion	0.23	−0.01	0.21	0.29*	0.05	0.28	−0.13
Impulsive or unpredictive behavior	0.04	−0.07	0.09	−0.12	0.02	0.26	−0.11
Intense but unstable relationships	0.20	−0.12	0.06	0.12	0.34 *	0.24	−0.02
Physically self-damaging acts	0.20	0.00	0.16	0.16	0.05	0.42**	−0.11
Efforts to avoid abandonment	0.19	−0.07	0.02	0.17	0.31*	0.13	−0.14
Chronic feelings of emptiness and boredom	0.25	−0.18	0.19	0.10	0.24	0.52**	−0.01
Total number of BD crieteria	0.29*	−0.10	0.20	0.21	0.20	0.56**	−0.04

(*) p < 0.05 (**) p < 0.001

ideas, and identity confusion more frequently than controls (Table 2). Some of these features were correlated with certain types of childhood trauma in this group, e.g., frequent mood swings with all types of childhood trauma except sexual abuse, and identity confusion was correlated with emotional abuse. Although at a subclinical level, these characteristics of family members suggest the presence of a hidden family pathology.

In order to describe the distinct behavioral states of a dissociative subject, Nijenhuis and Van der Hart (1999) have revived the terminology of Charles Samuel Myers (1940). Myers, a combat physician, described the behavior change which he repeatedly observed among traumatized soldiers as a shift from an 'apparently normal personality' to an 'emotional personality' and vice versa. Steele, Van der Hart, and Nijenhuis (2005) elaborated this simple model to a comprehensive theory for dissociative disorders: "Structural Dissociation of Personality." One of the advantages of this model and terminology is its coverage of subclinical (everyday) dissociation. Our findings suggest that families of many dissociative subjects may be seen as 'apparently normal' at least for a limited period of time. However, this observation does not eliminate the possibility of a pathogenic influence of these families. In fact, we hypothesize that the 'apparently normal family' is itself a contemporary agent of transgenerational childhood trauma and dissociation. We have demonstrated in two clinical studies that a subgroup of patients with trauma-related disorders had clearly ambivalent attitudes about the environments of their first-degree family members whereas they tended to minimize their trauma histories (Sar, Akyuz, Kundakci, Kiziltan, & Dogan, 2004; Sar, Akyuz, & Ozturk, 2004;).

In a family with subclinical dissociation, individuals can interchange their social roles over time, the available roles being a victim, abuser, or rescuer. Depending on their own traumatic past, or on their current interaction between each other and with their children, the parents may maintain trust and present themselves in a postive role ('angel,' affectionate/compassionate parent), but they can turn to an abusive parenting style (angry, aggressive, insistent) at any time. The changing attitudes of their parents and the marital discord will often cause contradicatory feelings within the children. Family members often feel trapped, first being unable to leave in the midst of a crises as it is not safe. Second- arely, a person doesn't leave the family when the atmosphere has turned positive as the crises is over and the need to escape has vanished. In an atmosphere of neglect, chaos may be an opportunity for making contact with each other. Family members, who restrict/dissociate their feelings and appear calm (apparently normal personality) can turn to a new personality state with flooding emotions (emotional personality) temporarily. Sometimes, the dissociative member of the family appears as the emotional member of the family, whereas remaining members stay apparently normal. Adjustment to this system would only be possible when all family members participate in this pattern.

In a comparison between Turkish and Dutch dissociative subjects, Sar, Yargic, and Tutkun (1996) demonstrated that the two studied groups endorsed different borderline personality disorder criteria whereas their dissociative symptom scores were similar. It is no wonder that borderline personality disorder criteria seem to be more sensitive to cultural influences than dissociative symptoms per se. The borderline characteristics may in fact be seen as relational aspects of dissociation (Blizard, 2003; Howell, 2003), i.e., interpersonal projections of hidden/subclinical dissociation. As such, we consider the elevated presence of subtreshold borderline criteria among family members in this study as a reflection of hidden dissociative psychopathology.

Types and Dynamics of Apparently Normal Family

Despite many disturbing characteristics described below, the first impression of an "apparently normal" family, by an outside observer is usually positive. This positive impression may even cause the observer to wish for more contact with the family. It is only after more long-term observations that a person may comprehend an obscure dysfunctional system. In extrapolation of our present findings, we will now describe eight family types in this realm of an "apparently normal family."

Extratensive family. There is a dominant parent who has an active egoistic attitude against his or her partner and children in this type of family. This active egoism can reach the level of sadistic behavior. All norms at home are determined by this parent. Disobedience of a family member is indemnified by all family members. The passive parent is not able to save himself or herself and the children from his or her partner's unfair attitude. Peace at home depends on obedience to the instructions of the dominant parent. There is only one leader role in this type of family, i.e., the dominant parent; all remaining family members are auxiliary. The dominant parent usually has mood fluctuations, intense anger and the lack of control of anger, transient dissociative and paranoid ideas, and symptoms of identity confusion. The passive parent is inconsistent, conformistic, and suggestible in his/her behavior, and lacks social skills. Nevertheless, he or she may also become abusive when he/she gains control in the family temporarily. The passive parent is not introversive but he or she is in a "latent extratensive" position due to the excessively dominant attitude of her/his partner. He or she tries to take control during his/her partner's weak moments.

Children brought up in an extratensive family participate in the dominance struggle at home even before adolescence and tend to behave in an extratensive manner. The dysfunctional family environment may lead them to develop an explosive behavior pattern. This is the most dysfunctional family type in the context of childrearing and internal family dynamics. Neither parents nor children are ready to accept that they personally have behavioral deficits or problems with each other. On the contrary, the atmosphere at home tends to be explosive and the intense verbal arguments may end up in violence. There is a failure of intimacy and emotional mutuality at home, and the individual members of the family are unable to feel like or perceive themselves as a true family.

Introversive family. Both parents are introversive in this type of family. They rarely communicate and intimacy is not displayed. Both parents are usually prescriptive in their parenting style. In fact, they have obsessive tendencies and may even be seen as obsessive-compulsive. There are no frank and serious arguments at home, because the children are brought up in this environment to not be argumentative. Differentiated social roles do not exist in this family, the boundaries are firm; distance and temperance problems do not exist. This is a family type with less intrafamilial chaos and few relationship traumas. The children tend to also become introversive. High emotional expression and impulsive behavior are not allowed. Emotionality is restricted and is allowed only as a collective experience. The mother is usually moralistic in character. Delegation (Stierlin, 1978) and the commission of the delegated actions are expected and usually delivered. The rather rigid cognitive style of the parents tends to nourish agression in the family, which ends up in negative mutuality. Family members can not be flexible and their adaptability to novel situations is limited. This family type is, however, welcomed by society. As such, this family style (not having conflict) serves the child for (over) adjustment to the social environment.

Mixed family. One of the parents is extratensive and the other one introversive. The introversive one is usually the mother. She and the children are constantly abused, sometimes sadistically, by her partner. This is the family type where most intense intrafamilial traumas happen, even up to the level of family terror. The abusive behavior of the dominant and extratensive parent can not be prevented by the remaining family members. The extratensive parent utilizes his/her empathy about family members to further abuse those family members and does not compromise. The intrafamilial traumatic experiences are kept as a secret. The children brought up in this atmosphere may become either extratensive or introversive.

Reversible family. In this type of family there is uncertainty about which parent is introversive or extratensive. The roles in the family are exchanged repeatedly (Blizard, 2003). There are no apparent cause or significant time period for a role exchange. A parent who is dominant in a certain context may become passive at another time or in a similar event. The behavior and attitudes of the parents are not consistent. A loving parental approach may turn to frank hatred in an instant or vice versa. Verbal discussions frequently happen where everybody is offended repeatedly, only to again be reconciled. There are no rules or norms in this family style. This type of family is not welcomed by the community and they may be even rejected. As stable communication does not exist in the family, the children remain unstable in their communications overall. Crises are usually provoked within the family. Friends that are included in the family system often attempt to help to solve the family problems. The number of friends associated with these types of familes diminish over time as they are unable to offer the family effective solutions. In the course of time, this family with its unstructured and variable characteristics will continuc to dcgcncratc. The parents believe that they can not leave each other, because, after a period of intense communication and discordance with other people, they basically are alone and only have each other.

Dissociative family. Any one of the family types defined above may cover the characteristics of a dissociative family. It is common in this type of family to have at least one family member with a dissociative disorder or subclinical dissociative experiences. Family secrets are sometimes discussed as an outburst in front of all family members, e.g., the existence of a previously unknown adopted or foster child, an unexplained death among relatives in previous years, hidden previous life experiences or life stories of the parents. The family is usually below or above a middle socioeconomic level. There are polarized roles in the family and a reversible abuser-victim cycle is common. The children are traumatized in this atmosphere, serving as "poison containers" (DeMause, 2002).

Schizoid family. The parents of the Schizoid family stylc have very limited social contacts. This type of family looks somewhat strange and the whole family seems to live in its own world ('aliens'). The relationship between the parents and children are seen as pathological. Children are typically physically and emotionally neglected the most in this type of family. The parents are behaviorally both infantile and immature. The children have either few responsibilities in the home or one of the children at a certain age takes overall responsibility of the home. Should the latter occur, the parents then take the role of the children (parent-ification). The life style of the family is disorganized, each member of the family seeming to live in his/her room. Regular meal times do not exist as each family member tends to eat on their own. The family members do not feel responsibility for each other. The family's physical self-care is seen as inadequate. They speak in short sentences, some-times hours can run without a word spoken. There are rituals at home. Guests are not invited into the home and a frequent behavior is looking out of the window and watching the neighborhood. Family members try usually to hide the strange characteristics of their family.

Depressive family. All family members live in depressive mood in this family style. In fact, several family members might have been diag-nosed as having clinical depression. They usually belong to a middle or low socioeconomic level. They maintain wrong beliefs and myths, such as they believe that everbody handled them unfairly and that something bad will happen to them. They blame themselves for adversities and they believe that everybody wishes evil for them. The children are frag-ile, depressive and inhibited without any ambitions in life. Lamenting and complaining are frequent at home.

Narcissistic family. The parents are arrogant, claiming, and exhibition-istic in their behavior in this style of family (Howell, 2003). Guests are invited frequently, and these parties often become feasts. Families with lower socioeconomic status than the host are preferred as guests. The parents talk about their successes, achievements, and possessions dur-ing these home parties. Communications between host and guests lack any mutuality. The families of so called "party" friends begin to sepa-rate from the "Narcissistic Family" after a while. The children may take either own family members or acquaintances as personal role models.

The Obscure Dysfunctional System

Research and conceptualizations about hidden dysfunctional com-munication styles in the families of psychiatric patients are not new. In North American psychiatry, many concepts have evolved to explain the psychopathogenesis of schizophrenia which may be of considerable in-terest for dissociative psychopathology today, e.g., pseudomutuality (Wynne, Ryckoff, Day, & Hirsch, 1958), double-bind (Bateson, Jack-son, Haley, & Weakland, 1956), schizophrenogenic mother (Fromm-Reichmann, 1950), marital schism (Lidz, Fleck, & Cornelison, 1965), and high expressed emotion (Brown, Monck, Carstairs, & Wing, 1962). These models collapsed in the face of evidence in support of a bio-genetic etiology for schizophrenia during the so-called neo-Kraepelinian period. However, while the models may not apply to biologically-determined schizophrenia, they may nevertheless apply to dissociative disorders (Spiegel, 1986). We would like to add the concept of an "apparently normal family" to this list as a further aspect of dysfunctional families. Inspired by Jung's (1912) words, we believe that many dissociative patients' tragedies can be formulated as a desperate effort to resolve a dysfunctional or "apparently normal family" and social context in their inner world (Sar, Öztürk, & Kundakci, 2002; Gold, 2004).

REFERENCES

Bateson, G., Jackson, D.D., Haley, J., & Weakland, J. H. (1956). Toward a theory of schizophrenia. *Behavioral Science*, 1, 251-264.

Bernstein, D. P., Fink, L., Handelsman, L., Foote, J., Lovejoy, M., Wenzel, K., Sapareto, E., & Ruggiero, J. (1994). Initial reliability and validity of a new retrospective measure of child abuse and neglect. *American Journal of Psychiatry*, 151, 1132-1136.

Bernstein, E. M., & Putnam, F. W. (1986). Development, reliability and validity of a dissociation scale. *Journal of Nervous and Mental Disease*, 174, 727-735.

Blizard, R. A. (2003). Disorganized attachment, development of dissociative self-states, and a relational approach to treatment. *Journal of Trauma and Dissociation*, 4, 27-50.

Braun, B. G. (1985). The transgenerational incidence of dissociation and multiple personality disorder: A preliminary report. In R. Kluft (Ed.) *Childhood antecedents of multiple personality* (pp. 127-150). Washington DC: American Psychiatric Press.

Brown, G. R., & Anderson, B. (1991). Psychiatric morbidity in adult inpatients with childhood histories of sexual and physical abuse. *American Journal of Psychiatry*, 148, 55-61.

Brown, G. W., Monck, E. M., Carstairs, G. M., & Wing, J. (1962). Influences of family life on the course of schizophrenic illness. *British Journal of Preventive and Social Medicine*, 16, 55-68.

Carlson, E. B., & Putnam, F. W. (1993). An update on Dissociative Experiences Scale. *Dissociation*, 6, 16-27.

Chu, J. A., & Dill, D. L. (1990). Dissociative symptoms in relation to childhood physical and sexual abuse. *American Journal of Psychiatry*, 147, 887- 892.

Chu, J., Frey, L. M., Ganzel, B. L., & Matthews, J. A. (1999). Memories of childhood abuse: Dissociation, amnesia, and corroboration. *American Journal of Psychiatry*, 156, 749-755.

Coskunol, H., Bagdiken, I., Sorias, S., & Saygili, R. (1994). SCID-II Türkce versiyonunun gecerlik ve güvenilirligi. (The reliability and validity of the SCID-II-Turkish Version). *Türk Psikoloji Dergisi*, 9, 26-29.

DeMause, L. (2002). *The emotional life of nations*. New York: Karnac Books.

Fromm-Reichmann, F. (1950). *Principles of intensive psychotherapy.* Chicago: University of Chicago Press.

Gold, S. N. (2000). *Not trauma alone. Therapy for child abuse survivors in family and social context.* Philadelphia: Brunner Routledge.

Gold, S. N. (2004). *Fight Club*: A depiction of contemporary society as dissociogenic. *Journal of Trauma and Dissociation,* 5, 13-34.

Howell, E. F. (2003). Narcissism, a relational aspect of dissociation. *Journal of Trauma and Dissociation,* 4, 51-71.

Jung, C.G. (1912). On the psychology of the unconscious. In *Collected works vol. 7: Two essays on analytical psychology* (p. 18). Princeton: Princeton University Press.

Kluft, R. P. (1984). Multiple personality in childhood. *Psychiatric Clinics of North America,* 7, 121-134.

Kundakci, T., Sar, V., Kiziltan, E., Yargic, L. I., & Tutkun H. (1998). The reliability and validity of the Turkish version of the SCID-D. *Paper presented at the 15th Fall Meeting of the International Society for the Study of Dissociation,* Seattle.

Lidz, T., Fleck, S., & Cornelison, A. R. (1965). *Schizophrenia and the family.* New York: International Universities Press.

Myers, C.S. (1940). *Shell shock in France 1914-18.* Cambridge: Cambridge University Press.

Nijenhuis, E. R. S., & Van der Hart, O. (1999). Forgetting and reexperiencing trauma. In J. Goodwin & R. Attais (Eds.), *Splintered reflections: Images of the body in treatment* (pp. 39-65). New York: Basic Books.

Nijenhuis, E. R. S., Van der Hart, O., & Steele, K. (1994). Strukturalle Dissoziation der Persönlichkeitssturktur, traumatischer Ursprung, phopische Residuen. (Structural dissociation of the personality structure, traumatic etiology and phobic residues) In L. Reddemann, A. Hofmann, & U. Gast, *Psychotherapie der dissoziativen Störungen* (Psychotherapy of dissociative disorders) (pp. 47-69). Stuttgart: Thieme.

Ogawa, J. R., Sroufe, L. A., Weinfield, N. S., Carlson. E. A., & Egeland, B (1997). Development and the fragmented self: Longitudinal study of dissociative symptomatology in a nonclinical sample. *Development and Psychopathology,* 4, 855-879.

Sar, V., Akyuz G., Kundakci, T., Kiziltan, E., & Dogan, O. (2004). Childhood trauma, dissociation, and psychiatric comorbidity in patients with conversion disorder. *American Journal of Psychiatry,* 161, 2271-2276.

Sar, V., Akyuz, G., & Ozturk, E. (2004). Axis-I dissociative disorder comorbidity of Borderline Personality Disorder and its impact on reports of childhood trauma. *Paper presented at the 21th Annual Conference of the International Society for the Study of Dissociation,* New Orleans, pp. 36-37.

Sar, V., Kundakci, T., Kiziltan, E., Bakim, B., Yargic, L. I., & Tutkun, H. (1997). Dissosiyatif Yasantilar Ölceginin (DES-II) Türkce Versiyonunun gecerlik ve Güvenilirligi. (The reliability and validity of the Turkish version of the Dissociative Experiences Scale [DES-II]). *Proceedings of the 33th national congress of psychiatry* (pp. 55-64), Antalya, Turkey.

Sar,V., Kundakci, T., Kiziltan, E., Yargic, L. I., Tutkun, H., Bakim, B., et al. (2003). Axis I dissociative disorder comorbidity in Borderline Personality Disorder among psychiatric outpatients. *Journal of Trauma and Dissociation,* 4, 119-136.

Sar, V., Öztürk, E., & Kundakci, T. (2002). Psychotherapy of an adolescent with Dissociative Identity Disorder: Change in Rorschach patterns, *Journal of Trauma and Dissociation*, 3, 81-95.

Sar, V., Tutkun, H., Yargic, L. I., Kundakci, T., & Kiziltan, E. (1996). DSM-IV Dissosiyatif Bozukluklar Icin Yapilastirilmis Görüsme Cizelgesinin Türkce Versiyonu (Turkish Version of the Structured Clinical Interview for DSM-IV Dissociative Disorders). Unpublished manuscript, Istanbul.

Sar,V., Yargic, L. I., & Tutkun, H. (1996). Structured interview data on 35 cases of dissociative identity disorder in Turkey. *American Journal of Psychiatry*, 153, 1329-1333.

Spiegel, D. (1986). Dissociation, double binds and posttraumatic stress in Multiple Personality Disorder. In B.G. Braun (Ed) *Treatment of multiple personality disorder* (pp. 61-77). Washington DC: American Psychiatric Press.

Spitzer, R. L., Williams, J. B.W., & Gibbon, M. (1987). *Structured Clinical Interview for DSM-III-R Personality Disorders*. New York: New York State Psychiatric Institute. Biometrics Research Department.

Steele, K., Van der Hart, O., & Nijenhuis, E. R. S. (2005). Phase-oriented treatment of structural dissociation in complex traumatization: overcoming trauma-related phobias. *Journal of Trauma and Dissocaition*, 6, 11-53.

Steinberg, M. (1994). *Structured Clinical Interview for DSM-IV Dissociative Disorders-Revised (SCID-D-R)*. Washington DC: American Psychiatric Press.

Stierlin, H. (1978). *Delegation und familie (Delegation and family)*. Frankfurt am Main: Suhrkamp Verlag.

Walker, C. E., Bonner, B. L., & Kaufmann, K. (1988). The physically and sexually abused child: Evaluation and treatment. New York, Pergamon Press.

Wynne, L. C., Ryckoff, I. M., Day, J., & Hirsch S. (1958). Pseudomutuality in the family relations of schizophrenics. *Psychiatry*, 21, 204-219.

Yargic, L. I., Tutkun, H., & Sar, V. (1995). The reliability and validity of the Turkish Version of the Dissociative Experiences Scale. *Dissociation*, 8, 10-12.

The History of Dissociation and Trauma in the UK and Its Impact on Treatment

Remy Aquarone
William Hughes

SUMMARY. The road to recovery from trauma cannot be seen in isolation. Isolation from self (self identity as well as self in the body) and from the world outside (family and society) is the tragedy of a survival system that kept hope and potential alive but extracts a heavy toll on living. In much the same way we, as facilitators on this journey of recovery, can no longer isolate ourselves as therapists from a world outside the consulting room. We have to take account of the real world outside, its particular culture as well as the reality of multi-professional involvement. Our clients/patients need encouragement to engage in the world of work, responsibilities and relationships alongside the therapeutic process. This piece examines the evolution of psychoanalysis and psychotherapy in the UK and the historic tensions between the National Health Service (NHS) and the private sector. It outlines a practice protocol that requires a diplomatic sensitivity to cultural differences within these two sectors. The approach mirrors the early dynamics between therapist and client/patient: developing a working alliance, recognising the power hierarchy, mapping the system. Thus, an audit (survey) of the acute wards

---

Address correspondence to: Remy Aquarone, 26 Princes Street, Norwich, Norfold, NR31AE, UK.

[Haworth co-indexing entry note]: "The History of Dissociation and Trauma in the UK and Its Impact on Treatment." Aquarone, Remy, and William Hughes. Co-published simultaneously in *Journal of Trauma Practice* (The Haworth Maltreatment & Trauma Press, an imprint of The Haworth Press, Inc.) Vol. 4, No. 3/4, 2005, pp. 305-322; and: *Trauma and Dissociation in a Cross-Cultural Perspective: Not Just a North American Phenomenon* (ed: George F. Rhoades, Jr., and Vedat Sar) The Haworth Maltreatment & Trauma Press, an imprint of The Haworth Press, Inc., 2005, pp. 305-322. Single or multiple copies of this article are available for a fee from The Haworth Document Delivery Service [1-800-HAWORTH, 9:00 a.m. - 5:00 p.m. (EST). E-mail address: docdelivery@haworthpress.com].

Available online at http://jtp.haworthpress.com
doi:10.1300/J189v04n03_07

in the locality was undertaken as a means of identifying levels of dissociative symptoms and potential for saving on unnecessary admissions. Finally the piece suggests that the Pottergate Model, as a practice protocol, aims to bridge the gap between these two vital sectors of the mental health system and at the same time keep the focus on the client/patient's need for both appropriate dependency and self responsibility throughout. *[Article copies available for a fee from The Haworth Document Delivery Service: 1-800-HAWORTH. E-mail address: <docdelivery@haworthpress. com> Website: <http://www.HaworthPress.com> © 2005 by The Haworth Press, Inc. All rights reserved.]*

KEYWORDS. Dissociation, history, UK, in-patient prevalence

Psychoanalysis and psychotherapy has followed a specific path in the United Kingdom (UK) that may well differ from many other countries. Its evolution needs to be understood if we are to comprehend the specific dynamics of the processes involved in working with trauma and dissociative clients.

Many of the early analysts and training analysts were people from non-medical backgrounds. The psycho-analytic training schools were, and have continued to be, virtually all in the private non-medical sector (The Institute of Psychoanalysis and the British Association of Psychotherapists, to name just two). The same has been true of other psychotherapy and counselling disciplines. Furthermore, there is still no statutory registration required in order to practice psychotherapy or counselling. Anyone can still call themselves a therapist and practice psychotherapy. This is fast changing as there are now three umbrella organisations that have been formed to regulate these practices within the private sector.

In the public sector, until very recently, consultant psychiatrists, clinical psychologists, occupational therapists and psychiatric nurses have gained their expertise without the need to undergo more specific training in psychotherapy or undergo personal therapy. So historically we have had a split between the psychotherapy and counselling mostly undertaken by the private non-medical sector (where adults are seen as clients) and the professional medical model within the public sector (where adults are seen as patients).

Twenty years ago, when dissociation was beginning to be encountered, the division between these two sections of the mental health field were well established. As knowledge and experience of dissociation and trauma began to grow in this country, it became clear that (with some worthy exceptions) virtually all the therapeutic work with dissociative clients was being undertaken by psychotherapists, counsellors, the clergy, rape crisis organisations and other voluntary organisations far removed from the public sector. These courageous people had to learn on their feet, were geographically fragmented, and exposed to attacks from the False Memory Syndrome Foundation (FMSF) and in some cases from individual psychiatric services. Those working with dissociative clients were generally unsupported but desperately sought to support their clients.

It became clear how alien the two languages were (public and private), with no attempt by either side to understand each other. Professionals within the public sector saw therapists in the private sector as "having the luxury of listening to middle-class neurotics who are able to afford this self-indulgence of hours of therapy, while managing adequately enough in the world outside." Meanwhile, medical professionals were under continual pressure to deal with the latest crisis, acting out or suicide with no adequate professional support or supervision. They were themselves struggling to survive and had to use dissociative mechanisms to make that possible. At the same time therapists working privately, in their own dissociative bubble protected from the real world, could moralise about the evils of medication and electroconvulsive therapy (ECT). The private therapists were also working alone, isolated and unconnected to the world outside.

TYPICAL NATIONAL HEALTH SERVICE (NHS) STRUCTURE

It is important to understand that when the NHS was established in 1948, the services for mental health were for the most part provided by the Asylum services, which were established during the 19th century. Some of these establishments had been started on a humane basis and some only were reluctantly provided by the County Asylum Act (Sivadon, 1952), which made a statutory order that each county in the UK provide safe and secure places for the containment of the mentally ill. Until 1948, there had been private houses set up for the mentally ill. After the NHS Act (Department of Health, 1948) all of that changed and services were provided by the medically dominated system of the NHS.

Some psychotherapy had been found to be of use in treating "shell shocked" or as we would know them Posttraumatic Stress Disorder

(PTSD) sufferers from the Second World War. In psychiatric circles, a conflict had grown between the group therapists, e.g., S.H. Foulkes and the physical therapists, e.g., William Sargent.

In the NHS it was the physical treatments that won the war over the treatment of PTSD types of disorders. Electroconvulsive therapy (ECT), medication and sedation with a kind of containment was the model that dominated and was promoted by the powerful Maudsley Hospital (in South London) as a pattern of high quality care. Psychotherapy was not an official part of provision but was represented by the Tavistock Clinic in London as a national resource and therapeutic communities such as the Cassell Hospital in London. There were other examples of psychotherapy programs/models in different parts of the country often directed by highly charismatic leaders. Gradually during the 1960s and 70s these psychotherapy programs were divested of power and authority, leaving a standard way of training psychiatrists in a strictly medical model of practice. This medical model was needed by psychiatrists to gain membership in the elite Royal College of Psychiatrists, without which a person could not be employed as a consultant psychiatrist within the NHS. Some psychiatrists persisted in psychotherapy training and were supported by a section of the Royal College, but remained small in number. These psychotherapy trained psychiatrists were largely concentrated in and around London because that is where the training institutions (privately owned and run) were based. In addition to typically being trained in the medical model, psychiatrists were not expected to have personal analysis or psychotherapy then or even to the present time.

Over the past fifty years of NHS psychiatry, clinical psychologists, occupational therapists, physiotherapists, art therapists, and psychiatric nurses have all been employed under different terms and conditions of employment and with different expectations for their work. These different groups of professionals were given no clear idea as to who should lead and direct the treatment team in any particular case except for an expectation that the consultant psychiatrist was "responsible." Different employee organisations represented the interests of the different professionals. The resulting different pay structures have created professional rivalry and enormous differences in benefits from employment when compared to the work actually undertaken. Until the care programme approach, which is a recent innovation, there was no one plan to which everybody involved in the care of a patient should adhere. The system was in fact dissociative in structure and in function.

Private psychotherapists had a vast body of information which was never incorporated in the training of future psychotherapists. Individuals had to seek personal analysis and psychotherapy training, paid for largely from their own pockets. A powerful example was the senior author's former teacher, Dr. Joe Redfearn. Dr. Redfearn published in 1985 (republished in 1994) a book with the title *My Self, My Many Selves*–a most helpful and straightforward account of the effects of trauma and dissociation in relation to subpersonality formation. It is doubtful that many health professionals in the UK or for that matter anywhere in the world have read this book, as he works in the private sector. A much better received book was published in 1996 by Dr. Phil Mollon as he was both a NHS psychologist and privately trained psychoanalyst. The book was entitled *Multiple Selves, Multiple Voices: Working with Trauma, Violation and Dissociation.*

Structurally, the health professions have been slowly growing together and can perhaps now begin to bring the wealth of experience of observed behaviour and patterns of dysfunctional thinking processes together with the feeling and meaning which has come from a split off private sector. The qualities of control, restraint, and public protection have come from a politically driven NHS; while containment, understanding, and interpretation with integration in the mind seem to come from the private sector.

In the last ten years, we have seen the development of hybrid clinics; Dr. Stuart Turner, for example, obtained funding from the NHS to set up a trauma centre in London, which also had an income derived from private earnings. Dr. Turner is a past president of the European Society for Study of Trauma. Dr. Valerie Sinason, a psychoanalyst, has established also in London a Clinic for the Study of Dissociation, again with public (NHS) and private money involved.

Where psychological therapy services are still viable in NHS mental health provision, some appointments of clinical psychologists have been dedicated to PTSD, but this is patchy and follows no set national pattern. There are no Statutory Guidelines except for those in connection with emergency services connected with large scale disasters and those are only short term services. It is as though all of the information from individual and group psychotherapy painfully gained and recorded largely in relation to large and small scale traumatic events has been ignored as far as mainstream psychiatry is concerned, within a State run NHS. A blind eye has been turned in favour of medications, ECT and social behavioural readjustment to fit in with a society that probably gave rise to the traumatic experiences in the first place. It would seem that the future opportunities for the treatment of PTSD and dissociative disorders in the UK are with voluntary and private institutions willing to negotiate for funding for services from the NHS and Insurance.

LEARNING THE LANGUAGE

The first author noted that after eight years of supervising a number of multi-disciplinary professional groups within the local psychiatric services, the level of projections, fragmentation, lack of containment and obvious presence of dissociative patients (though unrecognised) at both inpatient and outpatient level was revealed. For example, on several occasions two members of the same supervision group (sometimes from different professions) would find themselves presenting, over a period of time, the same patient but with no recognition of this. This was because the same patient would be experienced by each in a radically different way. It was only after a while that it became clear that both professionals were talking about the same person. One might see Patient A as strong, manipulative, acting out, provocative, a waste of space and deserving of being discharged; the other would talk of Patient A's vulnerability, terror and aloneness. Among the professionals involved, this could very easily lead to clashes, reinforcing patients' fear of their own destructiveness as well as lack of containment (reminiscent of the model of a dysfunctional family). The eventual containment and sense of self-worth and power within the supervision groups led to a diminishing of this acting out by both professionals and, eventually, by patients. To use dissociative language, you could say that the pro-bonding professionals began to outweigh the anti-bonding professionals within the institution and this inevitably began to improve the containment of these patients.

Though the examples quoted above were clearly triggered by dissociative patients, up to this point (about 12 years ago), no specific mention of dissociation had been used in exploring the dynamics of the group and the specific patients. It was too soon to bring in yet another consideration. It was felt that the work until then had been to consolidate a strong 'working alliance' (as with very fragmented clients) and incorporate an educational cognitive approach to the dynamics involved.

Some worthy professionals in the public sector were finding their own position hard to keep safe because of the climate that existed within the public sector and because they were in the minority. In much the same way, dissociative clients can only start to talk about the untellable when the inner system is co-operating and the therapeutic environment is sufficiently contained. The outcome of our experiences was to use the language of research to try to identify levels of dissociative symptoms among the local inpatient population and to use this as a tool to begin to educate the professionals in a less threatening way.

AUDIT

An audit or survey was conducted at a psychiatric hospital in Norfolk under the supervision of the second author and will be presented here to better understand the status of dissociation in the UK and demonstrate the effectiveness of an educational approach to complex trauma as far as the NHS is concerned.

Patients admitted to acute psychiatric units have clearly presented dissociative behaviours but, within a culture unaware of this phenomenon, they remain diagnosed. A point prevalence estimation using the Dissociative Experiences Scale-2 (DES-2, Carlson & Putnam, 1983; Carlson et al., 1993) and DES Taxon was undertaken in an acute psychiatric unit.

It was not possible to incorporate a diagnostic instrument (such as the Structured Clinical Interview for DSM-IV Dissociative Disorders, SCID-D [Steinburg, 1994]) into this study. The aim therefore of this audit was to raise awareness and interest in dissociation among the psychiatric professionals and identify possible links between undetected dissociation (both dissociative symptoms and dissociative disorders) and repeated hospital admissions. This would be a first step towards formulating a more appropriate treatment model at the outpatient level. The results of the audit have revealed a significant percentage of patients scoring over 30 on the DES with clear indications that some are likely to suffer from a dissociative disorder. Furthermore, some correlation has been demonstrated between the presence of dissociation and repeated hospital stays. This has helped staff to have a better understanding of slow responders or non-responders to standard biological treatment regimes.

Group supervision over a number of years at a local psychiatric hospital has highlighted clusters of patients clearly demonstrating dissociative symptoms, but within a culture unaware of this phenomenon. No study to date has been undertaken in the UK on the frequency of dissociation among the impatient population. Our objective was to identify dissociative disorders among the acute wards of this hospital and compare results from similar research in the United States of America (USA) and abroad.

It became clear that no research protocol involving a full diagnostic assessment (e.g., SCID-D) could be ethically undertaken without a treatment plan in place, if the postulated outcome of the research identified patients as having a dissociative disorder. The staff needed to implement such a treatment programme would have to be resourced within the psychiatric services. The type of staff needed for such a program was not available at the time of the audit. Furthermore, the proposal of such a research project had caused a dissociative reaction within the hospital. For instance, despite invitations to attend these early discussions, some of the key psychologists involved in work with abused patients were resisting any initiative outside their area of knowledge and authority. The compromise was to undertake a point prevalent audit on a specific day using the DES for which no outcome treatment plan was required and no ethical approval needed.

Our secondary objective was to look at possible links between multiple admissions and high dissociate symptoms. Strumwasser, Paranjpe and Udow (1991), when studying psychiatric admissions, found that a significant proportion of bed days (40%) utilised by general psychiatric patients were deemed to be inappropriate. In most UK acute psychiatric admissions units, routine evaluation of dissociate symptoms is not carried out. Our secondary objective was to find a marker that would correlate with poor response to conventional treatment and multiple admissions with the aim to undertake further research using a recognised alternative treatment model. We wanted to find out the number of patients with dissociate symptoms at a point in time on the acute admission unit and to correlate this with features that suggest that they may be inappropriately placed.

Dissociation

Dissociation, unlike many other mental processes, occurs in both minor non-pathological and major pathological forms. The creation of the dissociative disorders category in the Diagnostic and Statistical Manual of Mental Disorders, Third Edition (DSM-III, American Psychiatric Association [APA], 1980), followed by the DSM-III-R (APA, 1987) and DSM-IV (APA, 1994) has led to an increased interest in the nature of dissociation and its role in specific symptoms and syndromes. DSM-IV identified five "dissociative disorders," namely Dissociative Amnesia, Dissociative Fugue, Dissociative Identity Disorder [DID],

Depersonalisation Disorder and Dissociative Disorder Not Otherwise Specified [DDNOS].

Pathological dissociation is a post-traumatic defence mobilized by the patient as protection from overwhelming pain and trauma (Braun, 1990; Coons, Cole, Pellow & Milstein, 1990; Fine, 1990; Kluft, 1985; 1988; Kluft, Braun & Sachs, 1984; Putnam, 1985; Ross, Norton & Wozney, 1989; Spiegel, 1984, 1991; Spiegel & Cardena, 1991; Terr, 1991).

Dissociative symptoms occur within a variety of psychiatric diagnoses including personality disorders (such as Borderline Personality Disorder), eating disorders, anxiety disorders, depression and schizophrenia (Clary, Burstin & Carpenter, 1984; Fine, 1990; Fink & Goldinkoff 1990; Goff, Olin, Jenlike, Baer & Buttolph 1992; Havenaar, Boon & Tordoir, 1992; Kluft, 1988; Marcum, Wright & Bissell, 1985; Roth, 1959; Schultz, Braun & Kluft, 1989; Torem, 1986).

Recurrent to persistent dissociative symptoms occur in the dissociative disorders and may also be seen in PTSD (Blank, 1985; Bliss, 1983; Gelinas, 1984), and phobic disorders (Frankel & Orne, 1976).

METHOD

Participants

The study was carried out in an acute psychiatric unit in Norfolk. The unit has five wards with 20 patients in each, making a total of 100. There are ten consultant-led community mental health teams that have access to the acute admission unit. We decided to use the DES-2 as the screening instrument.

The Instrument

The DES is a 28-item self-report instrument that can be completed in 10 minutes, and scored in less than 5 minutes. It is easy to understand, and the questions are framed in a normative way that does not stigmatize the respondent for positive responses. A typical DES question is: *"some people have the experience of finding new things among their belongings that they do not remember buying. Circle the number to show what percentage of the time this happens to you."* The respondent circles a percentage ranging from 0% to 100%, at 10% intervals. Only one alteration was made to DES 2. In question 1, the word 'subway' was replaced by the word 'underground' to make the test more culturally appropriate.

The DES has very good validity and reliability, and good overall psychometric properties, as reviewed by its original developers (Carlson & Putnam, 1983; Carlson et al., 1993). It has excellent construct validity, which means it is internally consistent and hangs together well, as reflected in highly significant Spearman correlations of all items with the overall DES score. The scale is derived from extensive clinical experience with an understanding of DID. In the initial studies during its development and in all subsequent studies, the DES has discriminated DID from other diagnostic groups and controls at high levels of significance (Ross, 1997).

Scoring

DES scores over 30 are indicative of some dissociative symptoms and the possibility of a dissociative disorder (Ross, 1997). Follow up studies (Carlson et al., 1993) using a structured clinical interview (such as the SCID-D) generally confirm that 50% of such patients turn out to have a dissociative disorder. The DES Taxon consists of 8 of the DES questions: 3, 5, 7, 8, 12, 13, 22, and 27. These questions are familiar to clinicians who use the SCID-D (Steinberg, 1993, 1994) to evaluate the presence of a dissociative disorder. Steinberg's formulation is based upon 5 factors: depersonalization, derealization, amnesia, identity confusion, and identity alteration. The DES Taxon correlates roughly to these areas of inquiry, based on a spreadsheet by Waller and Ross, 1997. Calculations based on the article by Waller and Ross (1997).

Procedure

Six researchers were found among the psychiatric professionals, one for each of the six wards. On the day decided to conduct the point prevalence (Thursday, the 11th of December, 1997) all current inpatients were listed and allocated to a random number. The nurse in charge of each ward knew which patient had been allocated each number but referred to them only by number to the researcher who did not know the name of the patient. The questionnaire was administered on all six wards during the same day, collected and analysed.

RESULTS

Of 122 patients surveyed, 28 had been discharged on the day of the study and 19 were on leave. Ten patients were not well enough to take part, which gave us 59 completed questionnaires. Of the 59 question-naires, 18 (30.5%) scored over 30. It should be noted that none of the patients had been assessed for dissociative symptoms prior to this study. We also found in the study (Table 1) that frequent re-admission correlated with high dissociation scores. The results demonstrated that a third or more of patients with high numbers of admissions also has positive dissociation scores.

DISCUSSION

A paper published in the *Psychiatric Bulletin* by Peter Ellwood (1999) identified medical and socio-demographic characteristics of admissions considered inappropriate (25%) by psychiatrists. Ellwood's "twenty-five percent" of the admissions are approaching the fairly consistent one-third to two-thirds ratio found in this study. It would have been interesting to have had in Ellwood's study the dissociation scores of the patients found to be "inappropriate for admission."

This study revealed that a significant proportion of acute inpatients could be identified as having a possible dissociative disorder using a relatively simple dissociation test. It has also been presented that significant proportions of acute inpatients are reportedly inappropriately admitted. When we add to this mix the difficulty of multiple diagnosis and predictable responses to conventional (medication) treatment, serious questions are raised. The study supports the need for a research trial designed to test first, in a more detailed way, the precise nature of the dissociative symptoms recognised by the screening instrument. Further research using structured interviews such as the SCID-D are required, and the more accurate identification of dissociative disorder patients might result in differential treatment planning with behavioural management indices as treatment outcome variables, e.g., readmission/length of stay.

TABLE 1. Relationship of number of hospitalizations to mean DES score

Number of Patients	Number of Admissions	Number with DES Score over 30
42	2	16 [38%]
28	3 or more	9 [32%]
18	4 or more	6 [33%]

There are a high number of dissociators among inpatients in acute psychiatric units. Basic appropriate therapeutic principles are difficult to provide on a modern, acute psychiatric inpatient unit where bed occupancy rates are in excess of 100%. These raise challenges for those with responsibility for planning and maintaining services. This study suggests, however, that if more appropriate outpatient based "holding therapies" are provided, then at least a quarter and, perhaps, a third of inappropriate admissions could be reduced while, at the same time, providing more appropriate treatment with better outcomes. This, however, remains to be tested and there is an urgent need for such a project.

POSITIVE FAMILY MODEL

There is a growing awareness of the dynamics of the two very different worlds of mental health in the UK and confirmation that the levels of dissociative symptoms and likely dissociative disorders were very similar to levels experienced in other countries (The Ross Institute). The question remains as to how we could begin to address these splits and help bring about a more integrated approach to treatment and positive outcomes.

The first task was to identify the differences between the roles, the advantages and disadvantages of the two worlds of mental health. The advantages of working in the private sector involve being able to tackle dissociation and having a contained environment. The disadvantages of working in the private sector are that you tend to work in a "bubble" unrelated to the outside world and you may function as the client's "rescuer" in regards to the client's family, psychiatric or social services, or in court appearances.

The advantages of working in the public sector may include having a safe haven in times of emergency and having a range of therapies offered "in-house." The disadvantages include having no link with a private therapist and having an over reliance on medication for patients.

The first step in healing this split between the private and public sector of mental health is to learn the language of the dissociative patient. The first author was taught in his analytical training that it was up to the patient to learn the language of psychoanalysis. If they didn't they were either resisting or their condition was not suitable for therapy! When confronted with what turned out to be his first MPD client (as it was called in those days), the author had to radically change this prosaic attitude. It was up to the therapist to learn her language, not the other way around. The author's language of interpretations of fantasies was completely out of place at a starting point. A grounding into reality became the cornerstone of an early working alliance. In the same way, if a productive relationship was going to be developed with psychiatry then we would need to learn their language, the language of screening instruments and assessments and the DSM IV.

There are strong parallels between the work we do with individual clients at a micro level, and its mirroring within the UK psychiatric system. Dissociation, when no longer needed as a survival defensive mechanism, can become an enslaving entanglement within the interior world of the client whose default position is the "entrapment and infantalisation" of the individual's capacity to be a self-regulating independent and creative individual.

A second step in bridging the gap between the two mental health systems in the UK is to better understand a patient's behaviour when they are needing an emergency admission to the acute ward of a psychiatric hospital. There are at least three patterns of behaviour to be aware of. First, the new patient may lose "a sense of self." This loss of a sense of self leads to either a negative attention or compliant victim role. It doesn't take that much for any of us to lose a sense of self when we are away from our own environment. We generally revert to one of two primitive responses, to become compliant or to fight. It makes it understandable why some people taken hostage choose to make trouble for themselves, as it prevents their loss of self.

The second pattern of behaviour is that of a loss/abdication of responsibility for decisions taken. If you fight, decisions can be taken for you in actions that can lead to sectioning (compulsary admission to hospital under Mental Health Act). If you act in a compliant mode, you give over responsibility to authority and look to them to tell you what to do and behave in a childlike way. The third pattern of behaviour is illustrated by patients having their "antennae finely tuned" to splits/discords within the system and capitalising on these opportunities. This is such familiar territory for someone from a dysfunctional family.

The following is a example of a typical pathway for someone with DID when admitted to hospital: (1) crisis leads to hospital admission; (2) diagnosis is given which naturally can contradict an earlier diagnosis (in DID, etc.); (3) CPA (Care Plan Assessment) team is set up which can encourage splits in both the team and the patient; and (4) in general circumstances changes are made, often unilaterally by individual professionals involved, according to the patient's perceived behaviour and interpretation according to the professional involved. The patient will on the one hand quickly adapt to fit into the perceived role but then change behaviour according to the next professional or peer person they come in contact with.

This typical pathway for the DID patent in hospital admission can lead the patient to having difficult behaviour/acting out in the wards, self harm, and regression. This typically produces a "them/us culture" by both patient and professional. The patient can end up being discussed in either a derogatory or combative way.

With an understanding of the patient's language, the aforementioned possible patient behaviours at admission and the typical pathway for an admission, the authors offer an alternative, the "Positive Family Model." Appropriate responsibility by parental authority (professionals) and patient is encouraged in this model. All discussions and decisions should be taken at CPA meetings with the patient present. The views of the patient should be elicited respectfully as they know themselves at some level better than you do. When things "go wrong," view it as a group problem: "We have a problem." The more the patient is brought into solutions, problems, etc., the less likely acting out or self harm will take place. The hospital is not to become the equivalent of a child minder, wherein the children are dumped to be picked up again at the end of admissions. So right from the start we are encouraging the adult patient to take responsibility for the child within. It is a creative flow between dependency and independency.

POTTERGATE MODEL FOR LOCALITY MANAGEMENT SUPPORTIVE CONSULTATION

What steps have we taken, at the Pottergate Centre, to facilitate internal dialogue between professionals both in the private and public sector and dissociative clients, to get this condition treated seriously and to get the right help? We started by focusing just in our own locality but have broadened this in the last three years to offer this evolving model nationally. There are now broadly speaking two pathways through which the Centre gets referrals: first, professional referrals for an assessment and recommendation for treatment. The second is where the client self-refers and self-funds as a first step to getting appropriate help.

Such referrals to our Centre via this route were unknown as of four years ago. It has begun to change in a significant way. Some of this is down to survivors (trauma patients) fighting to get recognition of their plight. Right from the start, the person referred is included in all correspondence and invited to contact us regarding any worries, etc. If a screening instrument has not previously been completed, then this is sent to them for completion if they are able to. Two assessments are undertaken: the SCID-D with myself and the psychiatric assessment with my colleague, William Hughes, who is a consultant psychiatrist. He will have received all the relevant medical notes from the services as his role is to identify the primary diagnosis. Very often people have been diagnosed with Borderline Personality Disorder and immediately any question of effective help had been dismissed in the past.

These two extensive reports are sent (including details of the results of the screening instruments unless insignificant) along with a recommended treatment plan which will include several elements if the person was diagnosed with a dissociative disorder. The recommendation of individual psychotherapy is first given with the understanding that it will be intensive individual therapy (2/week) with a therapist trained in working with dissociation. The prognosis is given as generally good, but requiring long term work. The advantages of providing treatment locally rather than from a specialised unit in another area is given to avoid further splits and the effectiveness of having a strong and contained multi-disciplinary team in place at the outpatient level. We offer to select/train either an in-house therapist or someone from the private sector, supervision for the therapist and consultancy for the team and we encourage the therapist's involvement in CPA meetings.

With a strong CPA team in place, Multi-agency involvement can be reduced (reduction in costs), and positive moves can take place to outpatient treatment (cost reduction).With a strong plan in place "in case" of a future admission, there less likelihood that this will restart the diagnostic roller coaster noted before. All along the patient is encouraged to take appropriate responsibility and appropriate use of help. All of this in our experience helps reduce self-harm, the over use of services (an inappropriate search for parenting) and an increase in self worth.

FUTURE LINKS

Through the development of the United Kingdom Society for the Study of Dissociation (UKSSD), with support from the International Society for the Study of Dissociation (ISSD), it has been possible over the past five years to establish a growing body of professionals willing to undertake further training to give a secure base to treating and supporting people with a variety of trauma based disorders including specifically dissociative disorders as defined within DSM IV. We have found people willing to give up their time for supervision and case discussion to keep standards high. It is exciting that NHS Primary Care (GP) practices may soon have "purchasing power" to buy services for their patients because very often it is at the GP level that the most priority is given because outpatients turn up week after week with undiagnosed somatic and or psychological symptoms. Patient self-help groups such as First Person Plural are arranging national level interest and, as a recent conference demonstrated, are a voice that is reaching throughout the UK to unify understanding. European colleagues are increasingly interested to join with us in the UK to understand our own dissociation, as we come to a better understanding about our own divisions and chaotically organised services so we grow closer to helping the disorganised and fragmented inner world that we are striving to heal. It is difficult to find other than a powerful reflection that the divisions within Europe and within our UK NHS give us an incentive to work very hard to create a container that is worth internalising.

REFERENCES

American Psychiatric Association (1980). *Diagnostic and statistical manual of mental disorders (3rd ed.)*. Washington, DC: Author.

American Psychiatric Association (1987). *Diagnostic and statistical manual of mental disorders-revised (3rd ed.)*. Washington, DC: Author.

American Psychiatric Association (1994). *Diagnostic and statistical manual of mental disorders (4th ed.)*. Washington, DC: Author.

Blank, A. S. (1985). The unconscious flashback to the war in Vietnam veterans: Clinical mystery, legal defence, and community problem. In S. M. Sonnenberg, A. S. Blank, J. A. Talbot (Eds.), *The trauma of war: Stress and recovery in Vietnam veterans* (pp. 239-308). Washington, DC: American Psychiatric Press.

Bliss, E. L. (1983). Multiple personalities, related disorders and hypnosis. *American Journal of Clinical Hypnosis, 26*, 114-123.

Braun, B. G. (1990). Dissociative disorders as sequelae to incest. In R.P. Kluft (Eds.) *Incest-related syndromes of adult psychopathology* (pp. 227-246). Washington, DC: American Psychiatric Press.

Carlson, E. B., & Putnam, F.W. (1983). An update on the dissociative experience scale. *Dissociation: Progress in the Dissociative Disorders, 6*, 16-27.

Carlson, E. B., Putnam, F. W., Ross, C. A., Torem, M., Coons, P., Dill, D. et al. (1993). Validity of the Dissociative Experience Scale in screening for multiple personality disorder: A multicentre study. *American Journal of Psychiatry, 150*, 1030-1036.

Clary, W. F., Burstin, K. J., & Carpenter, J. S. (1984). Multiple personality and borderline personality disorder. *Psychiatric Clinics of North America, 7*, 89-100.

Coons, P. M., Cole, C., Pellow, T., & Milstein, V. (1990). Symptoms of post-traumatic stress and dissociation in women victims of abuse. In R.P. Kluft (Ed.), *Incest-related syndromes of adult psychopathology* (pp. 205-226). Washington, DC: American Psychiatric Press.

Department of Health (1948). NHS Act. Acts of Parliament, UK Government.

Ellwood, P. Y. (1999). Characteristics of admissions considered inappropriate by junior psychiatrists. *Psychiatric Bulletin, 23*, 1, 34-37.

Fine, C. G. (1990). The cognitive sequelae of incest. In R.P. Kluft (Ed.), *Incest-related syndromes of adult psychopathology* (pp. 161-182). Washington, DC: American Psychiatric Press.

Fink, D., & Goldinkoff, M. (1990). Multiple personality disorder, borderline personality disorder and schizophrenia: A comparative study of clinical features. *Dissociation, 111*(3), 127-134.

Frankel, F. H., & Orne, M. T. (1976). Hypnotizability and phobic behaviour. *Archives of General Psychiatry, 33*, 1259-1261.

Gelinas, D. J. (1984). The persisting negative effects of incest. *Psychiatry, 46*, 312-332.

Goff, D. C., Olin, J. A., Jenlike, M. A., Baer, L., & Buttolph, M. L. (1992). Dissociative symptoms in patients with obsessive-compulsive disorder. *Journal of Nervous and Mental Disease, 180*(5), 332-337.

Havenaar, J. M., Boon, S., & Tordoir, C. E. M. (1992). Dissociative symptoms in patients with eating disorders in the Netherlands: A study using a self rating scale (DES) and a structured clinical interview (SCID-D). In *Dissociative Disorders 1992: Proceedings of the Ninth International Conference on Multiple Personality/Dissociative States*. Rush Presbyterian St. Luke's Medical Centre, Rush North Shore Medical Centre, Skokie, IL.

Kluft, R. P. (1985). The natural history of multiple personality disorder. In R.P. Kluft (Ed.), *Childhood antecedents of multiple personality* (pp. 197-238). Washington, DC: American Psychiatric Press.

Kluft, R. P. (1988). The dissociative disorders. In J. Talbott, R. Hales, & S. Yudofsky (Eds.), *The American Psychiatric Press textbook of psychiatry* (pp. 557-585). Washington, DC: American Psychiatric Press.

Kluft, R. P., Braun, B. G., & Sachs, R. G. (1984). Multiple personality, intrafamilial abuse, and family psychiatry. *International Journal of Family Psychiatry, 5*, 283-301.

Marcum, J. M., Wright, K., & Bissell, W. G. (1985). Chance discovery of multiple personality disorder in a depressed patient by amo-barbital interview. *Journal of Nervious and Mental Disease, 174*, 489-492.

Mollen, P. (1996). *Multiple selves multiple voices. Working with trauma violation and dissociation.* John Wiley and Sons.

Putnam, F. W. (1985). Dissociation as a response to extreme trauma. In R.P. Kluft (Ed.), *Childhood antecedents of multiple personality* (pp. 65-97). Washington, DC: American Psychiatric Press.

Redfearn, J. W. T. (1994). *My self, my many selves.* London: H. Karnarc Books Ltd. (Original work published 1985)

Ross, C. A. (1997). *Dissociation Identity Disorder: Diagnosis clinical features and treatment of Multiple Personality (2nd Ed.).* New York: John Wiley & Sons, Inc.

Ross, C. A., Norton, G., & Wozney, K. (1989). Multiple personality disorder: An analysis of 236 cases. *Canadian Journal of Psychiatry*, 34, 413-418.

Roth, M. (1959). The phobic anxiety-depersonalization syndrome. *Proceedings of the Royal Society of Medicine*, 52, 587-595.

Schultz, R., Braun, B.G., & Kluft, R. P. (1989). Multiple personality disorder: Phenomenology of selected variables in comparison to major depression. *Dissociation*, 11(1), 45-51.

Sivadon, P. (1952). *County Asylum Act: The place of the psychiatric hospital in the mental health service united nations*, WHO/Ment/34.

Spiegel, D. (1984). Multiple personality as a posttraumatic stress disorder. *Psychiatric Clinics of North America*, 7, 101-110.

Spiegel, D. (1991). Dissociation and trauma. In A. Tasman & S. Goldfinger (Eds.), *American Psychiatric press review of psychiatry*, 10, pp. 261-275. Washington, DC: American Psychiatric Press.

Spiegel, D., & Cardena, E. (1991). Disintegrated experience: The dissociative disorders revisited. *Journal of Abnormal Psychology*, 100(3), 366-378.

Steinberg, M. (1994). Structured Clinical Interview for DSM IV Dissociative Disorders (SCID-D), Revised, Washington, DC: American Psychiatric Press.

Strumwasser, I., Paranjpe, N. V., & Udow M. (1991). Appropriateness of psychiatric and substance abuse hospitalization: Implications for payment and utilization management. *Medical Care 29 (supplement S77-S99)*.

Terr. L. C. (1991). Childhood traumas: An outline and overview. *American Journal of Psychiatry*, 148(1), 10-20.

Torem, M. (1986). Dissociative states presenting as eating disorders. *American Journal of Clinical Hypnosis*, 29, 137-142.

Waller, N.G., & Ross, C.A. (1997) The prevalence and biometric structure of pathological dissociation in the general population. *Journal of Abnormal Psychology*, 106(4), 499-510.

Index

T - #0472 - 101024 - C0 - 212/152/20 - PB - 9780789034083 - Gloss Lamination